MEDICAL PROCEDURES, TESTING AND TECHNOLOGY

THE I-GEL SUPRAGLOTTIC AIRWAY

Medical Procedures, Testing and Technology

Additional books in this series can be found on Nova's website under the Series tab.

Additional e-books in this series can be found on Nova's website under the e-book tab.

Medical Devices and Equipment

Additional books in this series can be found on Nova's website under the Series tab.

Additional e-books in this series can be found on Nova's website under the e-book tab.

MEDICAL PROCEDURES, TESTING AND TECHNOLOGY

THE I-GEL SUPRAGLOTTIC AIRWAY

PAVEL MICHALEK
AND
WILLIAM DONALDSON
EDITORS

NOVA BIOMEDICAL
New York

For permission to use material from this book please contact us:
Telephone 631-231-7269; Fax 631-231-8175
Web Site: http://www.novapublishers.com

Library of Congress Cataloging-in-Publication Data

ISBN: 978-1-62417-897-9

Library of Congress Control Number: 2012956338

Published by Nova Science Publishers, Inc. † New York

CONTENTS

PREFACE

The i-gel supraglottic airway is a disposable, latex-free device for airway management during anesthesia. The design of this device is significantly different from the previously used devices – laryngeal mask airways. Its bowl is made of a soft, noninflatable thermoplastic elastomer, anatomically preformed to mirror the perilaryngeal structures. The i-gel contains an additional epiglottis rest, which helps to prevent the epiglottis from down-folding or obstructing the laryngeal inlet. The device also includes a gastric channel, allowing drainage of air and gastric contents or passage of a gastric tube.

The first chapter of this book describes brief history of airway management, the second chapter overwievs the classification of supraglottic airway devices, the mechanisms and forces contributing to their seal and highlights the main differences between the devices.

In the following chapter the process of the i-gel development is described including an initial mannequin and cadaver studies. The other chapters involve a description of introduction of the i-gel into the clinical practice, indications and description of its use in the operating room, and use of the i-gel in different surgical subspecialities including laparoscopic procedures. Two chapters describe the i-gel use in a difficult airway scenario, including fibrescope guided tracheal intubation through the device. The i-gel may be also used in pediatric anesthesia, for airway management in pre-hospital and emergency departments and as an airway device in the Advanced Life Support.

In: The i-gel Supraglottic Airway
Editors: Pavel Michalek and William Donaldson
ISBN: 978-1-62417-897-9

Chapter 1

A Brief History of Airway Management

Jiri Malek*

Department of Anesthesia and Intensive Care Medicine,
3rd Medical Faculty of the Charles University and
University Hospital Kralovske Vinohrady,
Prague, Czech Republic

Abstract

The chapter is focused on the history of airway management from ancient times to the latest developments. The history of airway management is reviewed, with a special focus on primitive surgical techniques used for maintenance of a patent airway - tracheotomy and tracheostomy. The first part of this chapter also reviews the historical development of other airway management techniques - non-invasive approaches, different aids to maintain airway patency and the history of orotracheal and nasotracheal intubation.

The second part of the chapter describes the invention and development of the laryngeal mask airway and other supraglottic airway devices.

Early History of Airway Management

Breathing is a clear requirement for life, and in ancient civilisations any apparent obstacles to breathing were recognized as a threat to life and attempts were made to remove them. Invasive attempts involved cutting into the trachea and were perhaps the earliest methods used to obtain a clear airway. Procedures resembling a tracheostomy were depicted on Egyptian tablets dating back to 3600 BC [1] and descriptions concerning the treatment of a wound that could have been the result of a tracheotomy can be found in the Rig Veda, the ancient Hindu book of medicine that first appeared as an oral tradition around 2000 BC [2].

---

* E-mail: malekj@fnkv.cz.

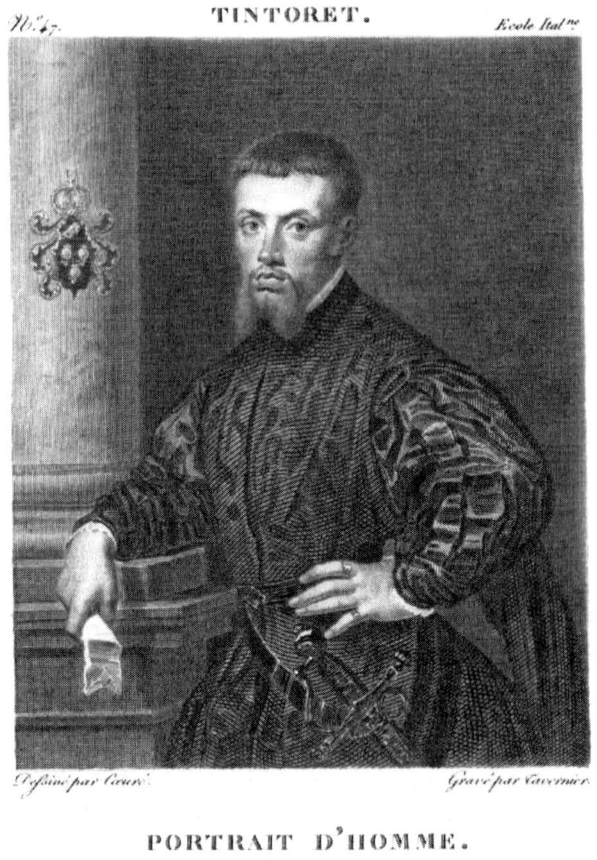

Source: public domain.

Figure 1. Andreas Vesalius, Belgian anatomist (1514-1564).

Centuries later, Alexander the Great (356-380 BC) was said to have used his sword to cut the throat of a soldier who was choking on a chicken bone [3]. The insertion of reeds into the trachea of newborns, to assist artificial breathing, was described in the Judaic Talmud some time between 200 BC and 400 AD [3]. Many Greek physicians (Hippocrates, Aesculapius, Aretanus) and the Roman anatomist Gallenus mentioned similar operations, so the tracheostomy can be regarded historically as a well-established method [2]. Tracheostomies seem to have been abandoned in the early Middle Ages, only to reappear again during the Renaissance. The great Flemish anatomist, Andreas Vesalius, passed a reed into the trachea of a dying animal whose thorax had been opened and maintained ventilation by blowing air into the reed (Figure 1). He noticed that the state of the animal improved [3]. In 1546 the Italian physician, Fabricius of Aquapendente, performed the first documented tracheostomy on a patient suffering from a tonsillar obstruction. Several other cases were published after this successful attempt. In 1667 Robert Hooke demonstrated, at a Royal Society meeting, with a bellows and an animal with an open chest, that a constant flow of fresh air was essential for life and not just the movement of the lungs themselves [3].

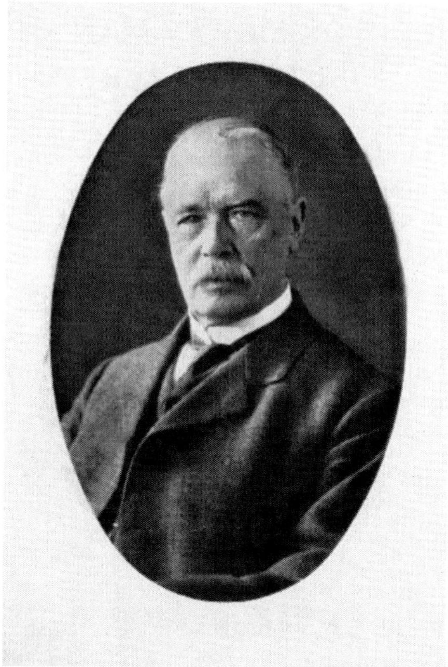

Source: public domain.

Figure 2. Friedrich Trendelenburg, German surgeon (1844-1924).

Artificial aids for securing patent airways were first used either to by-pass obstructions or to rescue drowning victims. Scientific societies for the resuscitation of drowning people were founded in Amsterdam, London, Paris, Venice and Philadelphia. In 1760 an opening in the "windpipe" for resuscitation was described by Buchan [3]. The use of tracheal intubation and ventilation, using bellows, for reviving the apparently dead, was recommended by Cullen (1776) and the use of the intralaryngeal cannula was introduced by Curry (1791). In 1774 Cogan and Hawes, from the Royal Rescue Society, advocated using tracheal intubation for resuscitation, instead of mouth to mouth ventilation [3]. Despite all these studies and publications, methods for securing a clear airway did not gain widespread use among physicians. George Washington died in December 1799; it is believed that he suffocated as a consequence of epiglottitis despite the presence of three physicians, who were with him at his death [4]. It is said that one of the physicians present at the scene was aware of the tracheostomy technique, but did not intervene since he believed the procedure to be futile. Increasing numbers of tracheostomies were performed in the 19th century, mainly to relieve obstruction in children caused by diphtheria. The best-known pioneers of this life-saving procedure are Armand Trousseau and Friedrich Trendelenburg (Figure 2). The tubes were usually made of silver and their shape was more similar to modern oral airways than to modern tracheostomy tubes [4]. Trendelenburg produced the first cuffed tracheostomy tube in 1869 and used it in 1871 to prevent aspiration of blood during surgery on the upper airway [2].

Techniques of Airway Management during the First 100 Years of Anesthesia

William Thomas Green Morton provided the first successful demonstration of ether anesthesia on the 16th October 1846. This anesthesia was probably in a superficial plane, so no airway problems occurred. However, over the next several years there were deaths reported that could be attributed to hypoxia caused by loss of the airway. Several other techniques were introduced to attempt to solve this problem, such as using forceps to pull the tongue out of mouth or even waking patients during surgery [5]. It is difficult to imagine that essential maneuvers such as backwards tilting of the head and lower jaw protrusion were not published until the late 1870s. The first publication concerning this, now universally used, technique is attributed to J. Heiberg, who published the article “A new expedient in administering chloroform“ in the *Medical Times*, in which he described “head extension and jaw thrust.” [5] The first scientific study concerning the etiology of manual techniques used to keep airways open can be attributed to B. Howard. Howard discovered and published (1880) that traction on the tip of the tongue relieved airway obstruction by moving the tongue away from the posterior pharyngeal wall, and not because it elevated the epiglottis as was generally believed [5]. In 1881 it was stated in Lyman´s textbook “Artificial Anaesthesia and Anaesthetics” that death by suffocation occured only as a result of great negligence or great ignorance of the operator [6]. Howard continued upper airway research and in 1888 published on the relationship between neck extension and the position of the epiglottis. Finally, in 1890, Hewitt published a review summarizing the causes and management of respiratory obstruction [6].

Clinicians also looked for instrumental methods of securing airways that were less-invasive than performing tracheostomy. Based on previous studies, several techniques were introduced. Joseph Thomas Clover (Figure 3), the famous English pioneer in the field of anesthesia, is thought to be the first to use a tube inserted into one nostril or a conic shaped rubber tube inserted through the nose into the oropharynx for administration of anesthesia during jaw surgery in early 1880s [5].

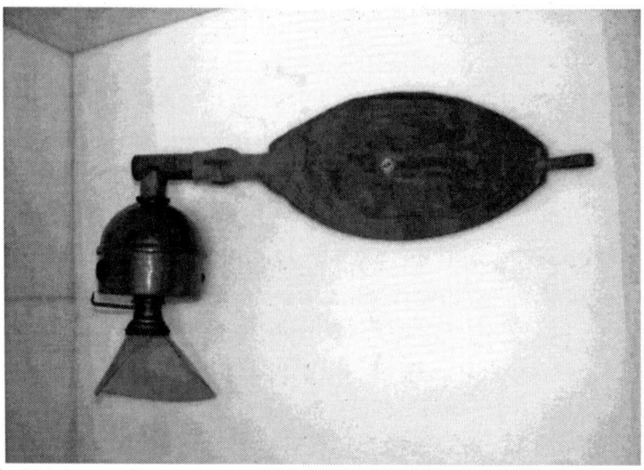

Courtesy of Anaesthesia Heritage Centre, London, UK.

Figure 3. Face mask and Clover´s portable regulating ether inhaler, invented in 1877 and modified by Hewitt.

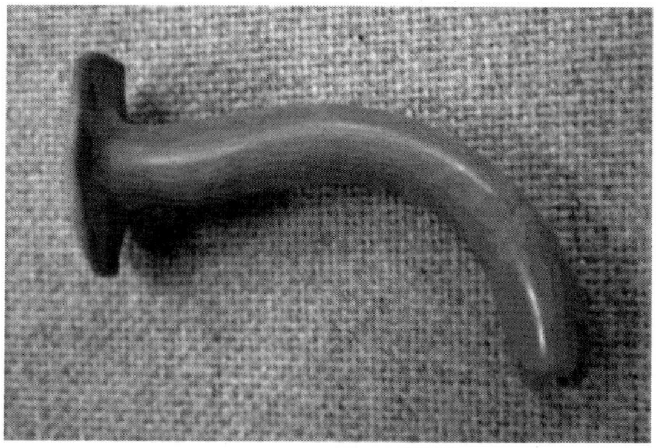

Figure 4. Guedel oropharyngeal airway.

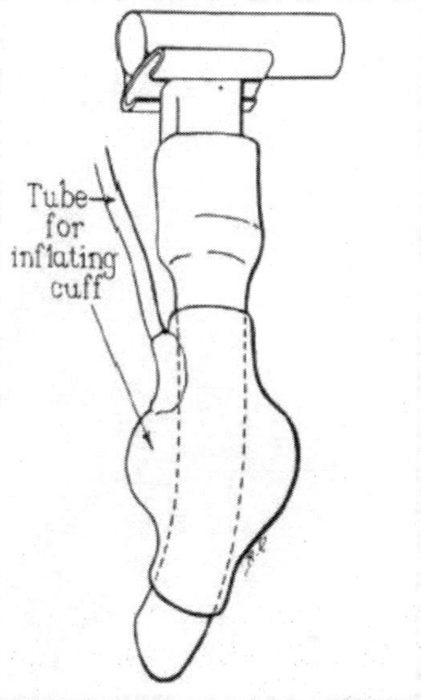

Source: public domain.

Figure 5. Shipway´s oropharyngeal airway (1935).

Nasopharyngeal airways became popular since they were more easily introduced than other devices, caused less irritation and in addition to providing a clear airway could also be used for inhalation of anesthetic agents in cases where access to the mouth was limited. In 1913 Karl Connell, from New York, described a technique for artificial ventilation using a nasopharyngeal airway. It required closing the lips and nostrils of the patient, to avoid air leakage, and compression of the cricoid cartilage [7].

Oral airways had a more difficult introduction. In 1908 Frederick Hewitt published a paper describing the forerunner of modern oral airways [6]. It was a straight short tube which proved not to be very effective. This model was later replaced by a longer curved tube, and many other modifications followed. In 1915, Joseph Lumbard developed an oropharyngeal airway constructed of a metal wire cage shaped like the upper airways [8]. It consisted of a double row of bent wires that were connected by wire bands. The Mayo oropharyngeal airway was also a metal open-cage airway, but more oval in cross-section. Other types combined metal and rubber, such as the Phillips airway [8]. Around 1930, Ralph Waters developed an anatomically curved metal oropharyngeal airway with a flattened cross-section and holes near the distal end which had a very similar appearance to Guedel´s airway [8].

The now most frequently used design was introduced in 1933 by Arthur Guedel (Figure 4) [8]. This moderately stiff, rubber airway, in the shape of the upper airways and flattened to be easily inserted between the teeth is still used. There were several other modifications of the oral airway including material, length and minor changes in shape, but the original design introduced by Guedel still persists.

In 1935, the airway was equipped, by Francis Shipway (senior anesthetist at Guy's Hospital), with an inflatable balloon to prevent aspiration during nasal surgery (Figure 5) [6]. This device was a forerunner of the cuffed oropharyngeal airway (COPA) that was patented by Robert S. Greenberg (Baltimore, United Kingdom) in 1990. Other cuffed oropharyngeal airways producing a seal without the use of a face-mask and without the use of intubation were produced by W.B. Primrose in 1934, S. Mehta in 1990 and S. Feldman in 1991 [6]. In 1937 Beverley Charles Leech described and patented a "Pharyngeal bulb gasway", based on his study of pharyngeal anatomy, which would fit snugly at the entry to the larynx [9]. It was mainly used during cyclopropane anesthesia. At first sight it resembled a laryngeal mask airway, but this airway was a rigid curved metal tube with a soft, non-inflatable rubber part on the distal end, which produced an airtight seal with the respiratory tract by forming a plug in the upper pharynx [10].

Factors which led to the decreased use of cuffed airways included the increased availability of:

a) tracheal intubating equipment,
b) anesthesiologists who were skilled in laryngoscopy,
c) the introduction of curare in 1942 and suxamethonium in 1951.

Younger anesthesiologists became uncomfortable administering anesthesia with a face mask, and the feeling developed that failure to intubate was a sign of sloppy practice, and if anything went wrong, it would be difficult to defend against a charge of malpractice.

The last model of the uncuffed oral airway seems to have been the Chou Airway, which was patented in 2004 by Takuma Norikata. This adjustable oropharyngeal airway apparatus includes a "rigid airway portion comprising a mouthpiece and a flexible airway portion frictionally engaging and slidably disposed in the mouthpiece. The overall length of the apparatus can be varied by sliding the flexible portion relative to the mouthpiece." [11]. The latest cuffed oropharyngeal airway, developed in the United Kingdom was, the Tulip® airway invented by Dr A. Shaikh in (2008) [12].

Tracheal Intubation Techniques

Before the advent of muscle relaxants, intubation was infrequently used compared to the years after their introduction. In 1880, William Macewen, a Scottish surgeon, described a blind digital intubation technique for relieving airway obstruction; first on cadavers, and later in clinical settings under chloroform anesthesia [2, 3]. Several years later, in 1885, the New

York physician Joseph O´Dwyer developed a system of metal tubes for the treatment of children suffocating from diphtheria or stenosis of the larynx; George Fell adopted and adapted this system for artificial ventilation [2]. The O´Dwyer tube was a combination of a supra- and intra- (infra-) glottic device. The oropharyngeal tube was rigid and shaped to match the anatomy of the upper airways. It also consisted of a conical distal end designed to produce an airtight seal in the larynx, which enabled artificial ventilation during resuscitation, together with a modified form for surgery. Further development of metal tubes introduced blindly to the trachea, using a curved introducer, was carried out in Germany by Hans Kuhn around 1900 [3]. His tube was partly flexible and caused lesser trauma to the upper airways. Packing of the hypopharynx with gauze was used to prevent pulmonary aspiration. Further progress followed after introduction of direct laryngoscopy.

The invention of laryngoscopy is attributed to Manuel Garcia, a voice teacher from Spain who, whilst working at the Royal Academy of Music in London in 1855, described the use of two small mirrors, one to direct sunlight to his mouth and the other to observe his vocal cords and their movements [2]. Alfred Kirstein from Berlin constructed in 1895 an "autoscop", a device for direct laryngoscopy with a handle, spatula and hood for observing the larynx and trachea. The source of light was provided by reflected light from a forehead mirror. Topical cocaine was used to provide anesthesia for the airways [2]. Chevalier Jackson improved Kirstein´s autoscop by adding a tungsten light bulb for illumination. During and after World War I, the number of patients with head and neck injuries demanded more frequent use of tracheal intubation. While Ivan Magill mastered blind nasal intubation using improved shapes and materials for tracheal tubes, laryngoscopy was, in the 1940s, facilitated by the introduction of 2 types of laryngoscopes that are still used in clinical practice. Robert Miller described a laryngoscope with a straight blade in 1941 and Robert Macintosh a laryngoscope with curved blade in 1943 [2]. The next step for the worldwide spread of tracheal intubation, as a gold standard for securing airways during anesthesia, was the introduction of curare into clinical practice by Harold Griffith from Montreal. Many types of laryngoscopes are used today, mainly to facilitate tracheal intubation in cases of difficult airways, including various types of blades, introducers, fiber-optic instruments and video-systems. The materials from which tracheal tubes are manufactured have also improved significantly.

Laryngeal Mask Airway Family and Other Supraglottic Airway Devices

The laryngeal mask airway (LMA) is the single most important device introduced for airway maintenance after tracheal intubation. This device gained a widespread use in 1990s, but development started in the 1980s. The inventor of the LMA, Dr Archie Brain (Figure 6), used a simplified scheme of the upper airways, which terminated at the glottis, and sought the best connection between this tube and the end of the anesthetic breathing system [13]. There are generally two possibilities. Facemasks can be used to maintain the airway but their shape can render maintenance of a reliable seal difficult and they demand that anesthesiologists use their hands to keep the airway open. The tracheal tube connects the trachea to a breathing circuit but is excessively long. The inflated cuff can harm the tracheal columnar epithelium and intubation has well known adverse effects. Brain concluded that the facemask is impractical and that tracheal tube is not physiological. The ideal artificial airway should rapidly overcome airway obstruction and be easy and atraumatic to use even when used by the unskilled operators.

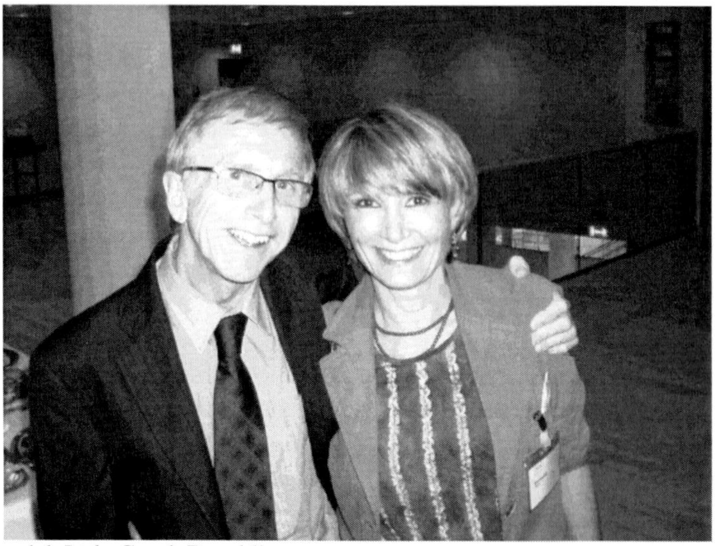

Courtesy of Chemelek Ltd., Czech Republic.

Figure 6. Archie Ian Jeremy Brain, the inventor of laryngeal mask airway (born 1942) with Milena Mountain, the LMA distributor in the Czech Republic.

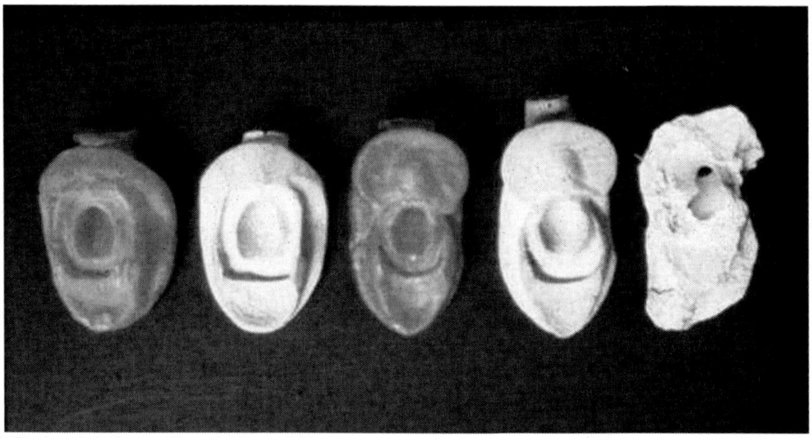

Courtesy of Chemelek Ltd., Czech Republic.

Figure 7. Prototypes of the Laryngeal Mask Airway demonstrating development of the cuff design.

Dr. Brain studied the anatomy of the upper airways and in 1981 made several plaster-of-Paris casts of cadaver pharynxes in order to visualize the shape around and posterior to the glottis [13]. This space is adapted to accept foreign bodies (i.e. food) and was likely to better tolerate the pressure of a cuff. Moreover, it was firm enough to form a seal. His observations led him to develop the first model of a supraglottic airway device made from a plastic tube with an attached rubber cuff from a Goldman Dental Mask, which had a shape very similar to the casts of the pharynxes (Figure 7). The first prototype was used successfully in the summer of 1981 [13]. It was introduced blindly under deep halothane anesthesia using a technique similar to the introduction of a Guedel airway and a tight seal was confirmed using gentle positive pressure artificial ventilation. Three more devices were made and used, but Dr. Brain discovered that the Goldman Mask did not fit perfectly against the laryngeal rim and leaks occurred, mainly in men. In spite of this problem, approximately 1000 patients were anesthetized using this design [13]. In February 1983 it was used for the first time in a case of a failed intubation in a 114 kg man [14]. Anesthesia lasted 3 hours and artificial ventilation without an air-leak was made possible by using a special clamping mechanism that applied pressure to the front of the neck. Dr. Brain noticed the absence of postoperative sore throat in this man and this encouraged him to pass the LMA prototype into his own pharynx, which hc did without any harm. Further attempts were made to solve the problem associated with the epiglottis, which sometimes folded over during insertion. A metal introducer was developed and successfully used in many cases, but was found not to be an optimal solution because of the risk of trauma. The second result was a change to the insertion technique to that which is used today, which is different from that used with the Guedel airway. Fiberoptic laryngoscopy had revealed that the orifice of LMA was located directly against the laryngeal inlet and that the LMA could be used as a guide for intubation. As a result the internal diameter of the incorporated tube was increased to 14 mm which enabled passage of a 9 mm tracheal tube (May 1983). Intubation through the LMA was carried out several times in 1983. In 1983/84, several prototypes were constructed with a double lumen for insertion of a gastric tube with the aim of reducing the risk of regurgitation [13].

New types, using a silicon mask instead of the Goldmann mask, were produced according to Dr. Brain's design by the Dunlop Rubber Company towards the end of 1985 [13]. They had a bar within the aperture to prevent the epiglottis from falling into the aperture and blocking it. Insertion of this design was significantly easier and the use of metal introducers was finally abandoned. Dr. Brain was now seeking the optimal shape of the inflatable cuff. He produced over 60 prototypes using moulds, again from cadaver casts. The cuffs and tubes had to be glued together manually, which was an arduous process. The aim of his research was to obtain the highest possible seal pressure against the laryngeal inlet, to avoid aspiration of gastric contents in the event of regurgitation, to avoid aperture obstruction by the epiglottis, to avoid misplacement after or during insertion, to avoid pushing the epiglottis into a downward folded position during insertion, and to make insertion easy and atraumatic. Many tests were carried out with these prototypes during 1986; the tests revealed that there was no optimal shape that met all demands. Finally, in December 1986, a silicon cuff version with improved characteristics was developed that could be produced in a small series and could be offered for tests by other medical professionals [13]. The manufacturing also enabled production of pediatric sizes. One year later, in December 1987, the first all-factory-made LMA was ready and in January 1988 three other sizes were ordered.

Dr. Brain's search for further developments continued. In 1987, a nasal laryngeal mask was tested. The tube could be detached and after normal oral insertion disconnected, introduced through the nose and again connected. This type was preliminary trialled, but not commercially manufactured. A flexible laryngeal mask airway with a narrower, metal-wire-reinforced connecting tube was introduced in 1989. An intubating laryngeal mask airway was released in 1997 and a disposable laryngeal mask airway manufactured from PVC was released in late 1997. The Proseal LMA, with a more effective seal and the ability to drain gastric contents (Figure 8), was released in 1999, the LMA-Supreme with an integrated drain tube and an improved curve for easy insertion, was introduced to clinical practice in 2005. The latest development in the LMA family is represented by the LMA CTrach, which was released in 2007. The CTrach is an LMA that is similar to the intubating LMA but with an integrated camera inside the bowl and an attachable monitor. This allows the process of insertion of a tracheal tube to be visualized, Other supraglottic airway devices with roughly the same shape as the LMA have been produced since Dr. Brain's original invention; for example, the Ambu-Aura laryngeal mask, Vital Seal, Portex Soft Seal Laryngeal Mask, Sheridan Laryngeal Mask, Intersurgical i-gel, Air-Q Laryngeal Mask and others. The Cobra Perilaryngeal Airway was invented by Dr. David Alfery and patented in 2001 [15]. This oral airway is composed of a breathing tube with a wide distal end and a cuff attached just proximal to the wide part. The distal end of the Cobra perilaryngeal airway airway is extended and shaped so as to be seated deep in the patient's hypo-pharynx and to surround the patient's epiglottis and glottis, thereby holding the patient's soft tissue away from the glottic opening of the patient [15].

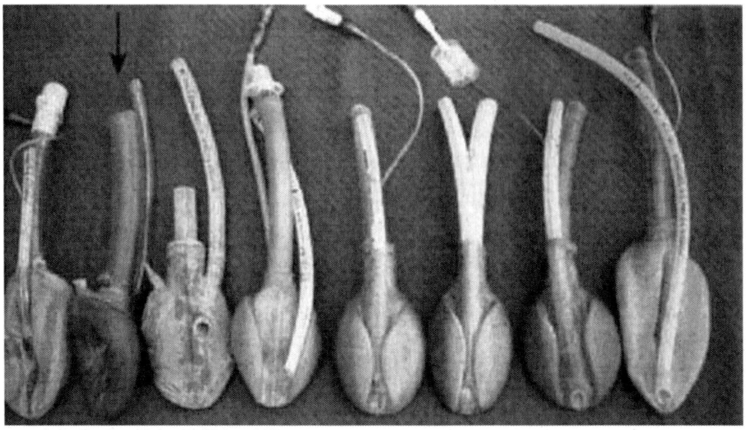

Courtesy of Chemelek Ltd., Czech Republic.

Figure 8. Prototypes of the ProSeal Laryngeal Mask Airway.

The Streamlined Liner of the Pharynx Airway (SLIPA) was invented by Donald Miller in 2003 (Figure 9). It is a disposable, cuffless, supraglottic airway designed to seal without the need for an inflatable cuff. It is comprised of a hollow blow-molded soft plastic airway shaped to form a seal with the pharynx. Being hollow, liquid entrapment is possible and this may provide effective protection against aspiration [16].

Several other alternatives to tracheal intubation have been introduced, mainly for use by emergency medical services. One of these was the Combitube, a double lumen double cuff device that could be blindly inserted into the esophagus. One lumen resembled a tracheal tube, the other an esophageal obturator-type tube with a distal blocked end and perforations at the pharyngeal level. Curiously, although it is thought that the device was developed in the early 1980s, a very similar device was developed in the 1960s by Drs. Don Michael, Lambert and Mehran [17]. These inventors designed this device because the mouth-to-mouth technique of resuscitation was felt to be unpleasant and inflated the patient's stomach. Their device, with some similarity to the modern Combitube, was inserted into the esophagus, had a balloon for establishing an esophageal seal, perforations along the oropharyngeal segment, a bite block, a mouth guard and a short tube for delivering air into and out of the patient's lungs [18]. A simplified device, the Laryngeal Tubus, was invented in 2001/2002.

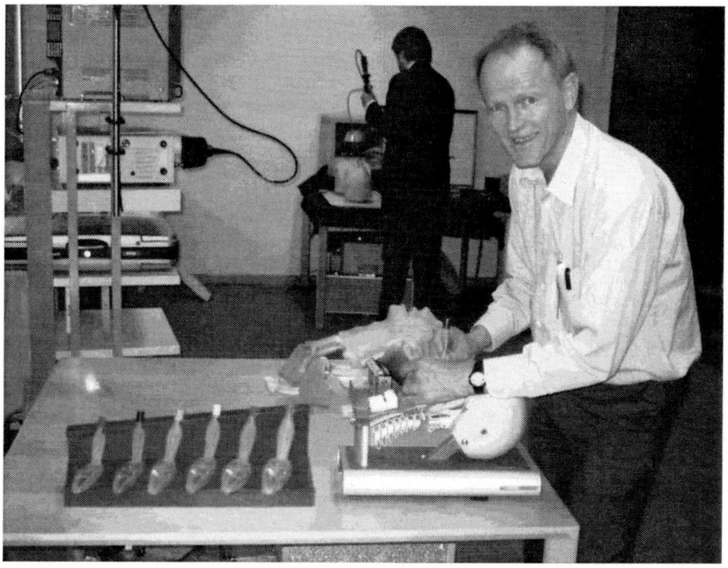

Figure 9. Donald M. Miller, Rhodesia-born anesthesiologist, the inventor of SLIPA (Streamlined Liner of the Pharynx Airway).

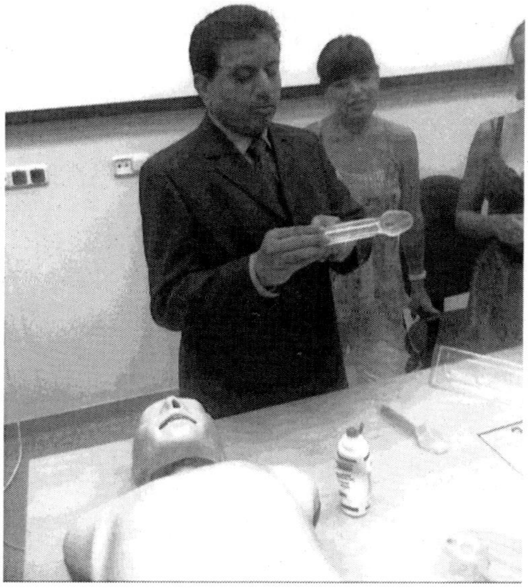

Figure 10. Muhammed A. Nasir, the inventor of i-gel supraglottic airway.

The most recent developments in supraglottic airway management involve two perilaryngeal sealers [19] - the i-gel supraglottic airway and the Baska mask. The i-gel airway was developed by Dr Muhammed Nasir (Figure 10) in cooperation with Intersurgical Ltd. (Wokingham, UK) and officially launched in London at the Annual Winter Meeting of the

AAGBI in 2007 [20]. The i-gel airway has been extensively used since, mainly in Europe, Japan and the United States.

The Baska airway was invented in Australia by a general practitioner with a special interest in airway management (Dr Meenakshi Baska) and by a specialist anesthesiologist (Dr Kanag Baska). The design of the device looks quite complicated and, so far, only two observational studies have evaluated its insertion parameters [21, 22].

Conclusion

Very much time has passed since the first documented attempts to secure a patent airway. History has seen advances and the revisiting of various techniques and aids. The invention of the LMA did not suppress further development. On the contrary, the apparent success of the LMA has resulted in increased attempts to invent new and even better products. The future may herald not only improvements to contemporary techniques, but novel approaches and equipment.

Conflict of Interest

None declared.

References

[1] L. Pahor, Ear, nose and throat in Ancient Egypt, *J. Laryngol. Otol.* 106: 773-9 (1992).

[2] J. J. Doyle, A brief history of clinical airway management, *Anesthesiology News, Supplement*, 9-14, (2008).

[3] P. Szmuk, T. Ezri, S. Evron, Y. Roth and J. Katz, A brief history of tracheostomy and tracheal intubation, from the Bronze Age to the Space Age, *Intensive Care Med.* 34, 222-8, (2008).

[4] S. E. Sittig and J. E. Pringnitz, Tracheostomy. Evolution of an airway, Available from: http://www.tracheostomy.com/resources/pdf/evolution. pdf.

[5] J. R. Brimacombe, Laryngeal mask anesthesia, principles and practice. 2nd edition, *WB Saunders*, Philadelphia, 2005, 1 – 40.

[6] J. W. McIntyre, Oropharyngeal and nasopharyngeal airways: I (1880-1995), *Can. J. Anaesth.*, 43, 629-35 (1996).

[7] K. Connell, Accuracy in anaesthesia: Advantage, technic and dosage in automatic insufflation of vapors and gases. Preliminary tables and charts of ether anaesthesia. *Ann. Surg*. 58, 877-90 (1913).

[8] E. Zadrobilek and G. Krystof, The Guedel oropharyngeal airway: seventieth anniversary of the first published description, *Internet Journal of Airway Management* 2, 2002-2003. Available from URL: http://www.adair.at/ijam/.

[9] C. Leech, The pharyngeal bulb gasway: a new aid in cyclopropane anesthesia, *Anesth. Analg.* (1937).

[10] R. P. Haridas, The Leech airway or pharyngeal bulb gasway, *Anaesth. Intensive Care* 39, S5-S10 (2011).
[11] United States Patent 6606991. Available from: http://www.freepatentsonline.com/6606991.html.
[12] S. Harrison, N. P. Robinson, A. Shaikh and S. M. Yentis, Manikin evaluation of the Tulip®, a new supraglottic airway, *Anaesthesia* 64, 807 (2009).
[13] A.I. Brain, The development of the laryngeal mask - a brief history of the invention, early clinical studies and experimental work from which the laryngeal mask evolved, *Eur. J. Anaesthesiol.* 4, S5-S17 (1991).
[14] I. Brain, Three cases of difficult intubation overcome by the laryngeal mask airway, *Anaesthesia*, 40, 353-5 (1985).
[15] United States Patent 6196224. Available from: http://www.freepatentsonline.com/6196224.html.
[16] D. M. Miller and D. Light, Laboratory and clinical comparisons of the Streamlined Liner of the Pharynx Airway (SLIPA) with the laryngeal mask airway, *Anaesthesia* 58, 136-42 (2003).
[17] T. A. Michael, E. H. Lambert and A. Mehran A, "Mouth-to-lung airway" for cardiac resuscitation, *Lancet* 2, 1329 (1968).
[18] A. Jarquin-Valdivia, A. Thompson, The origin of the Combitube, *The Internet Journal of Anesthesiology* 5 (2002). Available from : http://www.ispub.com/.
[19] D. M. Miller, A proposed classification and scoring system for supraglottic sealing airways: a brief review, *Anesth. Analg.* 99, 1553-9 (2004).
[20] R. M. Levitan and W. C. Kinkle, Initial anatomic investigation of the i-gel airway: a novel supraglottic airway without inflatable cuff, *Anaesthesia* 60, 1022-6 (2005).
[21] V. Alexiev, A. Salim, L. G. Kevin and J. G. Laffey, An observational study of the Baska® mask: a novel supraglottic airway, *Anaesthesia* 67, 640-5 (2012).
[22] T. van Zundert and S. Gatt, The Baska mask® - a new concept in self-sealing membrane cuff extraglottic airway devices, using a sump and two gastric drains: a critical evaluation, *J. Obstet. Anaesth. Crit. Care* 2, 23-30 (2012).

In: The i-gel Supraglottic Airway
Editors: Pavel Michalek and William Donaldson
ISBN: 978-1-62417-897-9

Chapter 2

RE-CLASSIFICATION OF EXTRAGLOTTIC/SUPRALARYNGEAL AIRWAY DEVICES

Donald M. Miller[1,*]
Department of Anaesthesia, Guys University Hospital,
London, United Kingdom

ABSTRACT

Classifications of supraglottic airways are presented to encourage good clinical assessment of a suitable choice of airway device appropriate for each clinical scenario and what to do in the event of failure. For example, the recognition of two different sealing sites amongst supraglottic/extraglottic airway devices (SADs/EADs) may alert departments to consider what aught perhaps to be made available. An extension of the classification by scoring each component also serves the role of providing a rational basis for quantifying the value for general or particular use and calculating cost effectiveness. It also demonstrates the progress that is taking place towards an ideal EAD and the move away from endotracheal anesthesia. A brief analysis to enhance understanding of the mechanics related to the different devices is presented. Such an approach is designed to equip anesthesiologists with their own reasoned thinking to make rational decisions.

INTRODUCTION

A classification of supraglottic airways should not simply be an academic exercise. It should encourage good clinical assessment of a suitable choice of airway device appropriate for each clinical scenario and good clinical practice in the event of failure. An extension of the classification by scoring each component could also serve the role of providing a rational basis quantifying the value for general or particular use and calculating cost effectiveness.

[*] E-mail: donald.miller@kcl.uk.

Such an approach is designed to equip anesthesiologists with their own reasoned thinking to make rational decisions.

The Laryngeal Mask Airway, ProSeal and i-gel are perilaryngeal sealing supraglottic airways. The CombiTube, SLIPA, CobraPLA, and Laryngeal tube with its variants are base of tongue sealing supraglottic airways. These two sealing sites represent the first division in a simple classification of supraglottic airway devices. This distinction provides a rational basis for switching devices to the other group if one is inadequate. On two occasions, this author tried three different perilaryngeal sealing supraglottic airways (not to be recommended), which failed and switching to a base of tongue sealing airway solved the problem. It is quicker, less traumatic and probably safer to try another supraglottic airway device of a different group with a known reliable success record, than to have to resort to a muscle relaxant followed by intubation of the trachea.

Intubation of the trachea is not as benign as we have thought in the past [1-3]. Delayed sequelae with manifestation of mild trauma to the cords can have disastrous consequences to people who depend upon their voice for their livelihood. It is preferable to avoid intubation, if there is a safer alternative. The incidence of permanent voice changes is of the order of 1 per 1000 routine cases that are intubated [3]. As a supraglottic airway device can prevent a sad outcome, this author thinks the acronym "SAD" is unfortunate. The term extraglottic airway (EAD) is therefore considered a better one. The ongoing pursuit of improvement in the design and availability of appropriate alternatives to the tracheal tube is important therefore, if we are to make good progress in airway management.

RE-CLASSIFICATION

One may classify SADs/EADs according to sealing site, sealing mechanism and/or other functional performance characteristics such as aspiration protection mechanisms and suitability as conduits for tracheal intubation. The latter characteristic becomes more important in relation to particular clinical scenarios for which the device may be required and so may be useful in decision making when an appropriate device is to be chosen.

A previous classification [4] of supraglottic/supralaryngeal airways could be improved by better separating sealing site and mechanism.

A sealing site classification:

This system has only 2 groups – "P" and "B".

"P" for Peri-laryngeal sealing in order of increasing effectiveness.

- Simple – e.g. LMA, -Sealing forces unbalanced and not perpendicular to expulsion direction.
- Wedge cuff improvement e.g. i-gel, LMA Supreme
- Rigid conduit – lever assistance e.g. iLMA, LMA Supreme
- Directional sealing – restores sealing forces perpendicular to direction of expulsion e.g. ProSeal
- 3rd Generation sealing mechanism e.g. Baska

"B" for Base of tongue sealing
Sealing forces perpendicular to direction of expulsion

- With oesophageal cuffs e.g. Combitube, LT, SLT.
- Without oesophageal cuff e.g.CobraPLA™
- Anatomical pre-shaped sealer e.g.SLIPA™

For a better understanding of the mechanics related to these two sealing sites, a series of Figures 1-5 is provided that contain vector forces that are thought to be operative at these two sites.

A sealing mechanism classification:

This system has 3 groups and may be referred to as first, second and third generation devices in order of their developmental history:

- "C" for cuff inflating mechanisms e.g. LMA and Combitube
- "W" for wedged sealing e.g. SLIPA and i-gel
- "S" for self-energizing sealing e.g. Baska

Other functional performance characteristics:

1. *Regurgitation protection mechanisms* (3 of them)

O) Obstruction (O) of the upper esophagus. Obstruction at the entrance to the esophagus is possibly not as effective as that which is lower in the esophagus unless there is a self-energizing sealing mechanism. A fixed rigid obstruction is less effective than an air inflatable mechanism.
High obstruction e.g. LMA™, ProSeal, i-gel.
Low obstruction e.g. CombiTube, LT, LTS.

D) Drainage (D) from the esophagus is effective in a way that depends upon the effectiveness of the obstruction. This is a pressure limited mechanism of proven effect in a cadaver model [5], lung model [6] and case reports. The effectiveness of this mechanism in preventing aspiration must be dependent upon the reliability of the esophageal seal. e.g. Combitube, LTS better than ProSeal or LMA Supreme with seal site at the entrance to the esophagus. That includes the i-gel with fixed volume obstruction. The Baska airway has an active suction aspiration mechanism with aspiration protection advantages and mucosal drying disadvantages.

S) Storage (volume in ml) within a chamber has direct bearing upon its effectiveness. A volume limited mechanism of proven effect in a laboratory lung model [6] and case reports e.g. SLIPA. LT is better than LMA [7].

A score for each may be provided in relation to effectiveness.

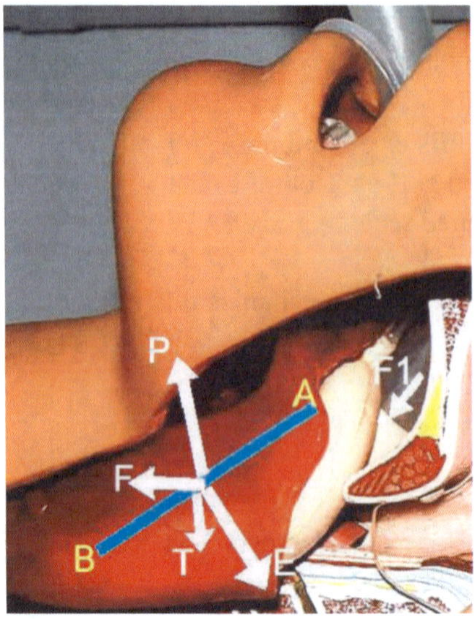

Figure 1a. The laryngeal mask airway is inserted into an Ambu manikin trainer. AB represents the side view of the axis of the bowl of the laryngeal mask, which comprises the area over which the sealing force is exerted. The expulsive force E will be exerted at right angles to this plane (AB). To prevent the airway from being expelled at the peak inflation pressure, equal and opposite forces need to be exerted. These comprise a force vector P from the posterior pharyngeal wall and T from the base of the tongue with resultant frictional force F that resists expulsion. If F is insufficient, then strapping or tying of the silicone tube at the mouth may be necessary to provide an additional force F1 that is transmitted via the tube to increase the total force vector F. Notice that the laryngeal mask tends to kink in the middle of its perilaryngeal cuff. This may alter the direction of the vector E in a more expulsive direction necessitating a larger value for F.

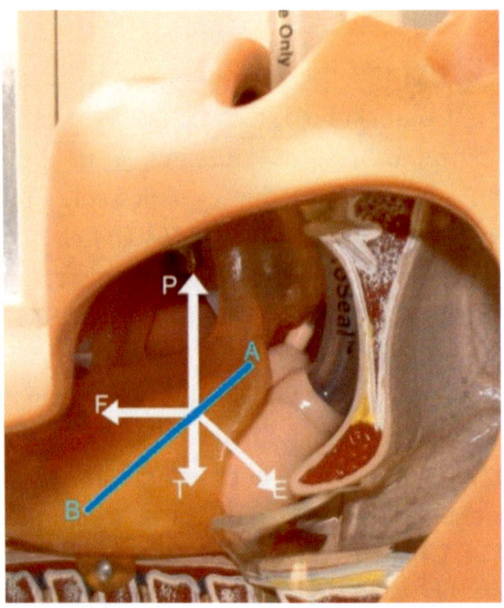

Figure 1b. The ProSeal LM is inserted into an Ambu manikin trainer. The ProSeal LM overcomes the limitations of the small value for the vector P **encountered in the LMA™ classic**. The directional sealing cuff that pushes against the posterior pharyngeal wall directly enhances the P vector and, by pushing the upper border of the perilaryngeal cuff more firmly against the base of the tongue, the T vector increases. A larger frictional force F results from enlarged opposing forces T and P.

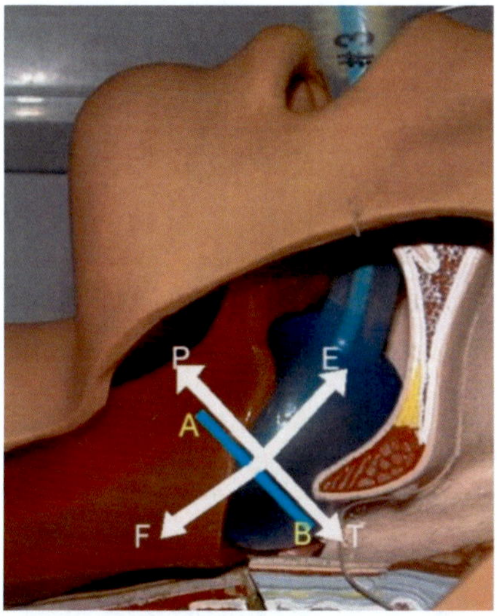

Figure 2. The laryngeal tube has been inserted into an Ambu trainer. AB represents the side view of the annular area where airway pressure exerts a force upon the sealing pharyngeal cuff producing an expulsive force E in the direction shown. The pharyngeal sealing cuff exerts pressure against the base of the tongue and the lateral and posterior pharyngeal walls in a direction that is approximately perpendicular to the expulsive force with the respective force vectors exerted upon the airway T and P. This in turn provides the frictional resistance force F to resist the expulsive force E.

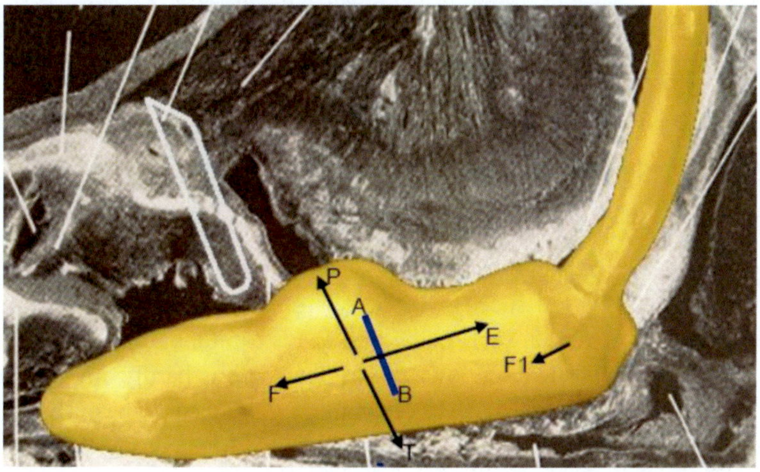

Figure 3. The soft palate of the Ambu trainer is rigid, so it cannot be used to illustrate the SLIPA™ airway where the "heel" of the airway normally fits snugly into the soft palate and nasopharynx as shown in the diagram. The SLIPA™ airway lines the pharynx sealing the escape of gas from the pharynx at the base of the tongue and posterior and lateral pharyngeal walls with sealing plane AB shown and the resultant expulsive force E perpendicular to the plane. Instead of an inflatable cuff in the pharynx, a soft plastic airway lines the pharynx with the resilience of the plastic maintaining a seal pressure gradient that is supported by the airway pressure itself as the pressure rises. The pharyngeal liner exerts pressure against the base of the tongue and the lateral and posterior pharyngeal walls shown by the respective vectors T and P. The resultant frictional force F is shown opposing E. Added to this and in the same direction is another force F1 that will resist the expulsive force E by virtue of its anatomical shape at the level of the "heel" of the SLIPA™ that should settle into the soft palate and nasopharynx.

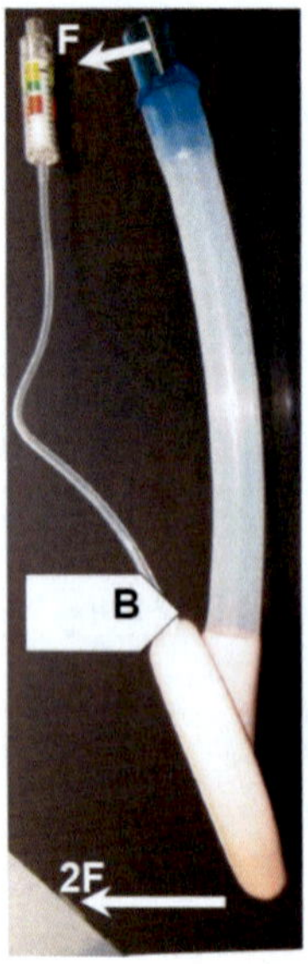

Figure 4. The natural curve of the laryngeal mask airway is insufficient to match the natural curve of the pharyngeal structures necessitating greater flexion when in use. To achieve this, forces about a pivot B are shown. In order to balance forces about the pivot B a force F will be balanced by a force 2F if the distance from F to B is double that of the distance between 2F and B. The base of the tongue becomes a pivot point B resulting in a levering moment in the opposite direction to the large arrow (2F) and resulting in a greater pressure in the posterior than anterior aspect of the laryngeal mask as it protrudes into the entrance of the esophagus. Therefore, regurgitation liquids are likely to go straight into the bowl of the LMA, which can only hold about 3.5 ml before aspiration is likely to occur [4].

The Use of a SAD/EAD for Intubation (Appropriate for Difficult Airway Scenarios)

This may be assessed by looking at the laryngeal view with a fiberscope or its use as a conduit for directing tracheal tubes into the trachea. A proposed gold standard for providing an objective figure must be the successful blind intubation using a tracheal tube with a tip located in the centre of the lumen such as the Parker Flextip tube or the Intavent tracheal tube designed to be used with the ILMA. However, as yet, there is hardly any data to give us this figure. Because of the bevel design of conventional tracheal tubes, their use for blind intubation is always an unreliable indicator because user skill plays such a large component in the success rate and articles that fail to consider this provide little useful information [8, 9]. Improved success with at least a 90 degree turn of a conventional beveled tracheal tube to the left improves the intubation success rate [10]. The use of the BURP maneuver (backward, upward right pressure) is another method of improving the success rate of intubation [11].

However, there are other ways that have been used that may give us a fairly good idea as to how good each device might be as a conduit for intubation. Criteria for excellence are a good laryngeal view that lines up with the cords. The ability to easily access the trachea using a fiberscope with minimal need to adjust the natural direction of the scope may be classed as excellent if this occurs over 90% of the time and good if over 50%. Without a precise percentage score perhaps we should limit the estimation to a simple three level estimation: ++ = Excellent, + = good, - = not ideal.

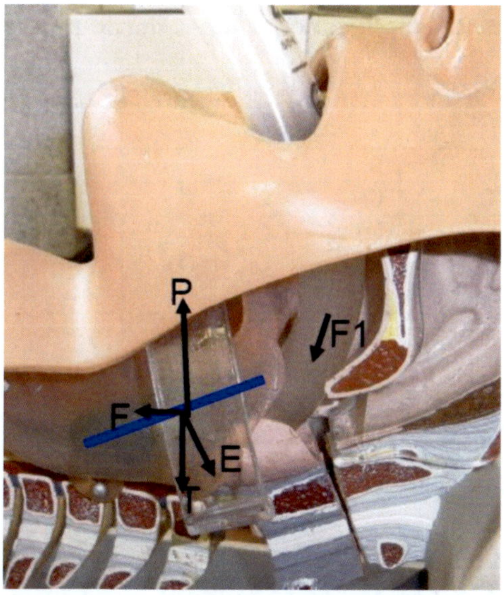

Figure 5a. This figure shows the forces that differ from the laryngeal mask in that the base of tongue force T is larger than with the LMA because of the greater forces required to bend the i-gel when in position. This **often increases the quality of the seal of "upward" escape of gases via the mouth.** The i-gel seal could be improved greatly by improvement of the downward seal via the oesophagus and the gastric tube, which limits the resultant seal pressure. Additional implications of bending of the i-gel are shown in Figure 5b.

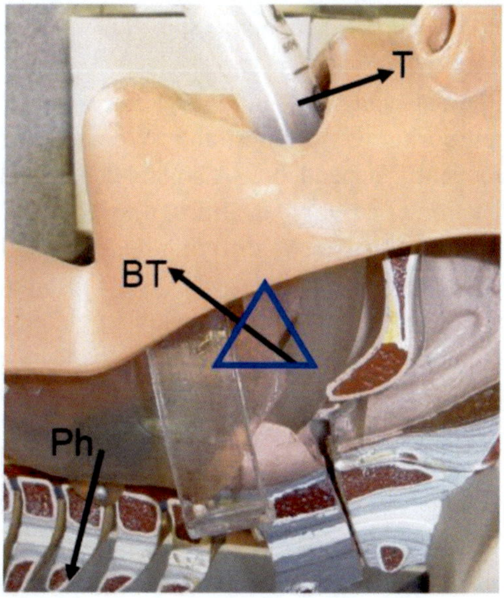

Figure 5b. The forces on the surrounding tissues as a consequence of the i-gel having to be bent in situ with a smaller radius of curvature than with which it is manufactured. There is a force against the teeth T and the posterior pharynx Ph and a force BT against the tongue. The force BT results in pressure against the tongue shown maximally at the pivotal point shown by the blue triangle. This causes obstruction of the venous drainage from the tongue and is a likely explanation as to the not-infrequent finding of a congested tongue and possible associated loss of sensation at the tip of the tongue.

Table 1. Re-classification o supraglottic airway devices

Airway Type	LMA	PLMA sLMA	Combi -tube	LT	SLT	Cobra PLA	SLIPA	i-gel	Baska
Site	P	P	B	B	B	B	B	P	P
Mechanism	C	C	C	C	C	C	W	W	S
Obstruction Drainage Storage	O2 D0 S0	O2 D2 S0	O3 D3 S1	O3 D0 S1	O3 D3 S1	O0 D0 S0	O1 D0 S3	O1 D1 S0	O3 D3 S1
Intubation	++	+ -	-	-	-	+	-	++	++

Table 1 provides a short hand summary of the above.

How Are We Going to Compare and Assess Old and New SADs/EADs ?

An extension of this classification may be able to provide us with a means of answering this question. As yet, there is no such thing as an ideal supraglottic airway. Nevertheless, it is a good exercise to imagine the ideal. It will focus priorities as to what to look for in a supraglottic airway. The three most prominent airway manufacturers for the European markets appear to be Intavent, Ambu and Intersurgical. All three manufacturers have opted to give us a whole range of products for different applications. The imagined objective is to not compromise in the quality of delivery.

All devices involve the balancing of features and compromises. Different circumstances will indicate which of the priorities is most desirable. We need to ask, which of the desirable qualities do we most frequently depend on? Also, related to safety is the question, how helpful is having a combination of desirable qualities in one device? These two questions both consider the priority of safety looking at two differing but potentially competing aspects. That raises a third question as to what is gained and what is compromised? An attempt to try and quantify these complex interactive factors is made below.

To relate these questions to specific situations will enhance the appreciation of the value of asking these questions. Higher seal pressures might be associated with a higher incidence of pressure damage [12-14]. The incidence of sore throats and dysphagia doubles when larger cuff volumes are used with the LMA. To incorporate intubation characteristics in the device might compromise on comfort, pharyngolaryngeal morbidity and ease of insertion [15]. So Intavent manufacture LMA Supreme that is really not good for accessing the trachea but Intavent decided that an LMA with a better seal, ease of insertion, and access to the stomach and protection from regurgitation were a higher priority. If you want to intubate a patient through the LMA, you should use an ILMA. The ILMA is an airway that has good seal characteristics and excellent blind intubating characteristics, 93-69% first time success [8, 16]. The compromises involved in the use of the device are an increase in sore throats, dysphagia and sometimes difficulty with insertion [12]. In addition, they are more expensive than standard LMA devices. Intubating characteristics are rarely needed. Price and sore throats are the main consideration here when it comes to the question whether they should become used as a routine device.

The i-gel is a device that is generally very easy to insert and gives a nice clear airway. However, the compromises associated with its use are the occasional low seal pressure, and although it has a gastric tube, it is not entirely risk free of aspiration with reflux because of a limited seal at the cricopharyngeus level [17]. In the event of regurgitation, it may be marginally safer than the standard LMA from an aspiration risk point of view. The gastric tube does allow for air to escape from the esophagus, so there is less risk of gastroesophageal insufflation than with LMA during IPPV. On the other hand, its features as a conduit for tracheal intubation are excellent, mainly with the use of an intubating bronchoscope.

The fact that i-gel has no cuff inflating mechanism may contribute to less risk of nerve damage that has been recorded occasionally with LMA. However, the injury rate appears to be too rare to feature as a consideration of importance in most people's estimates.

It may be concluded that the tendency to prefer to administer anesthesia with a supraglottic airway than with a tracheal tube is well founded on the available evidence [18, 19]. That is the case despite the fact that there are also serious side-effects using SADs/EADs. Brimacombe showed that up until 2005, there had been 10 published/reported cases of recurrent laryngeal neuropraxias, 4 hypoglossal, and 5 lingual neuropraxias [14]. Rujirojindakul et al. reported in total 13 cases of lingual nerve injury associated with various SADs/EADs in their review of literature [20]. The occurrence is fortunately rare, however, the incidence must exceed the published incidence by some margin. Many more have been reported since and many have not been reported. So although the evidence favours the use of an SAD/EAD in preference to a tracheal tube, it is still not free from the associated risk of serious side-effects.

Improvement in seal quality without the associated increase or preferably with a decrease in the risk of pressure damage to these vulnerable nerves in the pharynx is the future direction that we need to take in the development of EADs. In this regard there does appear to be a new device called the Baska airway with a cuff that is inflated by the airway pressure [21]. It supposedly has very good aspiration protection mechanism also.

The author's views of SAD/EAD characteristics are:

A) What are the most important and fundamental essential requirements in a supraglottic airway:-

1. Good quality seal pressure without the risk of pressure damage to recurrent laryngeal, hypoglossal nerves or lingual nerves.
2. A consistently clear reliable airway without airflow obstruction.
3. Minimal risk of trauma/damage/side-effects e.g. sore throat, hoarseness, dysphagia.

B) Highly desirable characteristics include:

1. Effective aspiration protection mechanism or mechanisms, with effectiveness being more important than the number of mechanisms.
2. A means of access to the esophagus from the point of view of surgical requirements (laparoscopic work) or monitoring requirements (esophageal doppler).
3. Alternative means of handling difficult airways – such as easy intubation or ease of access to the trachea with optical devices.

Table 2. Desirable features of the supraglottic airway devices

SAD/EAD	LMAu/c	LMAsup	ProSeal	LTSd/Ctube	SLIPA	i-gel
A1	1	3	5	5/5	5	3
A2	3	3	3	2/2	3	3
A3	1	1	1	2/0	2	2
B1	1	3	3	4/4	3	2
B2	0	1	1	1/1	0	1
B3	3	0	1	1/0	1	3
Total	9	11	14	15/12	14	14

SAD/ EAD	Cobra PLA	Air Q	ILMA	Baska	Aura Once (i)	COPA	Ideal
				Best/worst			
A1	4	1	5	6/5	2/3	1	6
A2	2	3	3	3/3	3/3	2	3
A3	2	1	1	3/1	1/1	2	3
B1	0	1	2	4/4	1/1	0	4
B2	0	0	0	1/1	0/0	0	1
B3	2	4	4	3/1	1/3	1	4
Total	10	10	15	20/15	8/11	6	21

The author´s personal view puts a weighting on the importance of each characteristic:

A1 – 6 points
A2 – 3
A3 – 3
B1 – 4
B2 – 1
B3 – 4

Total maximum score would be 21. A theoretical perfect SAD/EAD would score 21.

Information for completing these scores is based upon the following references [6, 7, 15-28].

Plus some theoretical considerations and preliminary results e.g. for Baska airway [29, 30] or AuraOnce (Aura-i) [31, 32] as we await the results of clinical trials.

Conclusion

General anesthesia with an endotracheal tube is associated with significantly greater morbidity than with the use of extraglottic airway devices. The inevitable improvement in extraglottic airway designs mean that the steady move away from tracheal tube anesthesia is inevitable for the benefit of patients. The systematic approach provides a framework for wise choices in their use. Sealing site, sealing mechanism and SAD/EAD functions have all been examined and we find that it is possible to attach to them a scoring system that provides a more rational approach to putting a relative value on these airways [33]. A brief repetition of the mechanics related to the functioning of these airways further enhances understanding. We can see from the scoring system, that progress towards an ideal EAD will eventually make tracheal intubation a rare event as opposed to an unnecessarily large proportion of what is current practice.

Conflict of Interest

Dr Donald M. Miller is the inventor of SLIPA and technical advisor to Curve Air Ltd. that manufactures supraglottic airway devices such as variants of the SLIPA and new variants of LM devices.

References

[1] M. A. Maktabi, R. B. Smith and M. M. Todd, Is routine endotracheal intubation as safe as we think or wish? *Anesthesiology* 99, 247-8 (2003).

[2] Tanaka, S. Isono, T. Ishikawa, J. Sato and T. Nishino, Laryngeal resistance before and after minor surgery: endotracheal tube versus laryngeal mask airway, *Anesthesiology* 99, 252-8 (2003).

[3] H. Yamanaka, Y. Hayashi, Y. Watanabe, H. Uematu and T. Mashimo, Prolonged hoarseness and arytenoid cartilage dislocation after tracheal intubation, *Br. J. Anaesth.* 103, 452-5 (2009).

[4] D. M. Miller, A proposed classification and scoring system for supraglottic sealing airways: a brief review. *Anesth. Analg.* 99, 1553-9 (2004).

[5] C. Keller, J. Brimacombe, A. Kleinsasser and A. Loeckinger, Does the ProSeal laryngeal mask airway prevent aspiration of regurgitated fluid? *Anesth. Analg.* 91, 1017-20 (2000).

[6] D. M. Miller and D. Light, Laboratory and clinical comparisons of the streamlined liner of the pharynx airway (SLIPA) with the laryngeal mask airway, *Anaesthesia* 58, 136-42 (2003).

[7] D. M. Miller and D. Light, Storage capacities of the laryngeal mask and laryngeal tube compared and their relevance to aspiration risk during positive pressure ventilation, *Anesth. Analg.* 96, 1821-2 (2003).

[8] L. Theiler, M. Kleine-Brueggeney, N. Urwyler, T. Graf, C. Luyet and R. Greif, Randomized clinical trial of the i-gel™ and Magill tracheal tube or single-use ILMA™ tracheal tube for blind intubation in anaesthetized patients with a predicted difficult airway, *Br. J. Anaesth.* 107, 243-50 (2011).

[9] J. K. Friis and I. Ahmad, Re: Randomized clinical trial of the i-gel™ and Magill tracheal tube or single-use ILMA™ tracheal tube for blind intubation in anaesthetized patients with a predicted difficult airway, (eLetter7749), *Br. J. Anaesth.* (2012). Available online on: http://bja.oxfordjournals.org/

[10] M. R. Rai, S. H. Scott, A. G. Marfin, M. T. Popat and J. J. Pandit, , A comparison of a flexometallic tracheal tube with the intubating laryngeal mask tracheal tube for nasotracheal fibreoptic intubation using the two-scope technique, *Anaesthesia* 64, 1303-6 (2009).

[11] O. Takahata, K. Mamiya, Y. Akama, T. Nozaka, H. Matsumoto, and H. Ogawa, The efficacy of the "BURP" maneuver during a difficult laryngoscopy, *Anesth. Analg.* 84, 419-21 (1997).

[12] J. Brimacombe, C. Keller and F. Puehringer, Pharyngeal mucosal pressure and perfusion: a fiberoptic evaluation of the posterior pharynx in anesthetized adult patients with a modified cuffed oropharyngeal airway, *Anesthesiology* 91, 1661-5 (1999).

[13] J. Zhang, Z. Zhao, Y. Chen and X. Zhang, New insights into the mechanism of injury to the recurrent larynygeal nerve associated with the laryngeal mask airway, *Med. Sci. Monit.* 16, HY7-9 (2010).

[14] J. Brimacombe, Laryngeal mask anaestheia, 2nd ed., WB Saunders, Philadelphia 2005.

[15] S. Kihara, Y. Yguchi, J. Brimacombe, S. Watanabe and N. Taguchi, Routine use of the intubating laryngeal mask airway results in increased upper airway morbidity, *Can. J. Anaesth.* 48, 604-8 (2001).

[16] Kapila, V. Addy, C. Verghese and A. I. Brain, The intubating laryngeal mask airway: an initial assessment of performance, *Br. J. Anaesth.* 79, 710-3 (1997).

[17] Gibbison, T. M. Cook and C. Seller, Case series: protection from aspiration and failure of protection from aspiration with the i-gel airway, *Br. J. Anaesth.* 100, 415-7 (2008).

[18] S. H. Yu and O. R. Beirne, Laryngeal mask airways have a lower risk of airway complications compared with endotracheal intubation: a systematic review, *J. Oral Maxillofac. Surg.* 68, 2359-76 (2010).

[19] K. B. Domino, K. L. Posner, R. A. Caplan and F. W. Cheney, Airway injury during anesthesia: a closed claims analysis, *Anesthesiology* 91, 1703-11 (1999).

[20] P. Rujirojindakul, C. Prechawaj and E. Watanayomnaporn, Tongue numbness following laryngeal mask airway SupremeTM and i-gelTM insertion: two case reports, *Acta Anaesthesiol. Scand.* (2012) [Epub ahead of print].

[21] Baska mask. Available online on: www.proactmedical.com.au.

[22] N. S. Gerstein, D. A. Braude, O. Hung, J. C. Saunders and M. F. Murphy, The Fastrach intubating laryngeal mask airway: an overview, an update, *Can. J. Anaesth.* 57, 588-601 (2010).

[23] L. G. Theiler, M. Kleine-Brueggeney, D. Kaiser, N. Urwyler, C. Luyet, A. Vogt, R. Grief and A. Unibe, Crossover comparison of the laryngeal mask SupremeTM and the i-gelTM in simulated difficult airway scenario in anesthetized patients, *Anesthesiology* 111, 55-62 (2009).

[24] M. Lange, T. Smul, P. Zimmermann, R. Kohlenberger, N. Roewer and F. Kehl, The effectiveness and patient comfort of the novel streamlined pharynx airway liner (SLIPA) compared with the conventional laryngeal mask airway in ophtalmic surgery, *Anesth. Analg.* 104, 431-4 (2007).

[25] T. Asai, A. Kawashima, I. Hidaka and S. Kawashi, The laryngeal tube in comparison with the laryngeal mask: insertion, gas leak and gastric insufflation, *Br. J. Anaesth.* 89, 729-32 (2002).

[26] K. Esa, I. Azarinah, M. Muhammad, M. A. Helmi and M. Z. Jaafar, A comparison between Laryngeal tube suction II airway and ProSeal laryngeal mask airway in laparoscopic surgery, *Med. J. Malaysia* 66, 182-6 (2011).

[27] J. Brimacombe and A. Berry, The cuffed oropharyngeal airway for spontaneous ventilation anaesthesia, *Anaesthesia* 53, 1074-9 (1998).

[28] T. Ezri, N. Ady, P. Szmuk, L. Glanz, B. Shklar, J. Katz and D. Geva, Use of cuffed oropharyngeal vs. laryngeal mask airway in elderly patients, *Can. J. Anaesth.* 46, 363-7 (1999).

[29] V. Alexiev, A. Salim, L. G. Kevin and J. G. Laffey, An observational study of the Baska® mask: a novel supraglottic airway, *Anaesthesia* 67, 640-5 (2012).

[30] T. van Zundert and S. Gatt, The Baska Mask® - a new concept in self-sealing membrane cuff extraglottic airway devices, using a sump and two gastric drains: a critical evaluation, *J. Obst. Anaesth. Crit. Care* 2, 23-30 (2012).

[31] W. Donaldson, A. Abraham, M. Deighan and P. Michalek, i-gel™ vs. AuraOnce™ laryngeal mask for general anaesthesia with controlled ventilation in paralyzed patients, *Biomed. Pap.* 155, 155-64 (2011).

[32] F. McAleavey and P. Michalek, Aura-i laryngeal mask as a conduit for elective fibreoptic intubation, *Anaesthesia* 65, 1151 (2010).

[33] D. M. Miller, A conceptual ideal supraglottic airway, *Anest. Intenziv. Med.* 22, 149-52 (2011).

In: The i-gel Supraglottic Airway
Editors: Pavel Michalek and William Donaldson
ISBN: 978-1-62417-897-9

Chapter 3

DEVELOPMENT OF THE I-GEL SUPRAGLOTTIC AIRWAY

Amy L. Williams, Rebecca M. Anderson and Muhammed A. Nasir*
Intersurgical Ltd, Wokingham, Berkshire, UK

ABSTRACT

i-gel® is the result of over 19 years work by both the inventor and Intersurgical. It has been assessed visually, anatomically and clinically and has been shown to provide safe and effective airway management.

In the past, the majority of laryngeal masks used in clinical practice were manufactured from silicone, and were reusable, risking cross-contamination. This generation of SADs also lacked a mechanism for managing the regurgitation of gastric contents. There was, therefore, an opportunity to further advance airway management through the development of an innovative, unique and novel airway device to address the common complaints associated with laryngeal mask airways.

Sore throat is a common minor complaint after general anaesthesia, so the face of the device needed to be soft enough to reduce the number of postoperative complications and co-morbidity experienced by patients.

Dr Richard Levitan, carried out the first study on i-gel. Comprehensive and elaborate endoscopic, radiological, CT, MRI and neck dissection work on fresh cadavers allowed the production of a truly anatomical device. This data was extrapolated into 3D imaging for the development of the paediatric i-gel.

The i-gel development team is constantly working on modifications and improvements, and further extensions to the range. With the launch of i-gel, airway management has truly evolved.

* E-mail: awi@intersurgical.co.uk.

INTRODUCTION

In 1983 a new type of airway was described in a paper by Brain, known as the laryngeal mask [1], consisting of a tube opening at one end into the lumen of a miniature inflatable mask [2]. The laryngeal mask airway represented a compromise between the endotracheal (ET) tube and the facemask, which were the methods predominantly used at the time to maintain the airways of anesthetized patients. It was a technological leap forward for airway management.

The choice of airway management device has the strongest influence on the incidence of sore throat in anesthetized patients [3]. Sore throat is a common minor complaint after general anesthesia affecting as many as 60% of patients [4]. Postoperative sore throat may be the result of cuff pressure of a laryngeal mask exceeding pharyngeal mucosal perfusion pressure [5] and also appears to be related to the technique of insertion. High intracuff pressures seem to be associated with nerve palsies - due to neuropraxia and nerve compression [6]. Endotracheal tube cuffs increase the risk of airway mucosal injury; however they are not always necessary in children, because an appropriately sized uncuffed tube will seal the airway well [7].

In the past, the majority of laryngeal masks used in clinical practice were manufactured from silicone, and were reusable. Sterilization is expensive and the risk of cross-infection remains a potential issue. These supraglottic airway devices (SADs) were mostly effective, but did have the potential to become displaced, rotated, and cause compression trauma. This generation of SADs also lacked a mechanism for managing the regurgitation of gastric contents [8]. There was, therefore, an opportunity to further advance airway management through the development of an innovative, unique and novel airway device to address the common complaints associated with laryngeal mask airways.

EARLY DAYS

Muhammed Aslam Nasir, born in 1961, was an ambitious young student who excelled at school and won scholarships to pursue his chosen career in the medical profession. After graduating from Nishtar Medical College, Multan, Dr Nasir became a House Officer in surgery at the Lahore Hospital. It was during his time in Lahore he first became aware of some of the issues surrounding anesthesia, in particular the limited choice between face mask ventilation and ventilation through an endotracheal tube.

Dr Nasir started to look into the concept of a tube with an anatomically shaped soft interface at the distal end that mirrored the human pharyngolaryngeal anatomy. The thought was that this could be placed over the larynx and would maintain a reliable perilaryngeal seal, without the need for an inflatable cuff. As well as matching the anatomy of the laryngo-pharynx, the face of the device could be soft enough to reduce the number of postoperative complications and co-morbidity experienced by patients. Significant research was carried out on other supraglottic airways and it was concluded that they had some common limitations and failings, and that no device at the time had tried to mirror the perilaryngeal framework.

Dr Nasir started to develop his anatomical airway from information gathered by direct and indirect pharyngolaryngeal endoscopies, x-rays, computerised tomography (CT) and magnetic resonance imaging (MRI) data. This knowledge was utilised to ensure that the shape and contours of the airway concept accurately mirrored the pharyngeal, laryngeal and perilaryngeal framework and enabled a design model of the face of the device to be produced.

The next step was to investigate the concept using real human anatomy. Dr Nasir visited the Cambridge University Anatomy Department in the United Kingdom (UK), where plaster of paris impressions and models were made using human anatomy specimens from cadaveric sections.

The plaster of paris models were converted into three dimensional computer aided design (CAD) models (Figure 1). Design engineers initially found it extremely difficult to reinterpret the plaster models so they were given the opportunity to examine the cadavers and the relevant structures for themselves. The result of this work was a stereolithographic apparatus (SLA) model with three distal openings in its face. This early design also included a gastric opening, which allowed the venting of gas and liquid from the stomach.

The SLA model illustrated to Dr Nasir that the concept showed promise and in 2003 he obtained his first silicone prototype. This prototype enabled Dr. Nasir to discuss the concept and to seek out commercial partners to develop and commercialize the idea into an actual product with his idea of an anatomical fit supraglottic airway device and this silicone prototype.

INTERSURGICAL

Intersurgical® are a leading global designer and manufacturer of respiratory care products for use in anesthesia, intensive care and airway management. The company was established in 1982 and has developed a comprehensive and flexible range of products in response to changing clinical practice and user requirements. They are a fully integrated medical device manufacturer with their own in-house production facilities in Lithuania, Guernsey, USA, Italy, and headquarters in Wokingham, UK, with proven expertise in design, and manufacture of consumable medical devices.

All Intersurgical products meet the requirements of the relevant BS, ISO and EN standards. Compliance with the US Food and Drug Administration (FDA), ISO 9001: 2000, ISO 13485 and Annex ii of the Medical Devices Directive allows CE marking of all of their products enabling Intersurgical products to be traded throughout Europe and the world without restriction.

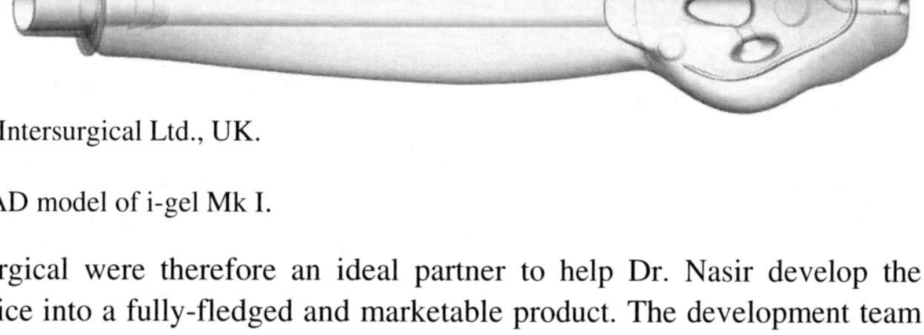

Courtesy of Intersurgical Ltd., UK.

Figure 1. CAD model of i-gel Mk I.

Intersurgical were therefore an ideal partner to help Dr. Nasir develop the prototype airway device into a fully-fledged and marketable product. The development team shared Dr

Nasir's enthusiasm and vision for the project, and he was confident that they were the right people to bring the product to the market.

Intersurgical took the opportunity and created a team of dedicated engineers, designers and material scientists to aid the design and development process. The team had a depth of knowledge, expertise and experience in the field that would complement Dr. Nasir's idea. The new partnership enabled an eight-member team, led by Dr. Nasir, to further develop the product through advanced research at the University of Maryland, Baltimore, Pennsylvania, USA. This signalled the start of a period of extensive evaluation and testing on the Nasir Airway Device.

INTERSURGICAL DEVELOPMENT

What's in a Name?

The concept prototype had been called a number of different names during its early development including the 'Nasir Airway Device' and the 'Cobra Mask Airway', so-called after its shape, which was contoured to follow the irregular anatomical landscape in the proximity of the glottis.

Over one hundred names had been put forward and one of the early front-runners was 'Remora' owing to the airway's unique shape resembling the distinctive head shape of this fish (Figure 2). However, in the end it was the material that gave Dr. Nasir and the Intersurgical® team the idea for the name 'i-gel®'- the *'Intersurgical Gel Airway'.* It was decided i-gel reflected both the physical and clinical characteristics of the device to achieve the most natural airway management possible.

First Steps

The first few prototypes were endotracheal tubes with plasticine and plaster moulded from cadavers, from which came the silicone model in 3 pieces (Figure 3). Originally the first few prototypes had a gastric channel, a syringe port at the proximal end to remove stomach contents rather than a port for a nasogastric tube.

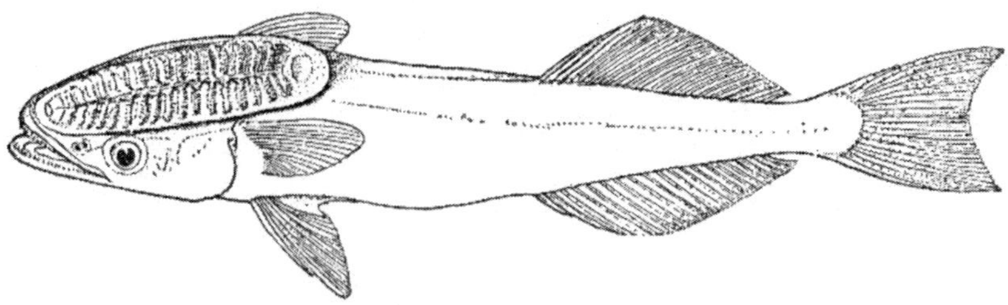

Courtesy of Intersurgical Ltd., UK.

Figure 2. Remora fish.

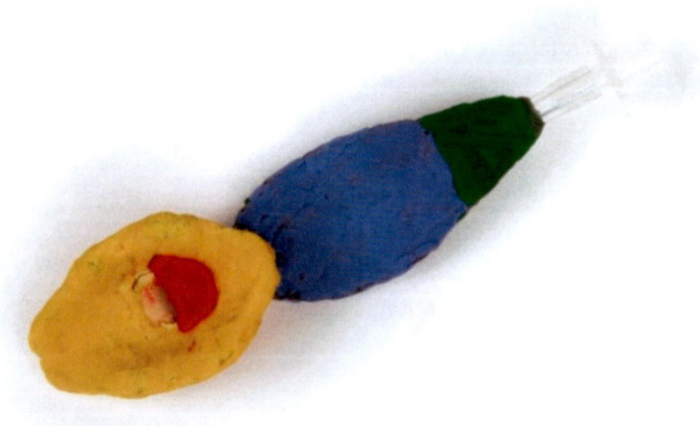

Courtesy of Intersurgical Ltd., UK.

Figure 3. Plasticine model of the first i-gel from cadavers.

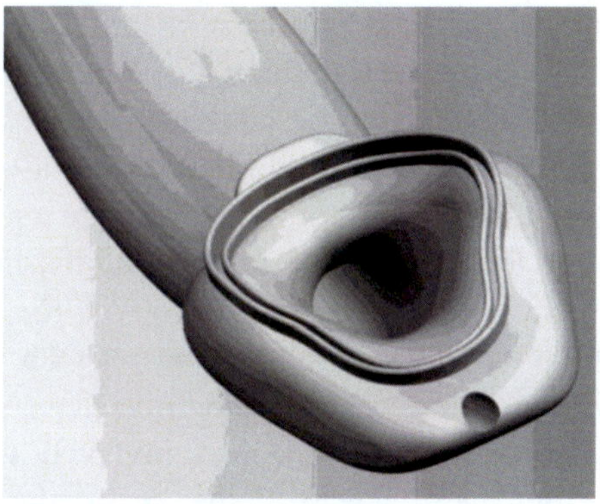

Courtesy of Intersurgical Ltd., UK.

Figure 4. This double seal around the cuff was subsequently removed.

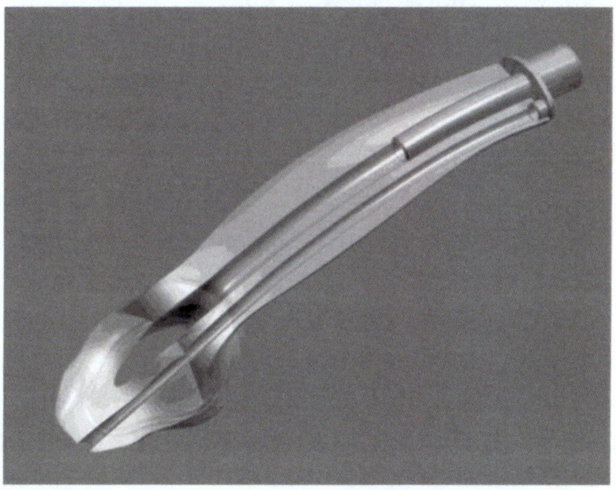

Courtesy of Intersurgical Ltd., UK.

Figure 5. Early position of the gastric channel. In later versions, the position was changed, so that the channel would exit centrally at the tip of the non-inflatable cuff.

Over the course of the device's development, changes were made to constantly improve upon the seal and the anatomical fit around the laryngeal opening and to improve the overall functionality of the product. The features that were optimized included:

- Body and cuff – Materials and double seal (Figure 4)
- Body - Injection moulding and tooling
- Gastric channel - Positioning and performance (Figure 5)
- Tip length
- Connector - Design and integration

Material World

The initial devices were made from a medical grade silicone material and the device proved a success not only in its ease of use but also its intra-operative and postoperative safety profile. However the product needed to be mass-produced and the material had to be economical enough for the product to be supplied as a single use device. Dr Nasir envisioned i-gel to be as soft as possible so that the device sat around the laryngeal inlet causing the least possible trauma. He also wished for it to be sterile and single-use to avoid cross-infection among patients. However, initial meetings in 2003 with Intersurgical® and their suppliers concluded that it was impossible to produce a grade of plastic as soft as Dr Nasir and Intersurgical required.

The cuff section was required to be soft and compliant with the anatomy of the laryngo-pharyngeal structures. The main body of the product needed to be of a stiffer material to provide strength and durability. Intersurgical was involved with sourcing the different materials from various companies, however the requirement for both softness and transparency was beyond the scope of materials available at the time. These characteristics provided a challenge for the research and development team to identify new and novel materials to meet the required product specification.

Eventually a supplier came forward with a bespoke ultra soft material that offered a viable solution and new prototypes were produced. The material selected was a thermoplastic elastomer (TPE) called styrene ethylene butadiene styrene (SEBS). The Shore Durometer scales are a measure of the hardness of a material. There are several scales, reflecting the wide range of materials that can be tested. Most soft gels and foam rubbers are measured using the 00 scale, for example a bicycle gel seat and chewing gum are measured on the 00 scale. Harder materials such as a hard hat or truck tires would be measured on the D scale. The materials developed for the i-gel were pushing the boundaries of softness with a double zero scale. The final material selected and validated gives the product its unique feel. It is malleable, soft and yet rigid and robust enough to perform effectively in the most testing clinical situations. The softness maximized safety, ease of insertion and comfort in patients.

Moulds and Tooling

Earlier models of the silicone i-gel were made in a more open casting process as opposed to the current injection moulding process. With the high variation in wall thickness it was seen as impossible to injection mould the i-gel as the plastic would freeze off before binding was complete.

To make the product more suitable for injection moulding air pockets were designed to go along the body of the i-gel. However this made it impossible to sterilize the product, as it had to pass through vacuum chambers. After the autoclaving cycle was completed some of the air pockets collapsed.

Currently, manufacturing of the i-gel is a two shot moulding process and both shots are soft plastic. The tool room at Intersurgical®, Lithuania is now able to use a single cavity two shot moulding process and the entire i-gel manufacturing process is completely automated.

The gastric channel of the i-gel curves around the buccal cavity to rest in the centre of the tip thus the demoulding process before automation was complicated. It could not simply be taken off; it had to be manipulated in a certain way. When cooling the mould it was found that water acted as a lubricant allowing the mould to be removed easily. Automation has proved an incredibly useful tool and a great achievement considering the complexity of the removal process.

Device Evaluations

With the revised models the next step in the project took place at the University of Maryland, Baltimore, USA, where there was access to fresh cadavers. Here it was possible to evaluate insertion, seal, function and positioning of the device. Dr Richard Levitan, a respected doctor in emergency medicine and airways, carried out training courses in advanced techniques at the University. Ultimately this work led to the first study on i-gel® by Levitan and Kinkle, published in Anaesthesia in 2005 [9]. Here, 65 non-embalmed fresh cadavers were used to study the positioning and mechanics of the new device (Figure 6).

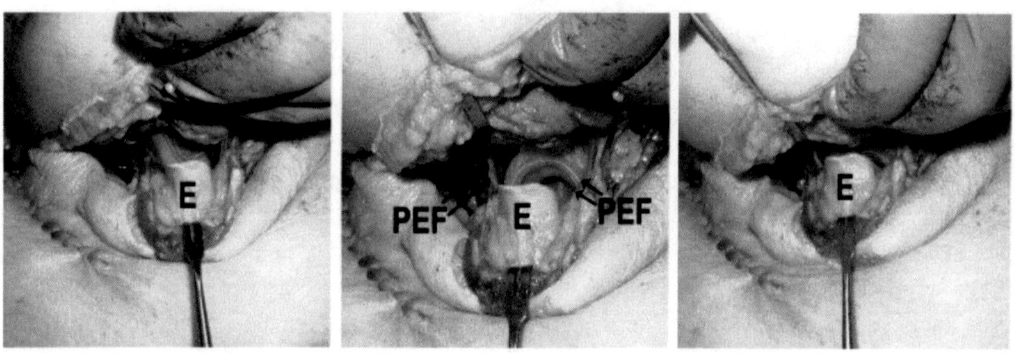

Figure 6. Sequential images from left to right of insertion of the i-gel after neck dissection at the level of the hyoid. The tip and distal section of the bowl of the i-gel is visible passing beneath the epiglottis in the image on the left; in the image on the right insertion is complete and the proximal portion of the bowl is barely visible. The sides of the bowl are seen passing beneath the pharyngoepiglottic folds in the middle image. The epiglottis is marked E, and the pharyngo-epiglottic folds are marked PEF.

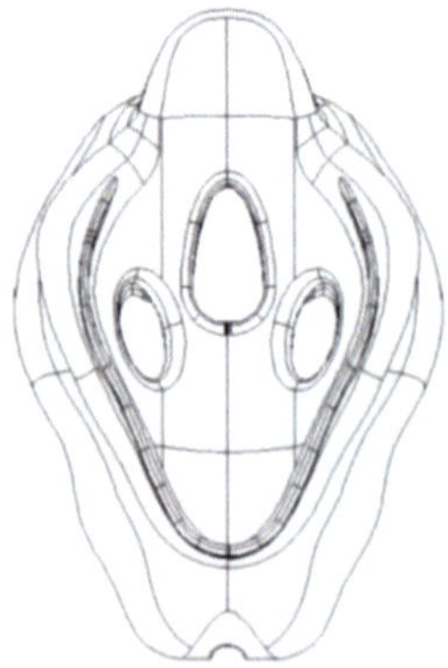

Courtesy of Intersurgical Ltd., UK.

Figure 7. Three openings on the distal face of the bowl.

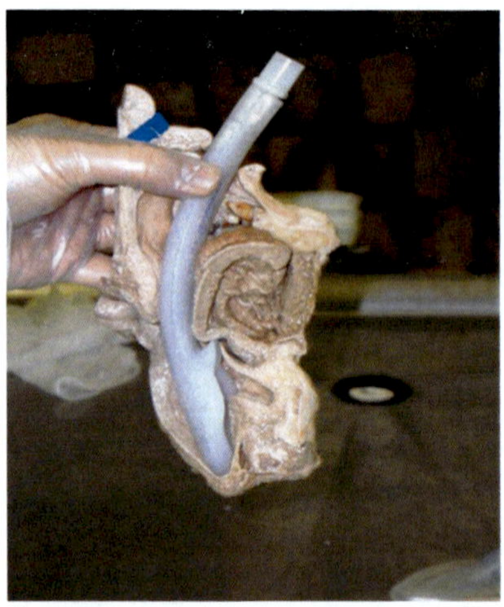

Courtesy of Intersurgical Ltd., UK.

Figure 8. i-gel inserted into a cadaver – lateral view.

Through the use of endoscopy, neck dissections and radiographs, Levitan showed the device had a mean percentage glottic opening (POGO) score of 82%. A 100% POGO score was achieved in 60% of the insertions. In each of the dissections and radiographs he saw that the bowl of the device covered the laryngeal inlet and his conclusions were that the device effectively conformed to the perilaryngeal anatomy and consistently achieved proper positioning for ventilation. Radiographic imaging of the device in comparison with other supraglottic airways and dissection were also undertaken. The confidence gained in the USA encouraged evaluation in a patient population. At the Difficult Airway Society's Conference in 2004 attendees were impressed with Intersurgical's ethos: to bring the device into the market only after proper investigative and research work had been undertaken.

Three teaching hospitals were involved in further evaluation of the device for the initiation and maintenance of anesthesia on voluntary patients. During this period, small changes to the design were made to improve performance including the removal of the three openings from the distal face (Figure 7). Initially, the reason for three openings was to provide a patent airway even if an occlusion occurred in one of them. However, in both the cadaver evaluations (Figure 8), and the clinical setting it was found that, when in-situ, the bowl of the device "tunnels" and deepens within the peri-pharyngolaryngeal pouch. This change, in combination with the epiglottic rest, prevents the epiglottis from down-folding and blocking the airway. As a result of these findings these distal openings were removed. It is seen as a milestone in the development of i-gel: with one opening it could now be used as a conduit for intubation. The team felt that the benefits of the deep open bowl and the ability to pass an endotracheal tube down it were more important than retaining the original design. This approach of steady evolution characterized the project and shows that nothing was taken for granted.

Evolution - Airway Management Has Evolved

In January 2007, the i-gel® supraglottic airway was released at the Winter Scientific Meeting of the Association of Anaesthetists in London. Speaking at the meeting, Dr Nasir said, "i-gel is a device that mirrors the anatomical landscape of the pharyngolarynx as nature might have intended". With the launch of i-gel, airway management had truly evolved (Figure 9).

i-gel is the result of over 19 years work by both the inventor and Intersurgical®. It has been assessed visually, anatomically and clinically and has been shown to provide safe and effective airway management. However, Intersurgical's development team are constantly trying to improve the i-gel where possible, whether it be sourcing different materials, complying with new medical guidelines or decreasing packaging for a more environmentally-friendly product.

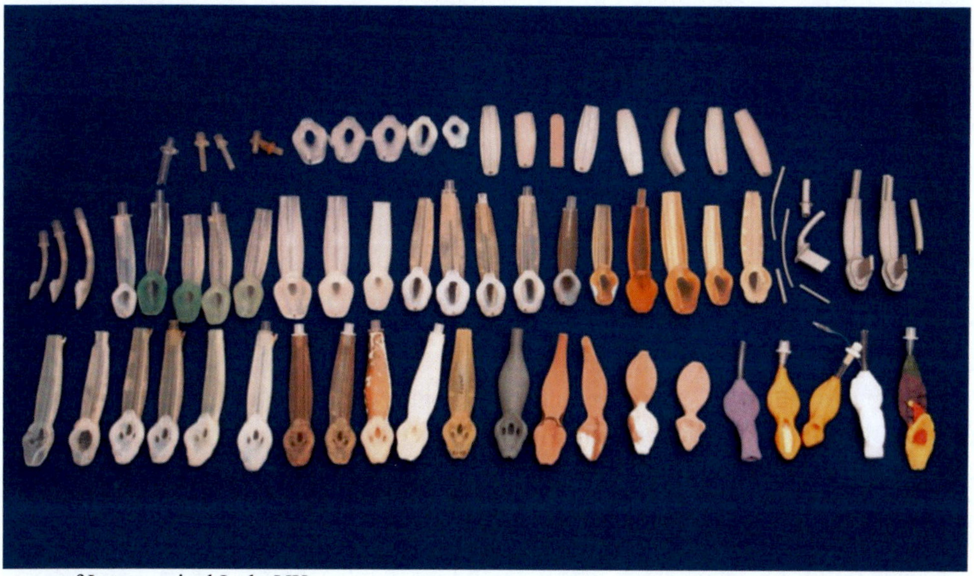

Courtesy of Intersurgical Ltd., UK.

Figure 9. The evolution of the i-gel supraglottic airway.

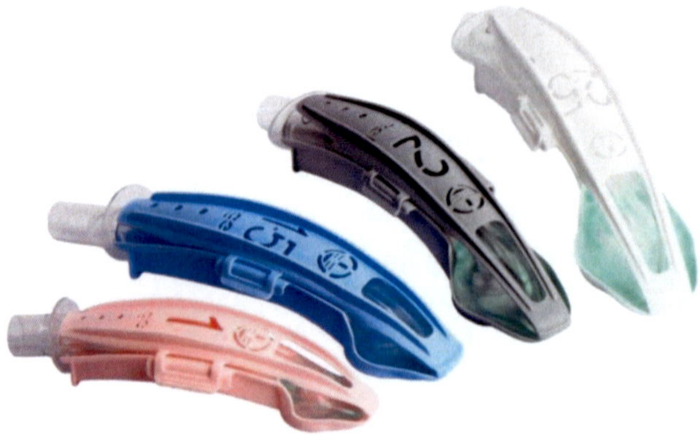

Courtesy of Intersurgical Ltd., UK.

Figure 10. Four pediatric sizes of i-gel.

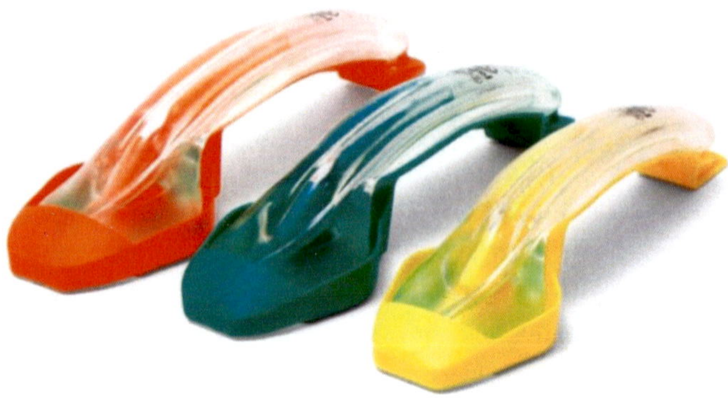

Courtesy of Intersurgical Ltd., UK.

Figure 11. Three adult sizes of i-gel.

I-GEL - FEATURES AND BENEFITS

The i-gel® is currently available in seven sizes (Figure 10) (Figure 11) and is supplied in a colour-coded polypropylene 'protective cradle'.

The absence of an inflatable cuff has several potential advantages including easier insertion, minimal risk of tissue compression and stability after insertion (i.e. no position change with cuff inflation). The i-gel is designed as a latex free, sterile, single patient use device. The buccal cavity stabilizer has a widened, elliptical, symmetrical and laterally flattened cross sectional shape (with a circular airway channel), providing good vertical stability and axial strength upon insertion. This houses a standard airway channel and a separate gastric channel. It has a built-in natural curvature and an inherent propensity to adapt its shape to the oropharyngeal curvature of the patient. It is anatomically widened and concaved to eliminate the potential for rotation, thereby reducing the risk of malposition. The risk of rotation and malpositioning leading to partial or complete airway obstruction is extremely low with the i-gel compared with other supraglottic devices [10].

The firmness of the tube section and its curvature allows the device to be smoothly, rapidly and reliably inserted by grasping the proximal end of the i-gel which helps glide the leading edge against the hard palate into the pharynx. It is not necessary to insert fingers into the mouth of the patient for achieving full insertion. The smooth contiguous under surface of the device, from the tip of the bowl and throughout the entire tube section, allows the device to easily slide posteriorly along the hard palate, pharynx and into the hypopharynx [10].

The novel soft non-inflatable cuff fits onto the perilaryngeal framework, mirroring the shape of the epiglottis, aryeptiglottic folds, piriform fossae, peri-thyroid, peri-cricoid, posterior cartilages and spaces. Each anatomical feature is met by an impression from the device, helping to support sealing by enveloping the laryngeal inlet. The tip lies in the proximal opening of the esophagus, isolating the esophageal opening from the laryngeal inlet. The outer cuff shape ensures that bloodflow to the laryngeal and perilaryngeal framework is maintained and helps to reduce the possibility of neurovascular compression. Sliding past the pharyngo-epiglottic folds it becomes narrower and deeper, creating an outward movement to fit snugly into the potential space of the perilaryngeal pouch [10].

The gastric channel runs through the device from its proximal opening at the side of the flat connector wing to the distal tip of the non-inflatable cuff. Since the distal tip of the device fits snugly and anatomically correctly into the upper esophageal opening, the distal opening of the gastric channel can provide an early warning of regurgitation, allows for the passing of a nasogastric tube to empty the stomach contents and can facilitate the venting of gas from the stomach [10].

The i-gel has its product information clearly displayed on the device including size and weight guidance. A horizontal line on the tube shows where the incisors should lie on all of the adult i-gels, providing easy confirmation of the optimum insertion depth. It is not present on the pediatric i-gel due to the large variations in infant sizes. With any airway device there is a risk of airway occlusion due to the patient biting down on the tube. The integral bite block reduces any possible risk of airway channel obstruction in the i-gel [10].

An artificial epiglottis and a protective ridge help prevent the epiglottis from down-folding or obstructing the distal opening of the airway. Down-folding of the epiglottis can occasionally occur and may be more common in children, but the i-gel's cuff and airway channel have been designed in such a way that the chance of obstruction to fresh gas flow (FGF) is minimal. The epiglottic ridge at the proximal end of the bowl rests at the base of the tongue, keeping the device from moving upwards out of position and the tip from moving out of the upper esophagus [9, 10]. The i-gel does not use aperture bars like some supraglottic airways. The cuff creates a deep tunnelling effect whilst in-situ, thus making it more difficult for a down-folded epiglottis to block the distal end of the airway channel.

I-GEL - CLINICAL STUDIES AND SUPPORT

Some inflatable/disposable SADs have been reported to cause postoperative morbidity (sore throat, dysphagia, dysphonia etc) in excess of 45% [11]. Most of the published and non-published clinical data shows a very low incidence of sore throat, dysphonia, dysphagia and blood on the device (mucosal damage) with the i-gel [12-14].

The correct inflation pressure can be difficult to achieve with the laryngeal mask, and there can be a fine line between the correct pressure and that, which causes damage to tissues. Too little pressure will prevent a seal from being formed and therefore increase the chances of regurgitation and aspiration greatly. Asai and Kawashima showed in their study that insertion of the i-gel was seen as easy in 106 out of 120 patients with no airway complications reported [15]. In the National census of airway management techniques, Woodall and Cook showed that i-gel was the most popular second-generation supraglottic airway device used [16].

The i-gel is indicated for use in anesthesia, resuscitation and can also be used as a conduit for intubation. Acott indicated its potential for a use in airway management of a patient in a diving bell or deck decompression chamber. Cuff expansion occurs with normal laryngeal masks when pressure decreases, a problem not associated with the i-gel [17]. Acott showed no changes in the consistency of the i-gel and it might therefore be preferred by Diving Medical Technicians due to its lack of an inflatable cuff. It was also deemed easier to insert from any position [17].

A proficient user can achieve successful insertion of the i-gel in less than 5 seconds. With no inflatable cuff, i-gel provides a safe and rapid airway management solution.

i-gel is usually easy to insert in both manikins and patients as shown in several experimental [18-21] and clinical studies [22-25]. The insertion time is usually around 10 seconds and in most clinical studies it is shorter for the i-gel than for other SADs [26-29]. The i-gel was introduced into clinical practice in Japan in 2010. In a study by Asai and Kawashima it was always possible to insert the i-gel at the first attempt in 120 patients. The authors state that the i-gel is useful in maintaining a clear airway during general anesthesia [15].

According to published evidence, the i-gel airway has the first attempt insertion rate between 85 and 95%, with an overall success rate over 96% [22, 23, 28-31]. The device is also more likely to be inserted in manikins and patients by inexperienced users (anesthesia novices, paramedics, nursing staff, medical students) at the first attempt than other supraglottic airway devices [21, 32].

In a number of studies on the i-gel the seal pressure varied from 20 cm H_2O [25] to 35.6 cm H_2O [33]. Most studies reported seal pressures over 25 cm H_2O. The i-gel proved to have a higher leak (seal) pressure than most 1st generation SADs [24, 25-27, 30, 35, 36] and comparable sealing parameters with the 2nd generation supraglottic airways [37].

More data related to the insertion parameters, seal pressure of the device, overall success rate and complications is provided in following chapters.

I-GEL - INDICATIONS FOR USE

The i-gel was initially indicated for limited application until there were appropriately robust clinical data to support other uses. Intersurgical® were diligent and responsible with the indications and were keen to assure the function of the device across all indicated clinical parameters. During the initial development of the i-gel it was only indicated for use in anesthesia. As the development process continued more clinical studies were performed suggesting that the i-gel could be indicated for use in resuscitation (see Chapter 10). Most recently, studies have indicated that the i-gel can be used as a conduit for intubation with fiberoptic guidance.

The i-gel is compatible with general anesthesia for relatively non-invasive diagnostic or therapeutic procedures such as MRI, CT scanning, cardiac catheterization, nuclear scans, and radiation therapy. The complications and side effects of tracheal intubation or non-compatible SADs can therefore be avoided for these types of procedures.

It is believed, that as a supraglottic device, the i-gel may be appropriate for use in areas where SADs have proved to be beneficial:

1. Use by paramedics in difficult or unexpectedly difficult intubations in a pre-hospital setting in order to quickly establish and maintain a clear airway.
2. In a known difficult or unexpectedly difficult intubation, to pass a fiberoptic scope through the device, to provide visualization of the glottic opening to aid intubation.
3. In the Intensive Care patients, for weaning a certain category of the population, in whom an endotracheal tube is not well tolerated.
4. In difficult mouth opening situations, the i-gel can also be inserted under direct vision with the help of a laryngoscope.

PEDIATRIC I-GEL

Development of the Device

The main impetus to designing the pediatric i-gel® was to provide an SAD, which would meet as many of the physiological, anatomical and clinical challenges likely to be encountered during anesthesia and resuscitation of the pediatric population as possible. There is no single device or technique that is suitable for every patient in every clinical situation, so every anesthesiologist needs to be able to apply his/her clinical knowledge to ensure the best outcome for the patient. The design of the i-gel has tried to address as many of these challenges as possible. The pediatric design came about several years after the development of the adult i-gel.

Since the early 1990s, pediatric anesthetic practice has been revolutionized by increasing use of the LMA Classic® and Flexible LMA®. Many new SADs, with the exception of the LMA-ProSeal®, appear to offer little or no benefit for clinician or patient, over existing ones; evidence supporting the efficacy and safety of such devices is often absent or inadequate. In 2009 the LMA-ProSeal® had yet to be outperformed by any other SAD making it the premier SAD in children and the benchmark to which newer 2nd generation devices were compared [38], however this was before the pediatric i-gel® had been released into the market.

In 2006, a study by Polaner et al showed that SADs were being used more frequently in pediatric anesthesia. The introduction of the LMA was followed by the development of several competing devices that were similar in concept but differed significantly in design [39].

For many SADs, with the exception of the LMA Classic® and LMA-ProSeal®, there is a lack of high-quality data of efficacy in children. The best clinical evidence requires conducting randomized controlled trials comparing a new device against an established alternative, properly powered to detect relevant differences in clinically important outcomes. Such studies in children are very rare. Safety data is even harder to establish particularly for rare events such as aspiration. Most safety data comes from extended use rather than high quality evidence, which inevitably biases against newer devices [38].

Initial Clinical Studies

A study presented at the ASA meeting in October 2009 by Bopp et al. described their initial experience with the pediatric i-gel after its introduction to clinical practice. The median age of the patients was 48 months (range: 6 months to 14 years). i-gels of sizes 1 up to 3 were successfully placed in 1 (80%) or 2 (20%) attempts [40].

A preliminary study by Vesselinova et al. suggested that the i-gel is a reliable airway device at five different head and neck positions in the pediatric population. This is of particular interest for pediatric anesthesiologists, since many of anesthetic techniques involve the carrying out a caudal neuraxial block with the child in the lateral decubitus position [41]. Ramesh and Jayanthi found that due to its stability, the i-gel allows the child to be placed in the lateral decubitus position to perform caudal anesthesia, without this causing a leak or displacement of the device [42]. The authors concluded that the i-gel is very easy to insert and appears to be safe for pediatric airway management.

The pediatric i-gel is suitable for ventilation of anesthetized children and offers the additional advantage of gastric access. Compared to the Ambu Aura Once, it shows higher airway leak pressures [43]. Similarly Beylacq et al. found that the i-gel has a very good insertion success rate with very few complications and seems to be an efficient and safe device for pediatric airway management [44]. The features of the i-gel supraglottic airway seem very attractive, especially for use in children. The security margin between the airway leak pressure and the level of controlled ventilation airway pressure is very good, even for the smallest sizes [45].

The angle between the cuff and the cervical spine is a common problem in all supraglottic devices as this is increased in small children. In a study by Monclus et al. radiological images were reviewed to determine this angle with the pediatric i-gel. The pediatric i-gel was found to be easy to insert and the drainage channel worked well. The authors conclude that the device proved to have a good clinical and radiological performance in pediatric patients [46].

Pediatric patients have relatively large heads and therefore, hyperflexion, extension or side-to-side movement and the drag effect from a breathing system that is not properly secured, increases the possibility of the SAD's malposition. Epiglottic downfolding causing partial or complete airway obstruction is a well-recognized complication. The buccal cavity stabiliser of i-gel reduces the risk of malposition. It also provides vertical strength to facilitate easy insertion. An artificial epiglottis and a protective ridge help prevent the epiglottis from down folding or obstructing the distal opening of the airway [8]. The epiglottic ridge at the proximal end of the bowl rests at the base of the tongue, thus keeping the device from moving upwards out of position and the tip from moving out of the upper esophagus. However, pediatric i-gel should always be secured in place, especially in very small children [45].

The larger tongue and tonsils in pediatric airways have relatively more lymphoid tissue and the tissue of the neck, pharynx and nasopharynx is softer. This increases the propensity for upper airway obstruction after sedation, general anesthesia or during respiratory arrest. The pediatric i-gel can overcome such physical obstructions and challenges with a clear and stable airway [15].

The pediatric airway is highly innervated, not well developed, hypersensitive and highly reactive to stimuli. The unique, streamlined back plate with a pharyngeal stabilizer and a very soft, gel-like non-inflatable cuff of the i-gel provides an easy, smooth and uninterrupted insertion with minimal stimulation to the patient [10, 31, 47]. The pediatric airway tends to be more vulnerable to airway trauma so the pediatric i-gel has a novel, soft non-inflatable cuff which is designed to cause the least possible compression trauma, stimulation or postoperative complications such as sore throat, dysphagia or dysphonia [11].

The ratio between minute alveolar ventilation and the functional residual capacity (FRC) is higher in pediatric patients. This reduces the oxygen reserve in the lungs should ventilation stop, thereby necessitating airway support. The pediatric i-gel has a large airway channel offering almost no resistance, with laminar flow of the fresh gas flow under anesthesia mimicking natural breathing.

Many SADs have a long learning curve for competent and safe use. In excess of 25 insertion techniques for the LMA have been described in the clinical literature [48] and anywhere between 15-60 insertions are recommended to achieve competency. The i-gel has a short learning curve for competent use in pediatric patients [32].

Deskilling is a well-known phenomenon among clinicians if a procedure is not practiced frequently enough. In a recent study, 41 paramedics attempted to insert the i-gel in a manikin. Three months later all participants were assessed without further training, showing no significant difference in success rates from their first attempts [20]. Medical students were given standardized training and inserted the i-gel in manikins. Twelve months later participants used the device again without further training and the i-gel was the most likely to be inserted successfully on the first attempt and was rated as the easiest to use, with the quickest time to successful ventilation [20].

The tip of an inflatable SAD residing in the upper esophagus can initiate a well known physiological response called “The Bolus Effect” that tends to reduce the lower esophageal sphincter pressure (The Barrier Pressure) thus rendering the patient prone to regurgitation and possible aspiration. The tip of the non-inflatable cuff of the pediatric i-gel lies in the proximal opening of the esophagus, isolating the esophageal opening from the laryngeal inlet [10].

Pediatric patients are well known to be the most unreliable patient group in respect of having an empty stomach, and therefore represent a higher aspiration risk than adults. Due to a lack of understanding of the potential consequences, parents sometimes allow their children to eat prior to surgery, despite warnings given to them not to do so. Parents then often hide this fact through fear of the operation being cancelled. The presence of the gastric channel of the pediatric i-gel permits insertion of a gastric tube (except in size 1). The gastric channel provides an early warning of regurgitation, allows for the passing of a gastric tube to empty the stomach contents and can facilitate the venting of gas from the stomach.

Some disposable/inflatable SADs can cause compression trauma and have low seal pressures. The pediatric i-gel is an anatomically contoured SAD that results in a better fit and seal of the airway and higher potential inflation pressures, thus providing a much improved seal at the glottis. The average seal pressure provided by paediatric i-gel is between 20-26 cm H_2O [43, 44, 49, 50].

The pediatric i-gel was recently released for wider clinical use; its inventive steps and design specifications were mainly based on the following considerations;

1. A comprehensive understanding of the physiological, anatomical and pathological characteristics and differences of the pediatric airway in relation to the use of SADs.
2. An extensive literature search of the issues surrounding the comprehensive airway management philosophy.
3. An extensive research on pre-dissected and preserved pediatric and adult models in various university departments of Anatomy in the United Kingdom and the USA.
4. Comprehensive and elaborate endoscopic, radiological, CT, MRI and neck dissection work on fresh cadavers in the USA and older cadavers in the UK to create a truly anatomical device, achieving a mirrored impression of the pharyngeal, laryngeal and perilaryngeal structures, without causing compression or displacement trauma to the tissues and structures in the vicinity. That knowledge was extrapolated into 3D imaging for the development of the pediatric i-gel.
5. Our comprehensive understanding and clinical knowledge of over 3 million adult uses.
6. The non-inflatable, super-soft cuff causing the least stimulus to the hypersensitive and highly reactive pediatric airway thus reducing the potential for laryngospasm, bronchospasm, breath holding, hiccoughing or retching.

As with the adult i-gel, Intersurgical are constantly trying to improve the pediatric product. Initially, the shelf life of the pediatric i-gel was 12 months, but this has now increased to 2 years, with the expectation of further shelf life progression. The final objective is to achieve a 5-year shelf life for both the adult and pediatric i-gels.

Conclusion

Both adult and pediatric sizes of i-gel are established 2nd generation SADs for a routine use in clinical anesthesia and with undisputable potential for insertion in cardiopulmonary resuscitation and difficult airway management.

Intersurgical are consistently developing their current product range and are always looking for opportunities to improve upon them. The Resus O_2 i-gel® is a product produced by Intersurgical that has a supplementary oxygen port along with other accessories available in a convenient pack (see Chapter 10). The i-gel development team is constantly working on modifications and improvements, and further extensions to the range.

Conflict of Interest

Amy L. Williams and Rebecca M. Anderson are employees of Intersurgical Ltd. Dr Muhammed A. Nasir is the inventor of the i-gel supraglottic airway.

REFERENCES

[1] I. Brain, The laryngeal mask – a new concept in airway management, *Br. J. Anaesth.* 55, 801-6 (1983).

[2] I. Brain, The laryngeal mask airway – a possible new solution to airway problems in the emergency situation, *Arch. Emerg. Med.* 1: 229-32 (1984).

[3] P. P. Higgins, F. Chung and G. Mezei, Postoperative sore throat after ambulatory surgery. *Br. J. Anaesth.* 88, 582-4 (2002).

[4] W. M. Splinter, B. Smallman, E. J. Rhine and L. Komocar, Postoperative sore throat in children and the laryngeal mask airway. *Can. J. Anesth.* 41, 1081-3 (1994).

[5] S. W. O'Kelly, K. J. Heath and E. G. Lawes, A study of laryngeal mask inflation, *Anaesthesia* 48, 1075-8 (1993).

[6] F. E. McHardy and F. Chung, Postoperative sore throat: cause, prevention and treatment, *Anaesthesia* 54, 444-53 (2002).

[7] H. H. Khine, D. H. Corddry, R. G. Kettrick, T. M. Martin, J. J. McCloskey, J. B. Rose, M. C. Theroux and M. M. Zagnoev, Comparison of cuffed and uncuffed endotracheal tubes in young children during general anesthesia, *Anesthesiology* 86, 627-31 (1997).

[8] M. A. Roomi, The hard road: steps on the entrepreneunial journey, *University of Bedfordshire* (2010).

[9] R. M. Levitan and W. C. Kinkle, Initial anatomic investigation of the i-gel airway: a novel supraglottic airway without inflatable cuff. *Anaesthesia* 60, 1022-6 (2005).

[10] Intersurgical, Intersurgical i-gel® User Guide, *Intersurgical Ltd.,* Wokingham, Berkshire, United Kingdom (2007).

[11] Keijzer, D. R. Buitelaar, K. M. Efthymiou, M. Sramek, J. T. Cate, M. Ronday, T. Stoppa, J. M. Huitnik and P. F. Schutte, A comparison of postoperative throat and neck complaints after the use of the i-gel® and the La Premiere® disposable Laryngeal Mask: A double blinded, randomized controlled trial, *Anesth. Analg.* 109, 1092-5 (2009).

[12] O. A. Bamgbade, W. R. Macnab and W. M. Khalaf, Evaluation of the i-gel airway in 300 patients, *Eur. J. Anaesthesiol.* 25, 865-6 (2008).

[13] A. Gabbott and R. Beringer, The i-gel supraglottic airway: a potential role for resuscitation? *Resuscitation* 73, 161-2 (2007).

[14] J. J. Gatward, T. M. Cook, C. Seller, J. Handel, T. Simpson, V. Vanek and F. Kelly, Evaluation of the size 4 i-gel® airway in one hundred non-paralysed patients. *Anaesthesia* 63, 1124-30 (2008).

[15] T. Asai and A. Kawashima, The i-gel: its efficacy in 120 patients undergoing general anaesthesia, *Masui* 60, 739-42 (2011). [Article in Japanese, English abstract].

[16] N. M. Woodall and T. M. Cook, National census of airway management techniques used for anaesthesia in the UK: first phase of the Fourth National Audit Project at the Royal College of Anaesthetists, *Br. J. Anaesth.* 106, 266-71 (2011).

[17] J. Acott CJ, Extraglottic airway devices for use in diving medicine – part 3: the i-gel®. *Diving Hyperbar. Med.* 38, 124-7 (2008).

[18] N. Castle, R. Owen, M. Hann, R. Naidoo and D. Reeves, Assessment of the speed and ease of insertion of three supraglottic airway devices by paramedics: a manikin study, *Emerg. Med. J.* 27, 860-3 (2010).

[19] N. Castle, Y. Pillay and N. Spencer, Insertion of six different supraglottic airway devices whilst wearing chemical, biological, radiation, nuclear-personal protective equipment: a manikin study, *Anaesthesia* 66, 983-8 (2011).

[20] K. Ruetzler, B. Roessler, L. Potura, A. Priemayr, O. Robak, E. Schuster and M. Frass, Performance and skill retention of intubation by paramedics using seven different airway devices – a manikin study, *Resuscitation* 82, 593-7 (2011).

[21] K. Stroumpoulis, C. Isaia, E. Bassiakou, I. Pantazapoulos, G. Troupis, A. Mazarakis, T. Demestiha and T. Xanthos, A comparison of the i-gel® and classic LMA insertion in manikins by experienced and novice physicians, *Eur. J. Emerg. Med.* (2012).

[22] Kannaujia, U. Srivastava, N. Saraswat, A. Mishra, A. Kumar and S. Saxena, A preliminary study of i-gel®: a new supraglottic airway device. *Indian J. Anaesth.* 53, 52-6 (2009).

[23] T Asai and E. H. Liu, The i-gel, a new supraglottic airway, Masui 59, 794-7 (2010). [Article in Japanese, English abstract].

[24] M. Helmy, H. M. Atef, E. M. El-Taher and A. M. Henidak, Comparative study between i-gel®, a new supraglottic airway device, and classical laryngeal mask airway in anaesthetised spontaneously ventilated patients, *Saudi J. Anaesth.* 4, 131-6 (2010).

[25] S. Amini and M. Khoshfetrat, Comparison of the Intersurgical Solus layngeal mask airway and the i-gel® supralaryngeal device, *Anaesthesia* 65, 805-9 (2010).

[26] U. Weber, R. Oguz, L. A. Potura, O. Kimberger, A. Kober and E. Tschernko (2011) Comparison of the i-gel® and the LMA Unique laryngeal mask airway in patients with mild to moderate obesity during elective short-term surgery, *Anaesthesia* 66, 481-7 (2011).

[27] V. Uppal, S. Gangaiah, G. Fletcher and J. Kinsella, (2009) Randomised crossover comparison between the i-gel® and the LMA Unique in anaesthetized, paralysed adults, *Br. J. Anaesth.* 103, 882-5 (2009).

[28] Cattano, L. Ferrario, V. Maddukuri, S. Sridhar, Y. Khalil and C. A. Hagberg, A randomized clinial comparison of the Intersurgical i-gel® and LMA Unique in non-obese adults during general surgery, *Minerva Anestesiol.* 77, 292-7 (2011).

[29] E.E. Chew, N. H. Hashim and C. Y. Wang, Randomised comparison of the LMA Supreme® with the i-gel® in spontaneously breathing anaesthetised adult patients, *Anaesth Intensive Care 38,* 1018-22 (2010).

[30] W. Donaldson, A. Abraham, M. Deighan and P. Michalek, i-gel® vs AuraOnce® laryngeal mask for general anaesthesia with controlled ventilation in paralyzed patients, *Biomed. Pap.* 155, 155-63 (2011).

[31] Richez, L. Saltel, F. Banchereau, R. Torrielli and A. M. Cros, A new single use supraglottic airway with a noninflatable cuff and an esophageal vent: An observational study of the i-gel, *Anesth. Analg.* 106, 1137-9 (2008).

[32] N. M. Wharton, B. Gibbison, D. A. Gabbott, G. M. Haslam, N. Muchatuta and T. M. Cook, i-gel insertion by novices in manikins and patients, *Anaesthesia* 63, 991-5 (2008).

[33] Sharma, R. Seghal, C. Sahai and J. Sood, PLMA vs. i-gel: a comparative evaluation of respiratory mechanics in laparoscopic cholecystectomy, *J. Anaesthesiol. Clin. Pharmacol.* 26, 451-7 (2010).

[34] J. Arevalo Ludena, J. J. Arcas Bellas, V. Lopez Perez, A. Cuarental Carcia and R. Alvarez-Rementeria Carbonell, Placement of a bronchial blocker through the i-gel® supraglottic airway device for single lung ventilation: preliminary study, *Rev. Esp. Anestesiol. Reanim.* 57, 532-5 (2010). [Article in Spanish, English abstract].

[35] Janakiraman, D. B. Chethan, A. R. Wilkes, M. R. Stacey and N. Goodwin, A randomized crossover trial comparing the i-gel® supraglottic airway and classic laryngeal mask airway, *Anaesthesia* 64, 674-8 (2009).

[36] H. Francksen, J. Renner, R. Hanss, J. Scholz, V. Doerges and B. Bein, A comparison of the i-gel® with the LMA-Unique in non-paralysed anesthetised adult patients, *Anaesthesia* 64, 1118-24 (2009).

[37] T. C. van Zundert and J. R. Brimacombe, Similar oropharyngeal leak pressures during anaesthesia with i-gel™, LMA-ProSeal™, LMA-Supreme™ laryngeal masks, *Acta Anaesth. Belg.* 63, 35-41 (2012).

[38] M. C. White, T. M. Cook and P. A. Stoddart, A critique of elective pediatric supraglottic airway devices, *Paediatr. Anaesth.* 19, 55-65 (2009).

[39] M. Polaner, D. Ahuja, J. Zuk and Z. Pan Z, Video assessment of supraglottic airway orientation through the perilaryngeal airway in pediatric patients, *Anesth. Analg.* 102, 1685-8 (2006).

[40] C. Bopp, G. Carrenard, C. Chauvin, C. Schwaab and P. Diemunsch, The i-gel in paediatric surgery: initial series, New Orleans, USA: American Society of Anesthesiologists (ASA) Annual Meeting, p. 147. A (2009).

[41] Vesselinova, E. Monclus, A. Sanchez, C. Roqueta and R. Banchs, Influence of five different head and neck positions on the perilaryngeal seal of the i-gel® device in paediatric patients, *Eur. J. Anaesthesiol.* 27, 155-6 (2010).

[42] S. Ramesh and R. Jayanthi, Supraglottic airway devices in children, *Indian J. Anaesth.* 55, 476-82 (2011).

[43] L. G. Theiler, M. Kleine-Brueggeney, B. Luepold, F. Stucki, S. Seiler, N. Urwyler and R. Greif, Performance of the pediatric-sized i-gel compared with the Ambu AuraOnce laryngeal mask in anesthetized and ventilated children, *Anesthesiology* 115, 102-10 (2011).

[44] L. Beylacq, M. Bordes, F. Semjen and A. M. Cros, (2009) The i-gel®, a single-use supraglottic airway device with a non-inflatable cuff and an esophageal vent: an observational study in children, *Acta Anaesthesiol. Scand.* 53, 376-9 (2009).

[45] T. Lehousse, A. Foucher-Lezla, A. Azau, J. P. Monrigal and J. C. Granry, Pediatric i-gel™ supraglottic airway: clinical experience and endoscopic data, American Society of Anesthesiologists (ASA) Annual Meeting, p. A947 (2010).

[46] Monclus, A. Garces, I. Vassileva, A. Sanches and R. Banchs, (2010) Paediatric i-gel® evaluation under nuclear magnetic resonance (NMR), *Eur. J. Anaesthesiol.* 27, 155 (2010).

[47] P. Jindal, A. Rizvi and J. P. Sharma, Is i-gel a new revolution among supraglottic airway devices? *Middle East J. Anesth.* 20, 53-8 (2009).

[48] J. R. Brimacombe, Laryngeal mask anesthesia. Principles and practice,.*2nd ed, W.B. Saunders,* Philadelphia (2005).

[49] C. Hughes, K. Place, S. Berg and D. Mason, A clinical evaluation of the i-gel™ supraglottic airway device in children, *Paediatr. Anaesth.* 22, 765-71 (2012).

[50] R. Goyal, R. N. Shukla and G. Kumar, Comparison of size 2 i-gel supraglottic airway with LMA-ProSeal™ and LMA-Classic™ in spontaneously breathing children undergoing elective surgery, *Paediatr. Anaesth.* 22, 355-9 (2012).

In: The i-gel Supraglottic Airway
Editors: Pavel Michalek and William Donaldson ISBN: 978-1-62417-897-9

Chapter 4

DESCRIPTION OF THE I-GEL AIRWAY

***Pavel Michalek*[1,2*] *and William Donaldson*[2]**
[1]Department of Anesthesia and Intensive Medicine,
First Medical Faculty of the Charles University and
General University Hospital, Prague, Czech Republic
[2]Department of Anaesthesia, Antrim Area Hospital, Antrim, UK

ABSTRACT

The i-gel® is a second generation, single-use, latex-free supraglottic airway device (SAD). It has a different design when compared with the cuffed laryngeal mask airways. Its cuff is soft and non-inflatable and anatomically mirrors perilaryngeal anatomy.

The cuff comprises an epiglottic rest and protective ridges which prevent the epiglottis from downfolding or causing airway obstruction. When classified according to its sealing mechanism, the i-gel is classified as a preshaped perilaryngeal sealer.

The stem of the device consists of a standard 15-mm connector, an integral bite block and a curved buccal cavity stabilizer. The airway channel of the i-gel is broad enough to pass a tracheal tube of a reasonable size and therefore the device may be used in difficult airway rescue situations. The i-gel incorporates an additional gastric channel which may be used for insertion of a gastric tube.

INTRODUCTION

Supraglottic airway devices (SADs) are considered the method of choice for airway management during elective procedures that do not require tracheal intubation [1]. According to published evidence, SADs are associated with a lower incidence of postoperative hoarseness, cough, laryngospasm and sore throat than tracheal intubation. The risk of gastric content aspiration is probably similar [2-3].

The first SAD was introduced to the clinical practice in 1988, when Dr Archie Brain developed his laryngeal mask airway (LMA Classic®, Intavent Direct, Maidenhead, UK) [4].

* Corresponding author: Pavel Michalek. E-mail address: pafkamich@yahoo.co.uk.

Currently, more than 50% of procedures in the United Kingdom performed under general anesthesia are managed using a supraglottic airway device. The first generation of SADs does not include an additional channel for drainage of gastric content or for a targeted insertion of gastric tube [1]. These devices are associated with some potential problems – intermittent positive pressure ventilation (IPPV) is sometimes not possible due to low pharyngeal seal pressures, and the respiratory and gastrointestinal tracts are not separated, which creates a potential for aspiration of gastric contents [4]. These possible downfalls of the 1st generation SADs led to development of the 2nd generation of supraglottic airway devices. The first 2nd generation device was the ProSeal laryngeal mask (LMA ProSeal®, Intavent Direct, Maidenhead, UK), which included an additional channel for drainage of gastric contents and featured some modifications to the cuff design. This new design helped to increase the pharyngeal seal pressure of the LMA ProSeal compared with the cLMA [5].

Further 2nd generation SADs were introduced in following years; LMA Supreme®, i-gel® supraglottic airway, SLIPA® and Baska® mask. The i-gel supraglottic airway, a single-use 2nd generation SAD with a different design to the laryngeal masks, was invented by Dr Muhammed Nasir and introduced into clinical practice in the United Kingdom in February 2007 [6, 7].

THE I-GEL AIRWAY

The i-gel supraglottic airway device consists of a soft non-inflatable cuff with an epiglottic rest, a stem with a breathing channel and integrated additional gastric channel, and a standard 15-mm connector for connection to a breathing circuit (Figure 1) [7, 8].

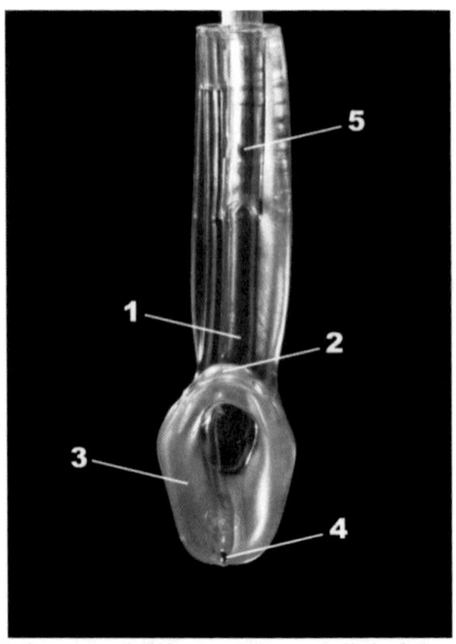

Reprinted with permission of Wolters and Kluwer from Michalek et al., Anesth. Analg. 2008;106: 1501-4.

Figure 1. The i-gel airway. Labelled features – 1 – buccal cavity stabilizer, 2- epiglottic rest, 3- noninflatable cuff, 4- distal opening of gastric channel, 5- integral bite blocker.

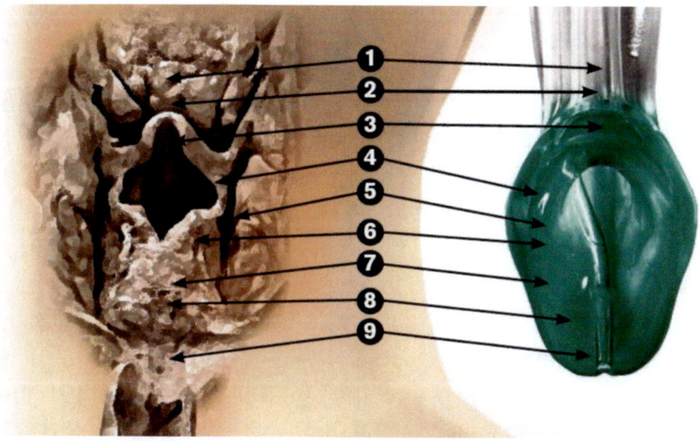

Figure 2. The i-gel cuff and its relation to the perilaryngeal structures (courtesy of Intersurgical Ltd., UK). Labelled features –1-tongue, 2-base of tongue, 3-epiglottis, 4-aryepiglottic folds, 5-piriform fossa, 6-posterior cartilages, 7-thyroid cartilage, 8-cricoid cartilage, 9-upper esophageal opening

Non-Inflatable Cuff

The bowl of the i-gel is made of soft, gel-like material. This material is a thermoplastic elastomer and its chemical structure is styrene-ethylene-butadiene-styrene [6, 7].

The cuff design is unique amongst supraglottic airway devices. Other perilaryngeal sealers are dependent on the inflation of the cuff and the pressure exerted by this cuff against the perilaryngeal tissue is responsible for the sealing mechanism of the device [1, 4].

The sealing mechanism of the i-gel is entirely different: the device mirrors the perilaryngeal structures, adhering to them and thus creating the seal. The i-gel cuff fits onto the perilaryngeal framework, with various parts of the device mirroring the shape of the epiglottis, aryepiglottic folds, piriform fossae, peri-thyroid structures, peri-cricoid cartilages and posterior cartilages (Figure 2) [6]. Contact between the cuff and its corresponding anatomical structures supports the seal of i-gel. The distal tip of the cuff should be placed in the proximal opening of the esophagus and separates the laryngeal inlet from the gastrointestinal tract [7]. The middle part of the cuff is broadest to mirror the pharyngoepiglottic folds whilst the distal part is narrower in both anterior-posterior and lateral diameters. The narrow distal part should fit into the perilaryngeal space.

Epiglottic Rest

This part of i-gel contains an artificial epiglottis with a protective ridge (Figure 3). This structure is not found in any of the laryngeal masks. Its purpose is to prevent epiglottic downfolding [6, 7]. The epiglottic rest also protects against malpositioning of the epiglottis into the laryngeal inlet (which may cause complete airway obstruction). The epiglottic ridge also helps to maintain the i-gel in its correct position.

Additional Gastric Channel

The i-gel, together with other 2nd generation SADs, has an additional channel designated for drainage of gastric content (Figure 3). The channel runs throughout the whole i-gel from the proximal opening of the bowl to the side part of the connector. Following correct insertion, this distal opening should correspond to the upper esophageal opening. A size 10F gastric tube may be inserted through a size 1.5 i-gel, while larger sizes may feed gastric tube size 12F (Figure 4) with the size 5 i-gel able to accommodate a size 14F gastric tube [7, 8].

The tube is inserted through the gastric channel (Figure 4) to drain stomach contents or air. The additional gastric channel may also help in recognizing regurgitation of gastric contents by the appearance of yellowish or greenish fluid in the channel [9]. The neonatal size of the i-gel (size 1) does not include a gastric channel whereas other pediatric sizes do [10].

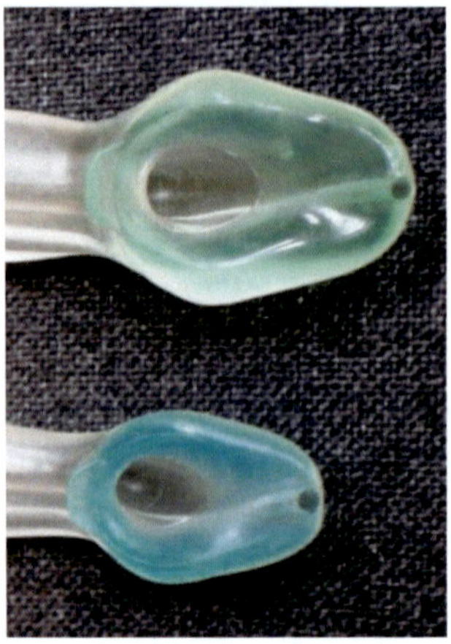

Figure 3. Detail of the i-gel cuff, distal opening of gastric channel and epiglottic rest (i-gel sizes 2 and 3).

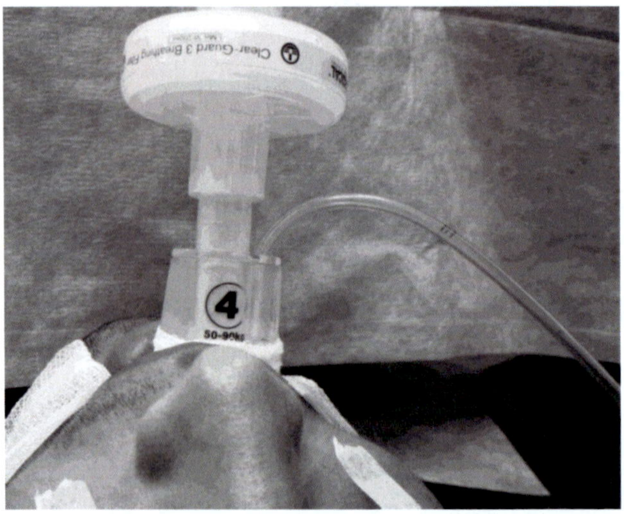

Figure 4. A 12F gastric tube inserted through the gastric channel of i-gel.

A gastric tube should not be inserted if there is a history of esophageal varices or upper gastrointestinal surgery, a recent history of upper gastrointestinal bleeding, presence of esophageal trauma and bleeding or clotting abnormalities. The tube also should not be inserted in presence of an excessive airway leak through the gastric channel which indicates incorrect (too shallow) positioning of the device [7, 11].

Stem of the Device

The stem of the i-gel is firmer than the soft cuff. The tube section of the device incorporates a 15-mm connector, an integral bite block and a curved buccal cavity stabilizer [6, 7].

The connector at the end of stem is multifunctional: It provides standard connection to the breathing circuits of an anesthetic machine or ICU ventilator. An entry point to the gastric channel is situated on the side of the wing close to the connector. The upper part of the stem below this connector serves as an integral bite block. This part of device is quite rigid when compared with laryngeal masks and even if patients bite upon it, obstruction of the airway channel should not occur.

The stem of the i-gel is marked with its size number, weight recommendation (Figure 5) and a horizonal black line that should lie, after insertion, just between the teeth. This rule is not always applicable to the pediatric sizes of the i-gel [7].

The buccal cavity stabilizer mimics the curved shape of the oropharynx. This part of stem is wider laterally and slightly narrower anteroposteriorly than the rest of the stem and serves to decrease the risk of malrotation and malpositioning. The stabilizer also helps to smooth insertion of device [6-8].

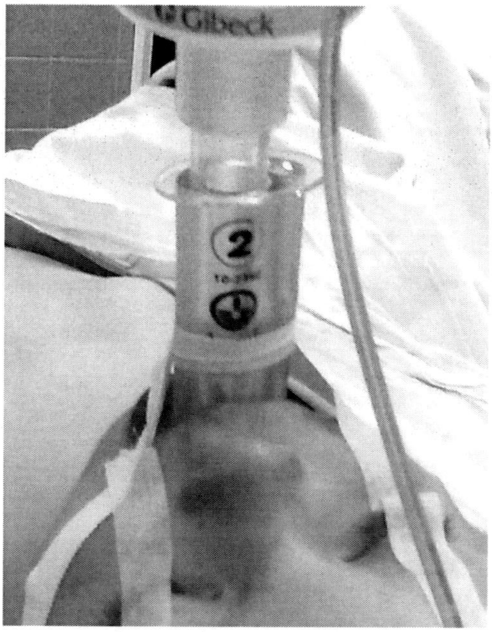

Figure 5. Integral bite block of the i-gel with its size, recommended weight and in adults also with black horizontal line showing the depth of device insertion.

Table 1. Size selection of the i-gel according to the patient´s weight and age [7]

Size of i-gel	Patient size	Recommended weight (kg)
1	Newborn	2-5
1.5	Infant/toddler	5-12
2	Small child	10-25
2.5	Large child	25-35
3	Small adult	30-60
4	Medium adult	50-90
5	Large adult +	90 +

Sizes of i-gel

The i-gel is available in seven different sizes: Sizes 1, 1.5, 2 and 2.5 are designated for pediatric patients while sizes 3, 4 and 5 are suitable for adult patients (Table 1). The size 3 i-gel may be used for children over 30 kg in weight. The size number and corresponding recommended weight range of the patient are written on the upper part of the integral bite block (Figure 5). Whilst size is usually selected according to the patient´s weight there are some exceptions related to head and neck anatomy or the patient´s Body Mass Index (BMI): Patients with wide thyroid or cricoid cartilages as well as those with a cylindrically shaped neck may require a larger size of device than predicted. Accordingly, patients with smaller perilaryngeal structures may require a smaller size of i-gel. Careful consideration must be exercised in obese patients and the device size should be selected according to the ideal weight rather than the actual weight [7, 8, 12, 13].

Sealing Mechanisms

SADs create their seal using different mechanisms: Perilaryngeal cuffed sealers rely on the pressure exerted by the inflated cuff of the device onto the surrounding anatomical structures. Typical examples of this category are laryngeal masks [1, 4].

Anatomically preshaped sealers do not include an inflatable cuff. The i-gel airway has a cuff which mirrors the perilaryngeal structures and its seal is created by tight contact of this cuff with the corresponding anatomical structures. Another example of the anatomically preshaped sealer is the Streamlined Liner of the Pharynx Airway (SLIPA) but its mechanism of seal is pharyngeal rather than perilaryngeal [1]. Seal pressures of the i-gel are generally slightly higher than seal pressures recorded with 1st generation SADs. They range between 20-30 cm H_2O according to most published studies [8, 12, 14-16]. However, other 2nd generation devices – mainly the LMA ProSeal, can achieve higher seal pressures than i-gel [17, 18]. Insertion of a gastric tube should not influence the seal pressure of the i-gel. This hypothesis was confirmed in a clinical study which assessed seal pressures of the device in 30 patients both before and after insertion of a gastric tube through the gastric channel of i-gel. The mean seal pressures were 23.3 mmHg before insertion of gastric tube and 24.4 mmHg after insertion [19].

Table 2. Guide for insertion of tracheal tube through the i-gel [7]

i-gel size	Maximum diameter of tracheal tube
1	3.0 mm
1.5	4.0 mm
2	5.0 mm
2.5	5.0 mm
3	6.0 mm
4	7.0 mm
5	8.0 mm

The mucosal pressures produced by the i-gel were measured in 15 patients under general anesthesia and muscle relaxation and compared with the LMA Supreme used in another fifteen subjects. Mucosal pressures were recorded by four silicone microchip sensors positioned on the external surface of the SADs – the sensors were located against the base of the tongue, in the distal oropharynx, in the hypopharynx close to the esophageal opening and in the piriform fossa.

i-gel mucosal pressures were low, varying between 5-8 cmH_2O and were equally distributed and similar in all four places. Pressures produced by the LMA Supreme were also low but higher in the distal hypopharynx (10.7 cmH_2O) than in the other locations. This study confirms that shape of the i-gel matching the surrounding anatomical structures is main mechanism of its seal [20].

Coverage of Glottic Opening

Following correct insertion, the i-gel provides very good coverage of the laryngeal inlet. Levitan and Kinkle evaluated the fiberoptic view through the i-gel in fresh cadavers. They found a full view of vocal cords in 60% of cadavers and a mean percentage of glottic opening (POGO) score of 82% [6].

Human trials assessing fiberoptic views through the i-gel have also found high coverage of the glottic opening. Theiler et al. found a full view of the vocal cords in a simulated difficult airway scenario (application of a neck collar) in 71% of patients [21]. Another trial found an even higher proportion of full view of glottic opening – 91% [14].

These studies together with several manikin trials and case reports highlighted a potential use of the i-gel as a device for difficult airway management. An endotracheal tube (preferably soft or armored) may be directly passed through the tube portion of any size of the device (Table 2).

Insertion Techniques

The i-gel should be inserted according to the guide provided by the manufacturer [7]. Manipulation with sterile gloves and proper lubrication [22] of device are key points in correct use of the i-gel. Insertion techniques are described in detail in Chapter 4.

PHYSICAL PROPERTIES OF THE I-GEL

The cuff of i-gel seems to be stable if exerted to high pressures or high altitude associated with lower temperatures and lower pressures than atmospheric.

Law et al. studied five different airway management devices for changes in the cuff volume in an altitude chamber [23]. The authors simulated ascent and descent conditions from ground level to 4572m above sea level. They found that in those devices with inflatable cuffs filled with air, the volume of the cuff increased significantly with increasing altitude (decreasing atmospheric pressure). The changes were less marked when these cuffs were filled with water. The cuff of the i-gel did not show any changes related to increased altitude and decreased atmospheric pressure and its volume remained stable. This feature of the i-gel could have importance for airway management during helicopter and aircraft medical transfers.

The i-gel airway has been also studied in simulated hyperbaric conditions and after rapid decompression. The device was exposed to 203kPa and 284kPa within a hyperbaric chamber and, in the second phase of this trial, exposed to a pressure of 608 kPa for six hours with rapid decompression. The operators did not find any changes in consistency of the cuff of the device following high pressure exposure and no air bubbles were detected with a magnifying glass inside the cuff of device following exposure to hyperbaric pressure and rapid decompression [24]. This trial demonstrated that the i-gel might be a useful airway device for use in diving medicine.

Initial expectations that i-gel may improve its seal after warming up to the body temperature have not been confirmed. Nishiyama et al. studied the effect of i-gel prewarming to 37 °C on its seal in 90 patients. Another 90 patients had inserted i-gels which were stored at a room temperature. There was no difference seen between the two groups in seal pressures, leak volumes or peak inspiratory pressures [26].

CONCLUSION

The i-gel is a 2nd generation SAD with some unique properties. Its cuff seals anatomically against the corresponding perilaryngeal structures exerting very low pressures on the pharyngeal mucosa. This feature should result in very low incidence of postoperative airway complications as postoperative sore throat, hoarseness and other complaints. Seal pressures of the device allow for volume controlled or pressure controlled ventilation during procedures under general anesthesia.

The broad diameter breathing tube of the i-gel and its good coverage of the vocal cords after insertion favour the i-gel as a useful tool in difficult airway management. Future directions of i-gel may be also in air transfers, hyperbaric medicine or diving medicine due to miminal changes of the cuff volume and physical properties following exposure to high pressure, altitude or low temperature.

The inventor of the i-gel device, Dr Nasir, is currently working in another fascinating area of airway management. He has invented, developed and introduced the first animal supraglottic airway devices for general anesthesia and resuscitation into veterinary practice. This device, the v-gel®, is currently available for cats and rabbits (Figures 6, 7).

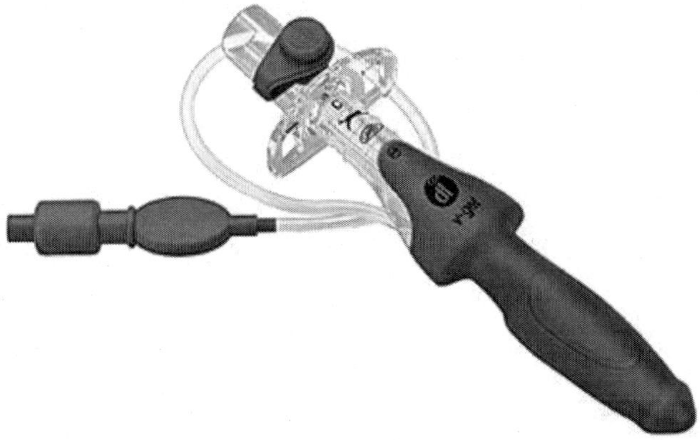

Figure 6. v-gel supraglottic airway device for cats (courtesy of Docsinnovent Ltd., UK).

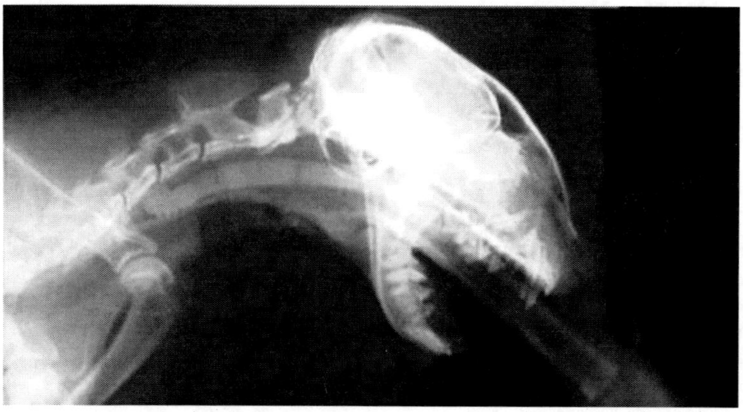

Figure 7. A lateral radiograph of the v-gel inserted into the cat (courtesy of Docinnovent Ltd., UK).

REFERENCES

[1] D. M. Miller, A proposed classification and scoring system for supraglottic sealing airways: a brief review, *Anesth. Analg.* 99, 1553-9 (2004).

[2] S. H. Yu and O. R. Beirne, Laryngeal mask airways have a lower risk of airway complications compared with endotracheal intubation: a systematic review, *J. Oral Maxillofac. Surg.* 68, 2359-76 (2010).

[3] E. Mizutamari, T. Yano, K. Ushijima, A. Ito, S. Anraku, H. Tanimoto, H. Terasaki, A comparison of postoperative sore throat after use of laryngeal mask airway and tracheal tube, *J. Anesth.* 18, 151-7 (2004).

[4] D. M. Miller, A conceptual ideal supraglottic airway, *Anest. Intenziv. Med.* 22, 149-52 (2011).

[5] B. Bein and J. Scholz, Supraglottic airway devices, *Best Pract. Res. Clin. Anaesthesiol.* 19, 581-93 (2005).

[6] R. M. Levitan and W. C. Kinkle, Initial anatomic investigation of the i-gel airway: a novel supraglottic airway without inflatable cuff, *Anaesthesia* 60, 1022-6 (2005).
[7] User guide, i-gel® single use supraglottic airway, available on: www.i-gel.com.
[8] B. Richez, L. Saltel, F. Banchereau, R. Torielli and A. M. Cros, A new single use supragottic airway device with a noninflatable cuff and an esophageal vent: an observational study of the i-gel, *Anesth. Analg.* 106, 1137-9 (2008).
[9] G. Liew, B. John and S. Ahmed, Aspiration recognition with an i-gel airway, *Anaesthesia* 63, 786 (2008).
[10] L. Beylacq, M. Bordes, F. Semjen, A. M. Cross, The i-gel, a single use supraglottic airway device with a non-inflatable cuff and an esophageal vent: an observational study in children, *Acta Anaesthesiol. Scand.* 53, 376-9 (2009).
[11] S. Baxter, Phenomenon with the i-gel airway? *Anaesthesia* 63, 1265 (2010).
[12] W. Donaldson, A. Abraham, M. Deighan and P. Michalek, i-gel™ vs. AuraOnce™ laryngeal mask for general anaesthesia with controlled ventilation in paralyzed patients, *Biomed. Pap.* 155, 155-63 (2011).
[13] W. Donaldson, P. Michalek, L. Pokorny and P. Leyden, An audit of the i-gel supraglottic airway for general anaesthesia with spontaneous and controlled ventilation – the effect of ventilation mode and operator experience on device performance, *Anest. Intenziv. Med.* 23, 63-8 (2012).
[14] J. J. Gatward, T. M. Cook, C. Seller, J. Handel, T. Simpson, V. Vanek and F. Kelly, Evaluation of the size 4 i-gel airway in one hundred non-paralysed patients, *Anaesthesia* 63, 1124-30 (2008).
[15] N. M. Wharton, B. Gibbison, D. A. Gabbott, G. M. Haslam, N. Muchatuta and T. M. Cook, i-gel insertion by novices in manikins and patients, *Anaesthesia* 63, 991-5 (2008).
[16] T. C. Van Zundert and J. R. Brimacombe, Similar oropharyngeal leak pressures during anaesthesia with i-gel, LMA ProSeal and LMA Supreme laryngeal masks, *Acta Anaesthesiol. Belg.* 63, 35-41 (2012).
[17] B. Sharma, R. Sehgal, C. Sahai and J. Sood, PLMA vs. i-gel: a comparative evaluation of respiratory mechanics in laparoscopic cholecystectomy, *J. Anaesth. Clin. Pharmacol.* 26, 451-7 (2010).
[18] R. Ragazzi, L. Finessi, I. Farinelli, R. Alvisi and C. A. Volta, LMA Supreme™ vs i-gel™ – a comparison of insertion success in novices, *Anaesthesia* 67, 384-8 (2012).
[19] S. Nawaz, A. A. Butter, A. Taqi and A. Shafique, A comparison of seal pressure of i-gel before and after insertion of a gastric tube, *J. Univ. Med. Dent. Coll.* 3, 12-15 (2012).
[20] S. Eschertzhuber, J. Brimacombe, M. Kaufmann, C. Keller and W. Kiefenthaler, Directly measured mucosal pressures produced by the i-gel™ and laryngeal mask airway Supreme™ in paralysed anaesthetised patients, *Anaesthesia* 67, 407-10 (2012).
[21] L. G. Theiler, M. Kleine-Brueggeney, D. Kaiser, N. Urwyler, C. Luyet, A. Vogt, R. Greif and M. M. Unibe, Crossover comparison of the laryngeal mask Supreme™ and the i-gel™ in simulated difficult airway scenario in anesthetized patients, *Anesthesiology* 111, 55-62 (2009).

[22] D. Chapman, Lubrication of the i-gel supraglottic airway and the classic laryngeal mask airway, *Anaesthesia* 65, 89 (2010).

[23] J. Law, A. Bair, J. Capra, A. Holder and R. Allen, Characterization of airway device cuff volumes at simulated altitude, *Aviat. Space Environ. Med.* 82, 555-8 (2012).

[24] C. J. Acott, Extraglottic airway devices for use in diving medicine – part 3: the i-gel^{TM}, *Diving Hyperbaric Med.* 38, 124-7 (2008).

[25] T. Nishiyama, Y., Kohno, H. J., Kim, W. J. Shin and H. S. Yang, The effects of prewarming the i-gel on fitting to laryngeal structure, *Am. J. Emerg. Med.* 30, 1756-9 (2012).

Conflict of interest: Prof. Pavel Michalek has lectured for several companies manufacturing supraglottic airway devices inluding Intersurgical Ltd., AMBU Ltd. and Intavent Orthofix Ltd.

In: The i-gel Supraglottic Airway
Editors: Pavel Michalek and William Donaldson
ISBN: 978-1-62417-897-9

Chapter 5

USE OF THE I-GEL FOR AIRWAY MANAGEMENT DURING GENERAL ANESTHESIA

William Donaldson*

Department of Anaesthesia, Antrim Area Hospital, UK

ABSTRACT

The i-gel® was initially indicated for elective and emergency surgery in fasted patients, although these indications have expanded to include resuscitation and use as a conduit for fiberoptic intubation. This chapter will focus only on the use of the i-gel for adults undergoing general anesthesia, children are discussed in detail elsewhere in the book. This chapter examines some of the features that a supraglottic airway device (SAD) should possess for use as an airway device for general anesthesia. Insertion technique, pitfalls and solutions are discussed and data from studies relating to insertion of the i-gel are presented. Sealing mechanisms and suitability of SADs, and the i-gel in particular, for spontaneous and controlled ventilation are also discussed. The chapter briefly touches on hemodynamic effects of the device and concludes with device removal.

INTRODUCTION

The i-gel® is a second-generation supraglottic airway device (SAD) invented by Dr Mohammed Nasir and manufactured by Intersurgical®. It is manufactured from a medical grade elastomeric polymer - Styrene ethylene butadiene styrene – and is composed of a stem with integral bite block, a non-inflatable cuff, an epiglottic rest and incorporates a gastric channel (Figure 1). Indications for its use include securing and maintenance of a patent airway, use under conditions of spontaneous or controlled ventilation and resuscitation. Its use is contraindicated in patients who are not adequately fasted or who are at risk of aspiration, patients who have trismus, patients with a Mallampatti classification of III or

* Corresponding author: William Donaldson. E-mail address: willdonaldson@mac.com.

greater, patients with limited mouth opening and patients who have trauma, abscesses or masses within the airway [1]. The principle use for the i-gel is for the maintenance of an airway during general anesthesia. In the United Kingdom it was estimated by the National Audit Project 4 (NAP4), a prospective project overseen by the Royal College of Anaesthetists and the Difficult Airway Society, that 120000 i-gels are inserted a year and that this represents 7% of SAD use. This figure from NAP4 is an underestimated, with the annual UK use being in excess of 350000 units – the worldwide use to date is over 7 million units (personal communication – D. Chapman, Intersurgical, Wokingham, UK).

REQUIREMENTS OF A SUPRAGLOTTIC DEVICE FOR USE IN GENERAL ANESTHESIA

There are several core features described by Miller that a SAD must possess to be suitable for routine use (Table 1) [2] SADs may be classified as first or second-generation. First generation devices, based largely on Brain's classic LMA, feature a stem with a 15mm connector that is attached to an inflatable elliptical mask. As a second-generation device, the i-gel features a separate gastric channel.

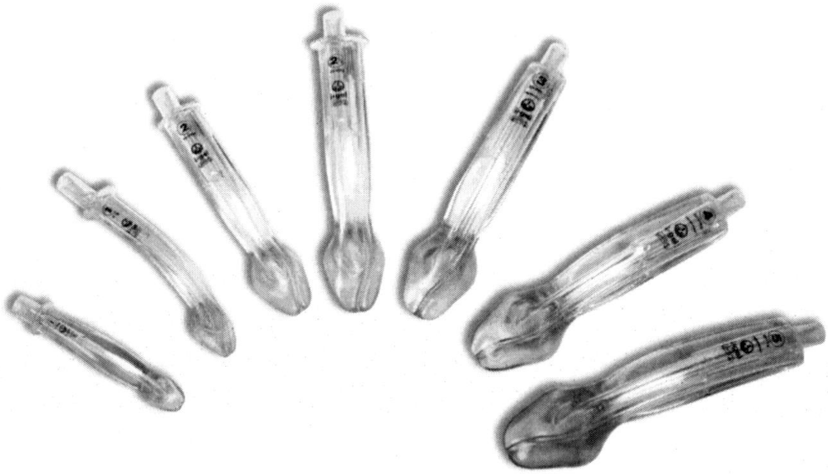

Figure 1. Seven sizes of the i-gel.

Table 1. Features which a SAD suitable for routine use should possess (after Miller[2])

1. A noninvasive (supraglottic) airway conduit.
2. Easy insertion, even by a nonspecialist.
3. Good first-time insertion success rate.
4. Stable airway once positioned, i.e., a reliable hands-free airway.
5. Sufficient sealing quality to apply positive-pressure ventilation.
6. Minimal associated risk of aspiration.
7. Minimal risk of cross-infection, i.e., a single-use device.
8. Minimal risk of serious side effects.

This, in common with other second generation SADs, is designed to separate the gastrointestinal and respiratory tracts. This is a feature that, with correct placement, limits the potential for aspiration of gastric contents.

Insertion

Size Selection

The i-gel should be selected based on the patient's weight, as per the manufacturer's guidelines [1] (Table 2). This advice comes with a couple of caveats:

- Anatomical considerations: Patients who have cylindrical necks or a wide thyroid/cricoid cartilage may require an i-gel a size larger. Conversely, a smaller sized i-gel may need to be inserted in those patients with short, stocky necks or narrow thyroid/cricoid cartilages.
- Obesity: Those patients with a central pattern of obesity may suit an i-gel that is sized based on their ideal, rather than actual, body weight.

Sizing has caused some issues in published studies. Note the overlap in weight guidance between sizes 3 and 4. Van Zundert reported that three devices in their study had to be upsized due to an unacceptable leak, which they blamed on this overlap [3]. Another study corrected leaks in 14/50 i-gels by inserting a larger size [4], and suggested a revision to the sizing guidance.

Insertion Technique

The device should be inserted once the patient is unconscious and with the patient's neck flexed and head extended: the 'sniffing the morning air' position (Figure 2). Depth of anesthesia should be such that the jaw is relaxed and there is no response to jaw thrust.

It can be helpful to have an assistant to open the mouth and/or provide jaw thrust. The mouth should be opened and the device introduced with the leading edge towards the hard palate. The i-gel should have been well lubricated in accordance with the manufacturer's guidance during preparation (Figure 3a-d): some of the difficulties encountered during insertion are due to inadequate lubrication. The i-gel should travel easily past the base of the tongue and come to rest with its tip at the level of the inferior constrictor muscles (Figure 4, Figure 5).

Table 2. i-gel size guide in adult patients

i-gel size	Patient size	Patient weight guidance (kg)
3	Small adult	30-60
4	Medium adult	50-90
5	Large adult	90+

This will be felt as a definitive resistance. There may be resistance felt before this stage, as the i-gel passes the tonsillar apparatus. This is distinguished from the resistance felt on correct positioning by the fact that the black marker line located on the dorsum of the i-gel will still be some distance from the incisors.

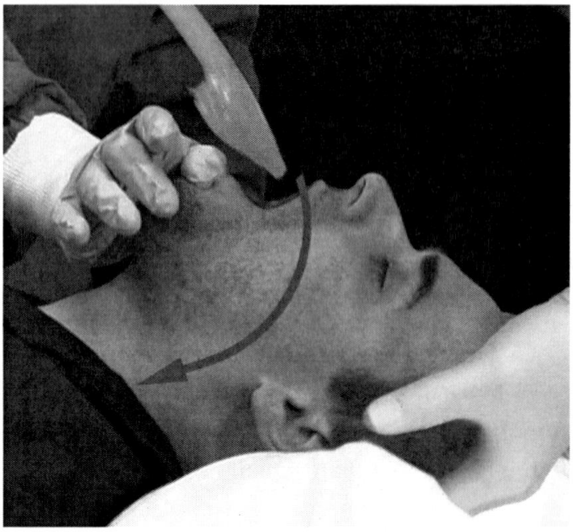

Figure 2. Insertion of the i-gel in a "sniffing morning air" position.

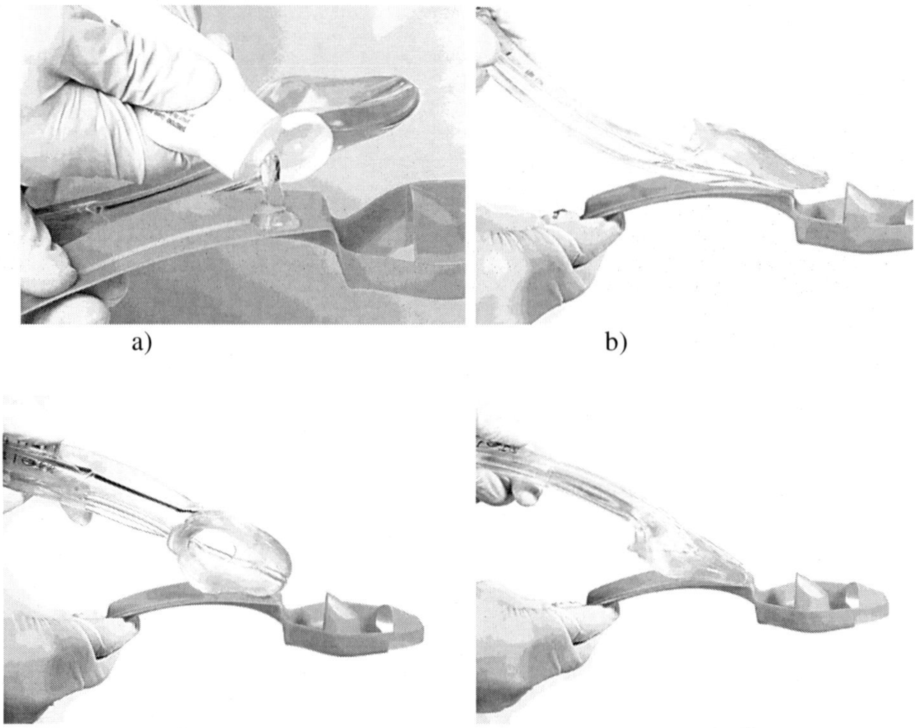

a) b)

c) d)

Figure 3a-d. Lubrication of the i-gel before insertion. (courtesy of Intersurgical® Ltd., UK).

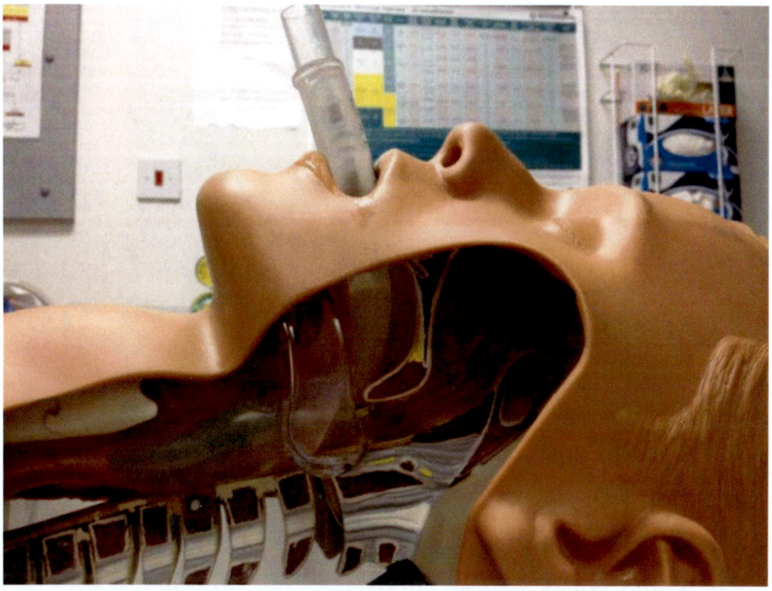

Figure 4. Ambu Airway Trainer™ with i-gel in situ. Note the position of the cuff at the level of the inferior constrictors

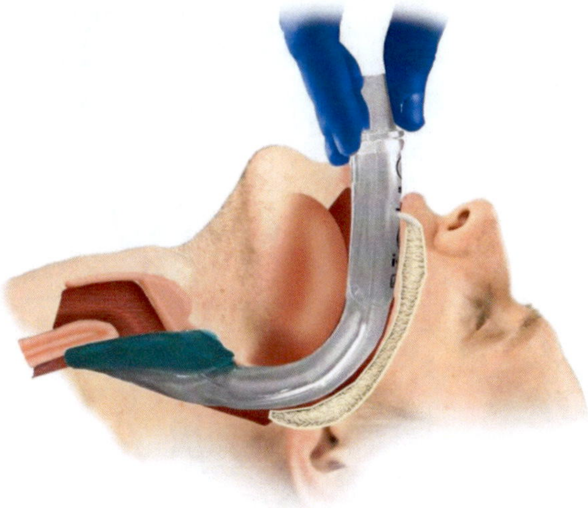

Figure 5. i-gel in its correct position (courtesy of Intersurgical® Ltd., UK).

Tackling Difficulties

In case of difficulty in insertion, there are a few techniques described that may help with placement of the device. These are jaw thrust, deep rotation, the triple maneuver and the thumb technique (Figures 6-9). Jaw thrust aids placement by lifting the mandible forward and with it the tongue to allow the i-gel to pass between it and the pharynx. Deep rotation involves passing the i-gel into the mouth rotated to 90°.

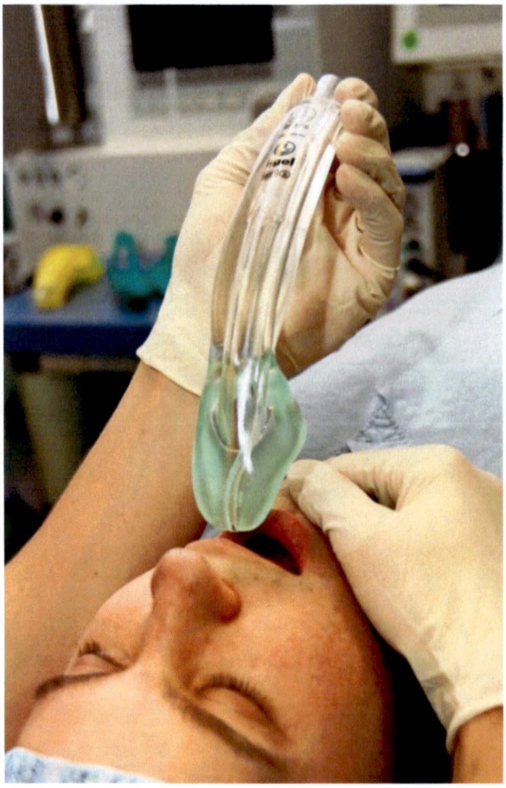

Figure 6. Jaw thrust as an aid to insertion (courtesy of Intersurgical® Ltd., UK).

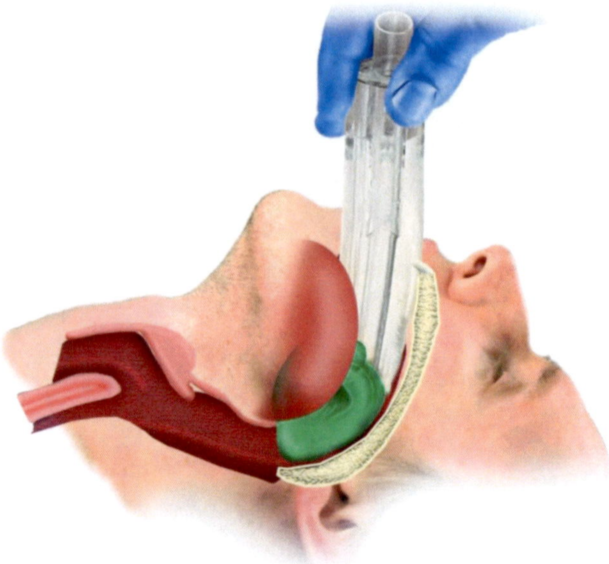

Figure 7. Deep rotation technique (courtesy of Intersurgical® Ltd., UK).

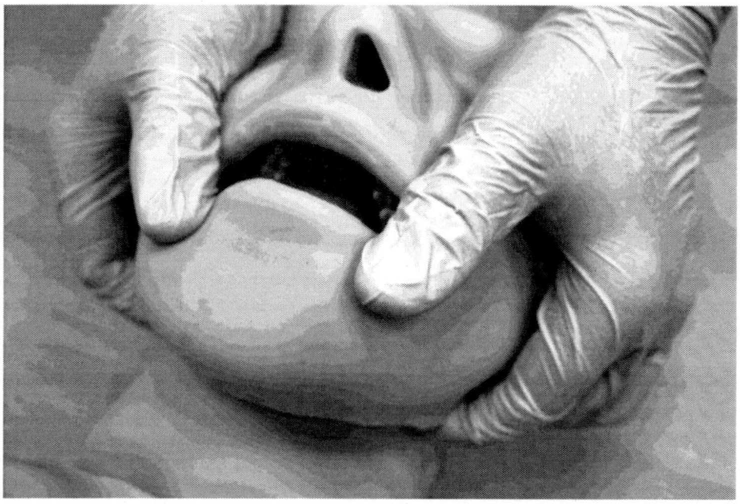

Figure 8. The triple maneuver.

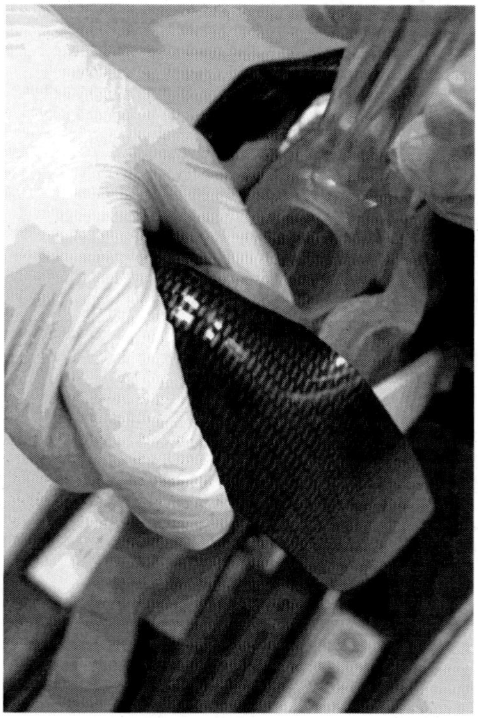

Figure 9. The thumb technique.

Once resistance is felt, the device is rotated back and advanced into place. The triple maneuver consists of jaw thrust, mouth opening and neck extension. The thumb technique requires the operator to place the gloved thumb of the non-dominant hand into the mouth. This acts to depress the tongue and can be used to pull the mandible forward [5]. It should be noted that the manufacturer does not endorse this technique but the author has found it to be of great use.

Some of the above differs from techniques that may be employed for other devices to which people are accustomed. In teaching those new to the device, it is important to remember this. Some of the complications that are described in the literature (see also Chapter 13) have resulted from user inexperience. As with other SADs training may be carried out on manikins and only after attaining a degree of competence in a non-clinical setting may the user move onto inserting devices into patients [6]. The use of the i-gel in experimental studies including manikins and its place in education are discussed in Chapters 16 and 15 respectively.

Table 3. i-gel insertion and leak data for published studies involving adult patients. Figures are medians (±SD) or (interquartile range). nr – not recorded. ‡Theiler defined primary success as success without changing size

Study	1st attempt success (%)	Overall insertion success (%)	Time for insertion (s)	Pharyngeal leak pressure (cmH_2O)
Theiler [8]	93‡	96‡	nr	26±8
Van Zundert [3]	80	100	44±2	34±9
Nishiyama [9]	90	100	15.6	29
Ragazzi [10]	54	85	28±13	24
Ali [11]	73.3	100	nr	25.5
Sanuki [12]	100	100	nr	25.8 (*)
Theiler [13]	90	98	33±18	26±8
Kleine-Brueggeney [14]	93.8	98.8	23±15	24±8
Weber [15]	92	100	18.3±6.5	23.7±9.2
Cattano [16]	68	100	nr	23.1±7.3
Donaldson [17]	85.6	96.3	10.6	30.4
Ibrahim [18]	86.7	100	nr	25.75
Teoh [19]	96	100	15.4±8.2	25±5.7
Sharma [20]	93.3	100	13.6±4.26	35.6±4.8
Jindal [21]	96	100	4.7±1.1	nr
Shin [22]	78.1	100	nr	27.1±6.4
Amini [23]	77	93.3	20±9.6	19.3±7.1
Helmy [24]	90	100	15.6±4.9	25.6±4.9
Uppal [25]	97.4	100	12.2(9.7-14.3)	25(22-30)
Keijzer [26]	nr	Nr	8.5±6.3	24
Francksen [27]	90	100	15(10-60)	29±5
Heuer [28]	82.5	100	13.9±3.6	nr
Theiler [29]	85	93	42±23	27±9
Janakiraman [4]	54	84	nr	20(14-24)
Singh [30]	100	100	nr	25.27
Uppal [25]	100	100	nr	28(20.35.5)
Bamgbade [31]	96.7	99.3	96.7% < 5s	≈33
Gatward [32]	86	100	15	24
Wharton [33]	82.5	100	17.5(7-197)	20(13-40)
Richez [34]	97	97	nr	30±7

*Sanuki's study measured pressures in various positions: neutral, flexion and extension of the neck. (*) neutral position.

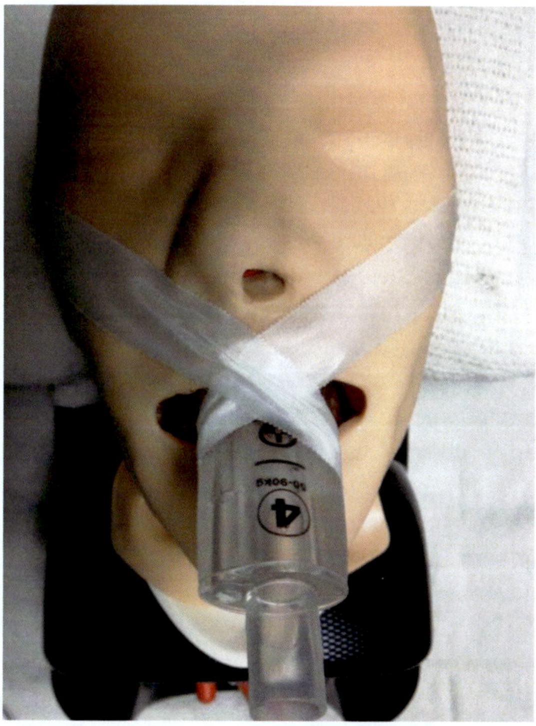

Figure 10. AirSim Cric™ (TruCorp, Belfast, UK) with i-gel in situ. Tape applied 'maxilla to maxilla'.

Once the device has been correctly placed, the black line on the dorsal surface of the i-gel should approximate to the incisors. The not infrequent phenomenon of an audible leak through the gastric channel on positive pressure ventilation signifies incorrect placement or device size selection [7].

In this case the device should be repositioned or reinserted until the leak disappears, or a different size selected. The gastric channel should not under any circumstance be occluded (with, for example, adhesive tape). Persistence of a leak despite the remedies above necessitates a change either to an alternative SAD or to an endotracheal tube.

The device should now be fixed in place. The recommended method is by using tape from one maxilla, around the stem of the i-gel, to the other maxilla: 'maxilla to maxilla'. This provides greater stability than taping to the mandible, which is mobile (Figure 10).

Insertion Attempts, Times and Success Rates

The median time taken for insertion of the i-gel varies in published studies from 4.7s [35] to 44s [3] with the majority of times between 10s and 20s (Table 3). The wide differences between reported insertion times may, in part, be explained by the differing definitions of insertion time. Some chose to define insertion time as the time to merely place the device [21, 26], others timed until connection of the breathing circuit [17] and others until establishment of ventilation as demonstrated by a capnographic waveform and/or movement of the chest (the effective airway time) [14, 29].

The number of attempts at insertion and first attempt success rates varies as well (Table 2). First time success rates vary, in adult patients, from 54% [4] to 100% [12, 25, 30]. Insertion success rates for the i-gel do appear to be overall lower than its comparators in many studies, which is dealt with in more detail in Chapter 14. There is a learning curve involved with any device, and this is perhaps more shallow in the case of the i-gel. This fact is alluded to by Nishiyama who commented that i-gel insertion success rates were higher in his second study [9] than the first i-gel study that he was involved [22].

Some studies used novices as test subjects to assess insertion when compared with more experienced operators [10, 33]. Wharton et al.'s study included only the i-gel and they found that the device was rapidly inserted and commented that it compared favorably with other devices available.

Ragazzi and his team compared the i-gel with the LMA-Supreme. They found the LMA Supreme to be easier to insert and that it provided a higher airway seal, concluding that it would be the better device for insertion by novices in emergency airway management. Jindal studied the device using first-time users and found that the i-gel was easier to insert than the cLMA and that insertion times were faster [21].

Theiler and colleagues have recently published the first large cohort study on the i-gel, involving 2049 patients [8]. They reported a 93.4% primary success rate (success without having to change size) and a 95.9% overall success rate. Of the primary success failures (135 cases), 31 (2% of all insertions) were due to impossible insertion and 103 (5% of all insertions) were due to impossible ventilation. These cases were resolved by a change in device size in 52 cases, by a change in SAD type in 34 cases, with tracheal intubation in 42 cases and facemask ventilation in 5 cases. Data were missing for two of the cases. What is of great interest is that the authors compiled risk factors for failure from the data that they had collected about patient characteristics (Table 4).

The study revealed one surprising finding: that there was a negative correlation between the experience of the experience of the operator and success rate. This was attributed to one of two things – either that less experienced providers dealt with easier airways, or that experienced providers took over the more difficult insertions (with the last person dealing with the airway being recorded as the responsible provider).

PATIENT POSITIONING AND TYPES OF SURGERY

The i-gel is indicated for securing and maintaining a patent airway in routine and emergency anesthetics of fasted patients, during spontaneous or intermittent positive pressure ventilation [1]. No mention is made of the types of surgery for which it is unsuitable although the contraindications state that it should not be left in situ for more than four hours.

Reports exist of the use of other SADs for prolonged periods of up to six hours [36, 37], and in one report for four days [38].

Sanuki et al. studied the effect that differing head and neck positions had on expired tidal volume with the i-gel [12]. They found that, when compared with the neutral position, flexion significantly decreased expired tidal volume (from 7.1 ± 1.2 $ml.kg^{-1}$ to 4.5 ± 2.1 $ml.kg^{-1}$). It is known that flexion of the neck narrows the laryngeal inlet [39] and the authors postulated that this narrowing caused compression of the i-gel cuff, hindering ventilation.

Table 4. Risk factors for i-gel failure. *Effect size given as odds ratio (frequencies) and as Cohen's *d* (interval data). CI – Confidence Interval [8]

	P-value	Effect size (95% CI)*
Males/ male sex	<0.001	2.25 (1.57-3.22)
Impaired mandibular subluxation	0.012	1.76 (1.12-2.79)
Rotten (poor) teeth	0.019	2.62 (1.34-5.10)
Older age	0.001	0.38 (0.21-0.56)

The i-gel has been used for patients operated on in the prone position [40, 41] and in the lateral position [31]. The use of the i-gel in positions other than supine and in different types of surgery is discussed in greater detail in Chapter 6.

Sealing Pressures

SADs may be classified, not only as 1st or 2nd generation devices but also according to their sealing mechanism [2]. Miller's classification divides SADs into:

- o Cuffed perilaryngeal sealers
  - Non-directional sealing: e.g. Classic LMA
  - Directional sealing: e.g. Proseal LMA
- o Cuffed pharyngeal sealers
  - Without esophageal sealing: e.g. Cuffed Oropharyngeal Airway
  - With esophageal sealing: e.g. Combitube
- o Cuffless anatomically preshaped sealers:
  - e.g. Streamlined Liner of the Pharynx Airway, i-gel

SADs airways must provide two seals with adjacent structures in order to function effectively: the esophageal seal and the pharyngeal seal.

Esophageal Seal Pressures

The esophageal seal pressure is determined by: the position of the tip of the device in the hypopharynx or proximal esophagus and the shape and size of the tip. It is one measure of the safety of a SAD – a high esophageal seal pressure both prevents the passage of gas into the gastrointestinal tract and stops regurgitated fluid from the esophagus from passing into the pharynx. Esophageal seal pressure can be evaluated using cadaveric models. Devices are inserted into a cadaver whose esophagus is exposed and connected to a column of fluid. The height of this column of fluid can be adjusted to represent different hydrostatic pressures within the esophagus. When studies have assessed the performance of SADs in such models, they have found wide differences between the performance of different devices [42, 43]. In one of these studies, the i-gel was found to perform poorly (under conditions simulating a slow release of pressure), achieving a seal pressure of 13 cmH_2O compared with 37 cmH_2O

for the cLMA and 58 cmH_2O for the PLMA. When a rapid release of fluid was tested, the authors noted that the devices with a gastric tube (PLMA, i-gel) drained the fluid rapidly and suggested that this may prevent tracheal aspiration [43].

Performance in cadaveric studies cannot, however, be directly related to performance in clinical scenarios. A novel method for assessing device performance in vitro has recently been published [44]. In this study, the authors instilled methylene-blue stained saline through the gastric channels of both the i-gel and the LMA-Supreme in patients under conditions of both spontaneous and positive-pressure ventilation.

They inspected both the gastric and airway tubes with fiberoptic scopes to assess regurgitation and transgression of fluid onto the bowls of the devices. They found no evidence of regurgitation in any of the patients. There was no evidence of fluid within the bowls of either device in the positive-pressure ventilation group. In the spontaneous ventilation group they noted blue staining (representing fluid ingress) in 2/36 of the i-gel group and none in the LMA-S.

There have been case reports regarding regurgitation and aspiration of gastric contents with the i-gel, and the subject is discussed in greater depth in Chapter 13.

Pharyngeal Seal Pressures

The pharyngeal seal pressure, also known as the leak pressure, is a measure of how well a SAD seals with the structures over which it comes to rest - these structures are often collectively termed the laryngopharynx. A higher leak pressure is an indicator of how well a device might perform during controlled ventilation. This can be tested using a number of methods (Table 4). Keller et al compared the four tests described in table 3 and found them all to be excellent for use in clinical practice [45]. The authors also stated that the manometric stability test might be more suitable for use when comparing sealing pressures in research settings. Airway leak pressure with the cLMA has a reported median value of 20cmH_2O, which is lower than that reported for the PLMA at 30cmH_2O [46]. The PLMA has been compared directly with the i-gel and cLMA, where it was found to have similar airway leak pressures to the PLMA [22]. In this study both devices had a higher airway leak pressure than that of the cLMA. Other studies have found the airway seal of the i-gel to be inferior to that of the PLMA [20,47] and some have found the i-gel to have a higher leak pressure [30]. Further work comparing these devices is expected, according to the clinical trails website (http://clinicaltrials.gov/ct2/show/NC T00624403?term=i-gelandrank=1).

Some authors have suggested that the thermoplastic nature of the material from which the cuff of the i-gel is manufactured may mold to match the laryngeal anatomy as it reaches body temperature [4]. This idea gained traction when Gabbott and Beringer published a letter in Resuscitation describing their experience with the i-gel in 100 patients [48]. They noted that the seal pressure appeared to improve over time, suggesting that the i-gel formed a more efficient seal around the larynx after warming to body temperature.

Nishiyama and colleagues tested this hypothesis in a study where i-gels were either inserted at room temperature or having been prewarmed to 37°C, using a water bath for 30 mins. Insertion time was faster in the warm group (12.9±9.3s) than the room temperature group (14.5±12.3s), but this result did not achieve statistical significance [9]. The leak pressure and leak fraction were not significantly different between the two groups.

Table 4. Methods of measuring pharyngeal sealing pressure. These methods are all performed with the expiratory valve closed with the fresh gas flow (FGF) set to 3 $l.min^{-1}$ [45]

Test	Method
Audible leak	Detection of an audible noise by listening over the mouth and noting the airway pressure at which this occurs
Oral capnography	Placing a capnography sampling line 5cm inside the mouth along the SAD stem and watching for the pressure at which carbon dioxide is first detected
Manometric stability	Observing an aneroid manometer dial monitoring breathing system pressure. Noting when the pressure reaches stability i.e. pressure at which leak is equal to FGF
Auscultation	Detection of a leak with a stethoscope placed lateral to the thyroid cartilage and noting the airway pressure at which this occurs

The material (styrene ethylene butadiene styrene) from which the i-gel cuff is made is stable over a wide range of temperatures and does not expand or contract across normal environmental or physiological temperature ranges.

Several studies have found the leak pressure to be higher with the i-gel than other supraglottic airway devices [4, 25, 27]. Weber conducted a study which involved mild to moderately obese patients, and they found that the difference in leak pressure between the i-gel and the LMA-Unique to be most marked in those patients whose body mass index was greater than 30 $kg.m^{-2}$ (i-gel 25.7cmH_2O v LMA-Unique 17.0cmH_2O; $p<0.0001$) [15].

Modes of Ventilation

The classic LMA was conceived as a device through which a patient could either breathe spontaneously or receive positive-pressure ventilation under general anesthesia [49].

In order to function well under conditions of both spontaneous and controlled ventilation, a supraglottic airway must both cover the larynx and form an adequate seal with the larygopharynx, as discussed above.

Positioning over the laryngeal opening may be checked with the use of a fiberoptic laryngoscope, as was first described through a cLMA by Payne [50]. Many studies of SADs now include a fiberoptic assessment of the view of the laryngeal inlet through the device. Whilst this is primarily with the aim of assessing the potential ease of passing a fiberoptic scope into the trachea for rescue intubation, it may also serve as a surrogate measure for correct positioning of the device.

Levitan and Kinkle carried out the initial investigations into the i-gel using cadavers [51]. They found, through taking lateral radiographs and by carrying out neck dissections, that the positioning of bowl of the device conformed to the laryngeal anatomy. They also carried out fiberoptic evaluation of the percentage of glottis opening (POGO) scores and found these to be consistently high. They concluded that the device consistently achieved proper positioning for supraglottic ventilation.

Spontaneous Ventilation (SV)

There are some important considerations in maintaining the airway with a SAD in a patient who is breathing spontaneously.

Depth of anesthesia: care must be taken to maintain a sufficient depth of anesthesia so that the device may be tolerated to avoid bucking, coughing, laryngospasm and device displacement. Too deep a plane of anesthesia may mean that the patient's minute volume is decreased and carbon dioxide levels may rise.

Development of atelectasis: General anesthesia is associated with the development of atelectasis [52]. PEEP applied through an endotracheal tube both limits the development of atelectasis and may help to resolve it. It might not be unreasonable to expect a similar effect with a SAD. It has been found, however, that that application of PEEP offered no improvement in spontaneously breathing patients' saturation levels when applied through a laryngeal mask [53]. The application of PEEP increases peak airway pressures and these may exceed seal pressures, increasing the chances of gastric insufflation.

The i-gel has been studied less often in spontaneously ventilating patients than in those under conditions of controlled ventilation. Gatward conducted one of the first studies into the i-gel. They found a first attempt insertion success rate of 86% (with no failures after three attempts), demonstrated a good view of the vocal cords in 91% of patients and achieved an expired tidal volume of 7 $ml.kg^{-1}$ in 96% of patients [32]. Apart from one episode of regurgitation, their complication rate was low. Janakiraman studied the i-gel and cLMA in a crossover study in patients undergoing spontaneous ventilation [4]. They reported a very low first time insertion success rate of 54%, which usually improved on upsizing the device. The i-gel had a higher leak pressure than the cLMA (20 cmH_2O v 17 $cmH_{2)}$) and provided a better fiberoptic view of the vocal cords. Chew et al. compared the device with the LMA-Supreme in spontaneously breathing subjects [54]. They found the LMA-Supreme to be easier to insert and to have a higher oropharyngeal leak pressure, although the i-gel yielded better fiberoptic views.

Positive-Pressure Ventilation

In an early study of the cLMA's performance under positive-pressure ventilation, Devitt et al concluded that the device was adequate for this purpose, provided that airway resistance and pulmonary compliance were normal [55]. It was comparable to the tracheal tube, which they also studied. They noted that gastric insufflation was more likely with the cLMA as airway pressures increased: in their study the cLMA had an incidence of gastric insufflation of 2.1% at 15cmH_2O and of 35.4% at 30 cmH_2O. Positioning of the cLMA is also crucial: in a study examining gastric insufflation, Latorre et al found 90% of cLMAs that caused the phenomenon were malpositioned [56].

The incorporation of a drain tube means that gastric distension should be less of an issue with the 2nd generation derivatives of the cLMA but it can still occur, especially with malpositioning of the device [57].

The i-gel has been found to cause no gastric insufflation at pressures of up to 25 cmH_2O [58]. Pharyngeal seal pressures in the majority of studies equal, or exceed this (Table 1). Schmidbauer's paper examining the performance of 2nd generation SADs in a simulated airway obstruction using cadavers found that none of the devices caused gastric insufflation at an airway pressure of 20 mbar (20.39 cmH_2O) [59]. There was gastric insufflation when the devices were subjected to pressures of 40 mbar and 60 mbar – more so in the Laryngeal Tubes that were tested. They recommended avoiding pressures higher than 20 mbar and also suggested that where a gastric channel was present, a gastric tube should be passed into the stomach.

The i-gel has been studied under conditions of both pressure and volume controlled ventilation. The i-gel has been compared with both a PLMA and tracheal tube in patients undergoing laparoscopic cholecystectomy. The study involving the PLMA and i-gel applied volume controlled ventilation at 10-12 $ml.kg^{-1}$ and found that the resistance, work of breathing, peak airway pressures and measured minute ventilation were similar for both devices [20]. Ibrahim et al. studied the i-gel and tracheal in patients undergoing the same operation [18]. They studied leak fractions at 6, 8 and 10 $ml.kg^{-1}$ and found that at the two higher tidal volumes, and especially after the commencement of pneumoperitoneum, the leak fraction of the i-gel was unacceptable. They had found the esophageal seal pressure of the i-gel to be 25.75 cmH_2O, which was exceeded at times by the peak airway pressure following pneumoperitoneum.

Uppal and colleagues found that, at 15 cmH_2O and 20 cmH_2O, there was no difference between the i-gel and tracheal tube in terms of leak fraction, but that at 25 cmH_2O there was a difference equivalent to 26.5 ml [58]. They found no evidence of gastric insufflation at any of the pressures studied and stated that the i-gel could be used as a reasonable alternative to the tracheal tube for pressure controlled ventilation with moderate airway pressures. The same group compared the i-gel and LMA-Unique under similar conditions and found no differences in leak fractions between the two devices [25]. In another study comparing the i-gel to the LMA-Unique [27] the seal pressures and fiberoptic postioning of the i-gel were found to be superior.

It would seem prudent given the information above to either ventilate with pressure controlled ventilation at pressures under 20 cmH_2O or to apply an upper pressure limit of 20 cmH_2O when using a SAD with volume controlled positive-pressure ventilation. If PEEP is to be used, it should be borne in mind that peak airway pressures may increase – and care must be taken to ensure that they do not surpass seal pressures.

HEMODYNAMIC EFFECTS

Insertion of the LMA is associated with a lower pressor response than that seen with tracheal intubation [60]. Any pressor response that is produced is maximal during stimulation of the epipharynx as the LMA passes through the pharyngeal space and is mediated through a direct pressure effect by the inflated cuff of the laryngeal mask. Marked pressor responses are undesirable in patients with cardiovascular disease – in particular those with coronary artery disease.

There is little published work that describes the hemodynamic effects of the i-gel. Jindal's group has published two studies that address this issue. In their study of the insertion of the i-gel by both first time and experienced users they also looked at the hemodynamic effects of device insertion [21]. They found that there was no difference in heart rate, systolic or diastolic pressures when the i-gel was inserted by both novices and experienced users. They found significant increases in all parameters when first time users inserted the cLMA. In a second study, the same group found that the i-gel caused less hemodynamic disturbance on insertion when compared with the SLIPA and the cLMA [35].

Ismail et al. studied the effect of device insertion on intraocular pressure (IOP), comparing the i-gel, cLMA and endotracheal tube in patients undergoing elective, non-opthalmic surgery [61]. They found that insertion of the tracheal tube and cLMA both increased IOP, but that the cLMA did not increase IOP above the pre-induction value. The i-gel was not associated with an increase in IOP, but was associated with a small and short-lived pressor hemodynamic response.

Removal of the i-gel

Removal of the cLMA is recommended in awake and cooperative patients, and this also the case, in most patients, with the i-gel. The manufacturer recommends suctioning gently around the airway device once consciousness has returned and protective reflexes have returned. When the patient is awake, or responding to voice, the i-gel should be removed after asking them to open their mouth. Oxygen via a facemask should be supplied for the recovery period.

Removal in a deeper plane of anesthesia is recommended in patients with the potential for an increased gag reflex, such as smokers, asthmatics and patients with chronic obstructive airways disease. In these cases, it may be necessary to maintain the airway with a facemask – and an oropharyngeal airway if required.

Safety Profile

Complications relating to the i-gel airway are discussed in detail in chapter 13. In general, the incidence of complications associated with the i-gel is low, and comparable with other supraglottic airways.

Conclusion

The i-gel is a suitable device for the airway management of patients undergoing general anesthesia for elective and emergency surgery providing the indications and exclusions described by the manufacturer are adhered to. Of particular importance is the correct sizing of the device and adequate lubrication.

It is rapidly inserted and has a reasonable first-attempt success rate that improves with user experience. Some maneuvers may be required after insertion.

It has an oropharyngeal leak pressure that compares favorably with other second-generation SADs. The drain channel of the i-gel allows the rapid drainage of gastric content and facilitates the passage of a gastric tube. Further, large, studies are required to elucidate how this might decrease the risks of regurgitation and aspiration.

REFERENCES

[1] i-gel user guide 2012, Intersurgical Ltd, Wokingham, UK.

[2] D. M. Miller, A proposed classification and scoring system for supraglottic sealing airways: a brief review, *Anesth. Analg.* 99, 1553–9 (2004).

[3] T. C. Van Zundert and J. R. Brimacombe, Similar oropharyngeal leak pressures during anaesthesia with i-gel, LMA-ProSeal and LMA-Supreme laryngeal masks, *Acta Anaesthesiol. Belg.* 63, 35–41 (2012).

[4] C. Janakiraman, D. B. Chethan, A. R. Wilkes, M. R. Stacey and N. Goodwin, A randomised crossover trial comparing the i-gel supraglottic airway and classic laryngeal mask airway, *Anaesthesia* 64, 674–8 (2009).

[5] P. Michalek, W. J. Donaldson and J. D. Hinds, Tongue trauma associated with the i-gel supraglottic airway, *Anaesthesia* 64, 692–3 (2009).

[6] K. M. Jackson and T. M. Cook, Evaluation of four airway training manikins as patient simulators for the insertion of eight types of supraglottic airway devices, *Anaesthesia* 62, 388–93 (2007).

[7] D. Chapman, Re: Phenomenon with i-gel airway, *Anaesthesia* 64, 228 (2009).

[8] L. Theiler, M. Gutzmann, M. Kleine-Brueggeney, N. Urwyler, B. Kaempfen and R. Greif, i-gel™ supraglottic airway in clinical practice: a prospective observational multicentre study, *Br. J. Anaesth.* (2012) [Epub. ahead of print].

[9] T. Nishiyama, Y. Kohno, H. J. Kim, W. J. Shin and H. S. Yang. The effects of prewarming the i-gel on fitting to laryngeal structure, *Am. J. Emerg. Med.* (2012). [Epub. ahead of print].

[10] R. Ragazzi, L. Finessi, I. Farinelli, R. Alvisi and C. A. Volta, LMA Supreme™ vs i-gel™- a comparison of insertion success in novices, *Anaesthesia* 67, 384–8 (2012).

[11] M. Z. Ali, R. S. Ebied, A. F. El-Tawdy, A. I. Refaat and N. M. Kamal, Controlled mechanical ventilation with LMA Sureme versus i-gel in anesthetized adult patients, *J. Egypt. Soc. Parasitol.* 41, 365–78 (2011).

[12] T. Sanuki, R. Uda, S. Sugioka, E. Daigo, H. Son, M. Akatsuka and J. Kotani, The influence of head and neck position on ventilation with the i-gel airway in paralysed, anaesthetised patients, *Eur. J. Anaesth.* 28, 597–9 (2011).

[13] L. Theiler, M. Kleine-Brueggeney, N. Urwyler, T. Graf, C. Luyet and R. Greif, Randomized clinical trial of the i-gel™ and Magill tracheal tube or single-use ILMA™ and ILMA™ tracheal tube for blind intubation in anaesthetized patients with a predicted difficult airway, *Br. J. Anaesth.* 107, 243–50 (2011).

[14] M. Kleine-Brueggeney, L. Theiler, N. Urwyler, A. Vogt, A. and R. Greif, Randomized trial comparing the i-gel™ and Magill tracheal tube with the single-use ILMA™ and ILMA™ tracheal tube for fibreoptic-guided intubation in anaesthetized patients with a predicted difficult airway, *Br. J. Anaesth.* 107, 251–7 (2011).

[15] U. Weber, R. Oguz, L. A. Potura, O. Kimberger, A. Kober and E. Tschernko. Comparison of the i-gel and the LMA-Unique laryngeal mask airway in patients with mild to moderate obesity during elective short-term surgery. *Anaesthesia* 66, 481–7 (2011).

[16] D. Cattano, L. Ferrario, V. Maddukuri, S. Sridhar, Y. Khalil and C.A. Hagberg. A randomized clinical comparison of the Intersurgical i-gel and LMA Unique in non-obese adults during general surgery, *Minerva Anestesiol.* 77, 292–7 (2011).

[17] W. Donaldson, A. Abraham, M. Deighan and P. Michalek, i-gel™ vs. AuraOnce™ laryngeal mask for general anaesthesia with controlled ventilation in paralyzed patients, *Biomed. Pap.* 155, 155–64 (2011).

[18] M. Ibrahim, A. Ragab and H. El Shamaa, i-gel vs cuffed tracheal tube during volume controlled ventilation in elective laparoscopic cholecystectomy, *Egypt. J. Anaesth.* 27, 7–11 (2011).

[19] W. H. Teoh, K. M. Lee, T. Suhitharan, Z. Yahaya, M. M. Teo and A.T. Sia, Comparison of the LMA Supreme vs the i-gel™ in paralysed patients undergoing gynaecological laparoscopic surgery with controlled ventilation, *Anaesthesia* 65, 1173–9 (2010).

[20] B. Sharma, R. Sehgal, C. Sahai and J. Sood, PLMA vs. i-gel: A comparative evaluation of respiratory mechanics in laparoscopic cholecystectomy. *J. Anaesthesiol. Clin. Pharmacol.* 26, 451–7 (2010).

[21] P. Jindal, A. A. Rizvi, G. Khurana and J. P. Sharma, Safety and efficacy of insertion of supraglottic device in anaesthetised patients by first-time users, *S. Afr. J. Anaesthesiol. Analg.* 16, 23-6 (2010).

[22] W. J. Shin, Y. S Cheong, H. S. Yang and T. Nishiyama, The supraglottic airway i-gel in comparison with ProSeal laryngeal mask airway and classic laryngeal mask airway in anaesthetized patients, *Eur. J. Anaesth.* 27, 598–601 (2010).

[23] S. Amini and M. Khoshfetrat, Comparison of the Intersurgical Solus™ laryngeal mask airway and the i-gel supralaryngeal device, *Anaesthesia* 65, 805–9 (2010).

[24] H. Atef, E. El-Taher, A. Henidak and A. Helmy, Comparative study between i-gel, a new supraglottic airway device, and classical laryngeal mask airway in anesthetized spontaneously ventilated patients, *Saudi J. Anaesth.* 4, 131-6 (2010).

[25] V. Uppal, S. Gangaiah, G. Fletcher and J. Kinsella, Randomized crossover comparison between the i-gel and the LMA-Unique in anaesthetized, paralysed adults, *Br. J. Anaesth.* 103, 882–5 (2009).

[26] C. Keijzer, D. R. Buitelaar, K. M. Efthymiou, M. Šrámek, J. ten Cate, M. Ronday, T. Stoppa, J. M. Huitink and P. F. Schutte, A comparison of postoperative throat and neck complaints after the use of the i-gel® and the La Premiere® disposable laryngeal mask: a double-blinded, randomized, controlled trial, *Anesth. Analg.* 109, 1092–5 (2009).

[27] H. Francksen, J. Renner, R. Hanss, J. Scholz, V. Doerges and B. Bein, A comparison of the i-gel™ with the LMA-Unique™ in non-paralysed anaesthetised adult patients, *Anaesthesia* 64, 1118–24 (2009).

[28] J. F. Heuer, M. Stiller, J. Rathgeber, C. Eich, K. Züchner, M. Bauer and A. Timmermann, Evaluation der neuen Kehlkopfmasken Ambu AuraOnce™ und Intersurgical i-gel™. *Anaesthesist* 58, 813–20 (2009). [Article in German, abstract in English.]

[29] L. G. Theiler, M. Kleine-Brueggeney, D. Kaiser, N. Urwyler, C. Luyet, A. Vogt, R. Greif and M. M. Unibe, Crossover comparison of the laryngeal mask supreme and the i-gel in simulated difficult airway scenario in anesthetized patients, *Anesthesiology* 111, 55–62 (2009).

[30] Singh, M. Gupta and M. Tandon, Comparison of clinical performance of i-gel with LMA-Proseal in elective surgeries, *Indian J. Anaesth.* 53, 302–5 (2009).

[31] O. A. Bamgbade, W. R. Macnab and W. M. Khalaf, Evaluation of the i-gel airway in 300 patients, *Eur. J. Anaesth.* 25, 865–6 (2008).

[32] J. J. Gatward, T. M. Cook, C. Seller, J. Handel, T. Simpson, V. Vanek and F. Kelly, Evaluation of the size 4 i-gel™ airway in one hundred non-paralysed patients, *Anaesthesia* 63, 1124–30 (2008).

[33] N. M. Wharton, B. Gibbison, D. A. Gabbott, G. M. Haslam, N. Muchatuta and T. M. Cook, i-gel insertion by novices in manikins and patients, *Anaesthesia* 63, 991–5 (2008).

[34] B. Richez, L. Saltel, F. Banchereau, R. Torrielli and A. M. Cros, A new single use supraglottic airway device with a noninflatable cuff and an esophageal vent: an observational study of the i-gel, *Anesth. Analg.* 106, 1137–9 (2008).

[35] P. Jindal, A. Rizvi and J. P. Sharma, Is i-gel a new revolution among supraglottic airway devices? --a comparative evaluation, *Middle East J. Anesthesiol.* 20, 53–8 (2009).

[36] J. Brimacombe and J. Archdeacon, The LMA for unplanned prolonged procedures, *Can. J. Anesth.* 42, 1176 (1995).

[37] J. Patki and C. N. Reddy, Six hours positive pressure ventilation with size 5 laryngeal mask in a 55-kg patient, *Indian J. Anaesth.* 54, 174–5 (2010).

[38] M. J. Bucx, W. Grolman, F. H. Kruisinga, J.A. Lindeboom and A. A. van Kempen, The prolonged use of the laryngeal mask airway in a neonate with airway obstruction and Treacher-Collins syndrome, *Pediatr. Anesth.* 13, 530–3 (2003).

[39] S. H. Park, S. H. Han, S. H. Do, J. W. Kim and J. H. Kim, The influence of head and neck position on the oropharyngeal leak pressure and cuff position of three supraglottic airway devices, *Anesth. Analg.* 108, 112–7 (2009).

[40] S. Taxak and A. Gopinath, Insertion of the i-gel airway in prone position, *Minerva Anestesiol.* 76, 381 (2010).

[41] M. Senthil Kumar, R. Pandey and P. Khanna, Successful use of i-gel airway in prone position surgery, *Pediatr. Anesth.* 19, 176–7 (2009).

[42] S. Bercker, W. Schmidbauer, T. Volk, G. Bogusch, H. P. Bubser, M. Hensel and T. Kerner, A comparison of seal in seven supraglottic airway devices using a cadaver model of elevated esophageal pressure, *Anesth. Analg.* 106, 445–8 (2008).

[43] W. Schmidbauer, S. Bercker, T. Volk, G. Bogusch, G. Mager G and T. Kerner, Oesophageal seal of the novel supralaryngeal airway device i-gel™ in comparison with the laryngeal mask airways Classic™ and ProSeal™ using a cadaver model, *Br. J. Anaesth.* 102, 135–9 (2009).

[44] S. G. Russo, S. Cremer, U. Mühlhäuser, C. Eich and M. Quintel, Investigating the fluid seal of supraglottic airway devices in humans using indicator dye via the drainage tube: a potential roadmap for future studies, *Open J. Anesth.* 2, 18–22 (2012).

[45] C. Keller, J. R. Brimacombe, K. Keller and R. Morris, Comparison of four methods for assessing airway sealing pressure with the laryngeal mask airway in adult patients, *Br. J. Anaesth.* 82, 286–7 (1999).

[46] T. M. Cook, G. Lee and J. P. Nolan, The proseal™ laryngeal mask airway: a review of the literature, *Can. J. Anesth.* 52, 739–60 (2005).

[47] L. Gasteiger, J. Brimacombe. D. Perkhofer. M. Kaufmann and C. Keller, Comparison of guided insertion of the LMA ProSeal vs the i-gel, *Anaesthesia* 65, 913–6 (2010).

[48] D. A. Gabbott and R. Beringer. The iGEL supraglottic airway: a potential role for resuscitation? *Resuscitation* 73, 161–2 (2007).

[49] A. I. Brain, The laryngeal mask—a new concept in airway management, *Br. J. Anaesth.* 55, 801–6 (1983).

[50] J. Payne, The use of the fibreoptic laryngoscope to confirm the position of the laryngeal mask, *Anaesthesia* 44, 865–5 (1989).

[51] R. M. Levitan and W. C. Kinkle, Initial anatomic investigations of the i-gel airway: a novel supraglottic airway without inflatable cuff, *Anaesthesia* 60, 1022–6 (2005).

[52] L. Magnusson and D. R. Spahn, New concepts of atelectasis during general anaesthesia, *Br. J. Anaesth.* 91, 61-72 (2003).

[53] B. Froessler, J. Brommundt, J. Anton, R. Khanduja, R. Kuhlen, R. Rossaint and M. Coburn, Spontaneously breathing anesthetized patients with a laryngeal mask airway: positive end-expiratory pressure does not improve oxygen saturation, *Anaesthesist.* 59, 1003-7 (2010). [Article in German, abstract in English.]

[54] E. E. Chew, N. H. Hashim and C.Y. Wang, Randomised comparison of the LMA Supreme with the i-gel in spontaneously breathing anaesthetised adult patients, *Anaesth. Intensive Care* 38, 1018–22 (2010).

[55] J. H. Devitt, R. Wenstone, A. G. Noel and M. P. O'Donnell, The laryngeal mask airway and positive-pressure ventilation, *Anesthesiology* 80, 550–5 (1994).

[56] F. Latorre, B. Eberle, N. Weiler, R. Mienert, A. Stanek, R. Goedecke and W. Heinrichs, Laryngeal mask airway position and the risk of gastric insufflation, *Anesth. Analg.* 86, 867–71 (1998).

[57] J. Brimacombe, C. Keller and A. Berry, Gastric insufflation with the ProSeal laryngeal mask, *Anesth. Analg.* 92, 1614-5 (2001).

[58] V. Uppal, G. Fletcher and J. Kinsella, Comparison of the i-gel with the cuffed tracheal tube during pressure-controlled ventilation, *Br. J. Anaesth.* 102, 264–8 (2009).

[59] W. Schmidbauer, H. Genzwürker, O. Ahlers, H. Proquitte H and T. Kerner, Cadaver study of oesophageal insufflation with supraglottic airway devices during positive pressure ventilation in an obstructed airway, *Br. J. Anaesth.* 109, 454–8 (2012).

[60] M. L. Wood and E. T. Forrest, The haemodynamic response to the insertion of the laryngeal mask airway: a comparison with laryngoscopy and tracheal intubation, *Acta Anaesthesiol. Scand.* 38, 510–3 (1994).

[61] S. A. Ismail, N. A. Bisher, H. W. Kandil, H. A. Mowafi and H. A. Atawia, Intraocular pressure and haemodynamic responses to insertion of the i-gel, laryngeal mask airway or endotracheal tube, *Eur. J. Anaesth.* 28, 443–8 (2011).

Conflict of interest: Dr William Donaldson has delivered lectures on the i-gel for Intersurgical®.

In: The i-gel Supraglottic Airway
Editors: Pavel Michalek and William Donaldson

ISBN: 978-1-62417-897-9

Chapter 6

USE OF THE I-GEL IN SPECIAL CONDITIONS - LAPAROSCOPIES, LATERAL OR PRONE POSITIONS, AIRWAY STENOSIS

Pavel Michalek [1,2,*]

[1]Department of Anesthesia and Intensive Medicine,
First Medical Faculty of the Charles University and
General University Hospital, Prague, Czech Republic
[2]Department of Anaesthesia, Antrim Area
Hospital, Antrim, UK

ABSTRACT

As a "second generation" supraglottic airway device (SAD), the i-gel® may be used not only for elective cases of extraperitoneal surgery but also in some extended or alternative indications. The use of SADs in laparoscopic procedures remains controversial because of the potentially increased risk of gastric regurgitation and pulmonary aspiration in comparison with tracheal intubation. The i-gel airway has been used in laparoscopic cholecystectomies and gynecological laparoscopies without any significant complications.

The i-gel may be used also in procedures performed in positions other than supine. For the surgery in the lateral position, the device may be inserted in the supine position and the patient turned afterwards. Alternatively induction of general anesthesia and insertion of the i-gel may be performed with the patient already in the lateral position. Isolated case reports also describe i-gel use in prone position surgery.

Other nonconventional indications for the i-gel insertion include use in patients with tracheal stenosis, as a conduit for bronchial blocker insertion in uncomplicated thoracic procedures or during tracheostomies.

[*] Corresponding author: Pavel Michalek. E-mail address: pafkamich@yahoo.co.uk.

INTRODUCTION

The popularity and use of supraglottic airway devices (SADs) is growing worldwide [1]. Initial indications for the use of classical laryngeal masks (1st generation SADs) involved only elective cases in patients without an increased risk of gastric content aspiration and for procedures outside the abdominal cavity. The main concerns were of regurgitation of gastric contents into the oral cavity and passage of these contents around the laryngeal mask into trachea, causing aspiration. Although the estimated incidence of gastric content aspiration with the classical laryngeal mask airway (cLMA) is very low – 0.02% (2:10 000 patients) [2, 3] or 0.01% (3:35 630 patients) [4] – investigators have tried to further decrease its risk. The second generation of SADs incorporates an additional channel designated for the passive drainage or active suctioning of gastric contents [5].

The ProSeal laryngeal mask (LMA ProSeal®, Intavent Direct, Maidenhead, UK) was the first second generation SAD and was introduced in 1999 [6]. Its design should decrease the risk of gastric content aspiration but this fact has not yet been confirmed in clinical studies. Due to the very low incidence of gastric aspiration associated with the classical laryngeal mask, a study recruiting more than 2 million people would be necessary to confirm or disprove any superiority of 2nd generation SADs.

However 2nd generation SADs, including the i-gel®, are considered to be safe devices for routine laparoscopic procedures [1]. High seal pressures, ease of insertion and other factors also helped 2nd generation SADs to find their way to less conventional areas of usage. The i-gel is routinely employed in some centres for procedures performed in lateral or semi-sitting positions or even in a prone-position surgery [7]. SADs may also be used as a conduit for a fiberscope for examination of the trachea or as conduit for the insertion of bronchial blocker in simple thoracic cases [8].

One case report describes the i-gel use for maintenance of airway patency in a patient with subglottic stenosis [9].

THE I-GEL AIRWAY IN LAPAROSCOPIC SURGERY

The last twenty years of the 20th century were characterized by significant changes in surgical operative strategies. Open laparotomies were replaced by less invasive approaches – laparoscopic operations. The first laparoscopic cholecystectomy was performed in France in 1987. Laparoscopic and retroperitoneoscopic techniques were developed and have been introduced into clinical practice in other surgical disciplines – gynecology, urology and vascular surgery [10]. The main benefits of laparoscopic surgery are: less surgical trauma, decreased intensity of postoperative pain, decreased postoperative inflammatory response and a better cosmetic effect [11].

Pathophysiological Changes Associated with Laparoscopic Surgery

The pneumoperitoneum required for laparoscopic surgery may affect different organs and systems. Those most important for the anesthesiologist are respiratory and hemodynamic changes. Insufflation of carbon dioxide (CO_2) into the abdominal cavity is associated with complex pathophysiological changes of which the anesthesiologist must be aware (Table 1, Table 2) [11].

Following CO_2 insufflation, intraabdominal pressure increases and, due to an expansion of the abdominal cavity, pulmonary compliance decreases by 30-50%. CO_2 is relatively quickly absorbed into the blood and its partial pressure ($PaCO_2$) increases [11]. Those patients with chronic cardiac conditions (e.g. coronary artery disease, congestive heart failure) have a high risk of developing atelectatic changes at the bases of the lungs even at relatively low levels of intraabdominal pressure (13-15 mmHg). Laparoscopic surgery also affects the cardiovascular system through a combination of CO_2 insufflation, patient positioning, hypercarbia and general anesthesia itself [11-13].

Elevation of the intraabdominal pressure above 10 mmHg may induce significant hemodynamic changes: mean arterial pressure (MAP) increases, as well as pulmonary (PVR) and systemic (SVR) vascular resistances. Cardiac output is usually decreased depending on the patient´s cardiac function and reserve [14, 15].

Both cerebral blood flow (CBF) and intracranial pressure (ICP) are elevated. Neurohumoral responses are activated – laparoscopic surgery is associated with elevated plasma levels of renin, angiotensin, aldosterone and vasopressin due to activation of the renin-angiotensin-aldosterone axis. The sympathetic nervous system is also activated due to elevated plasma levels of endogenous catecholamines [11, 12].

Table 1. Important factors for anesthesia during laparoscopic procedures [11, 12]

• CO_2 insufflation associated with pathophysiological changes (hemodynamics, respiratory system, neuroendocrine functions), increased intraabdominal pressure • Patient position ("head down" vs. "head up") • Coexisting disease (cardiovascular, respiratory) • Duration of procedure (prolonged surgery)

Table 2. Patient position during laparoscopy and its influence on hemodynamic and respiratory parameters [11]

"Head down" (Trendelenburg) position	"Head up" (anti-Trendelenburg) position
↑ CVP, ↑ venous return	
↑ CO	↓ CVP, ↓ venous return
↑ hydrostatic pressure	↓ CO
↓ SVR (↑ receptor irritation)	↓ hydrostatic pressure
↓ HR	↑ SVR (↓ receptor irritation)
↓ transmural pressure of pelvic organs	↑ HR
↓ bleeding	↑ transmural pressure of pelvic organs
↑ ICP	↑ bleeding
↑ incidence of gas embolism	↓ ICP
↓ FRC, ↓ pulmonary compliance	

Laparoscopic Surgery and Gastric Regurgitation

The risk of regurgitation of gastric contents increases significantly during laparoscopic procedures. The main determinants of gastric regurgitation are the balance between lower esophageal sphincter pressure (LESP), barrier pressure (BrP) and intragastric pressure (IGP). Following CO_2 insufflation into the abdominal cavity during laparoscopy, both lower esophageal and intragastric pressures rise. Barrier pressure usually remains relatively stable [16]. Two studies have evaluated the incidence of gastric regurgitation during elective laparoscopic procedures. Duffy found regurgitated gastric content inside the hypopharynx in two patients in his cohort (total 93 patients – incidence 2.2%) anesthetized for laparoscopic gynecological surgery [17]. Another trial evaluated the incidence of regurgitation in 100 females scheduled for gynecological laparoscopies with cLMA. Patients swallowed capsules containing methylene blue dye 10-15 min before induction to general anesthesia. The authors found signs of dye within the bowl of the LMA in one patient – 1%. They concluded that the true rate of regurgitation in laparoscopic gynecological procedures (95% CI) is less than 4.1% [18].

Supraglottic Airway Devices in Laparoscopic Surgery

Many studies have evaluated SADs as an alternative to endotracheal intubation in laparoscopic cholecystectomies and laparoscopic gynecological procedures.

Published evidence shows that the LMA ProSeal is a good alternative to tracheal intubation for gynecological laparoscopies [19, 20] and that it is associated with less hemodynamic changes during insertion and removal than the tracheal tube [19]. Other studies have even recommended the cLMA as an alternative to intubation [20, 21]. Maltby et al. compared the LMA ProSeal with endotracheal intubation in elective non-obese patients scheduled for laparoscopic cholecystectomies and found that both devices performed equally [22]. The LMA Supreme has also been trialled in patients undergoing laparoscopic procedures: Belena et al. inserted the LMA Supreme in 100 patients scheduled for elective laparoscopic cholecystecomies and did not find any serious complication associated with this SAD [23]. Success rates and postoperative complications between LMA Supreme and endotracheal tubes were compared in gynecological laparoscopies. Postoperative complaints were significantly higher in intubated patients, whilst other evaluated parameters were without any difference [24]. Viira and Myles performed a literature search for laryngeal mask usage in laparoscopic surgeries. They concluded that there is no robust evidence to either support or refute its use for this indication. The reported incidence of regurgitation and gastric content aspiration was extremely low [25]. There is very little evidence supporting the use of SADs during laparoscopic procedures in children [26].

The i-gel Airway in Laparoscopic Procedures

The first descriptive study of the i-gel was performed by Richez et al. in France [27]. The authors prospectively assessed use of the i-gel in female patients undergoing gynecological surgery. They did not mention if any of the procedures in their cohort were performed using laparoscopy.

Teoh and colleagues compared the i-gel and LMA Supreme in 100 female patients scheduled for gynecological laparoscopic operations [28]. Patients were paralyzed and ventilated using volume-controlled positive pressure ventilation (VCV). All procedures were performed using capnoperitoneum and a steep Trendelenburg position was employed. The authors did not find any differences between the two SADs in oropharyngeal seal pressures (26.4 ± 5.1 cmH_2O for LMA Supreme and 25.0 ± 5.7 for i-gel) or in first-attempt insertion success rates (94% in the LMA Supreme group and 96% in the i-gel group). Gastric tube insertion was easier and faster in the LMA Supreme group. After CO_2 insufflation, there was a smaller difference between expired tidal volumes in the LMA Supreme group than in patients studied in the i-gel group.

Another study assessed i-gel airway in laparoscopic cholecystectomies and compared it with the cuffed endotracheal tube [29]. Volume controlled ventilation was used in both groups of patients. The authors assessed the leak volumes and leak fractions (leak volume/inspired tidal volume) in both devices. Leak volumes and leak fractions increased in the i-gel group after establisment of capnoperitoneum, when higher volumes (8-10 $mL.kg^{-1}$) were used.

Based on these findings, the authors conluded that the i-gel should only be used in laparoscopic cholecystectomies as an alternative to tracheal intubation if peak pressures do not exceed leak (seal) pressures.

Sharma et al. compared the i-gel with the ProSeal LMA in 60 patients undergoing elective laparoscopic cholecytectomy [30]. They evaluated oropharyngeal seal pressure (OSP) and respiratory mechanics (dynamic compliance, respiratory system resistance, work of breathing, peak airway pressures and expired tidal volume/minute ventilation) in both SADs. The oropharyngeal seal pressure was higher in the ProSeal group (38.9 ± 3.2 cmH_2O) than in the i-gel group (35.6 ± 4.8 cmH_2O, $p = 0.007$). Dynamic compliance was higher in the i-gel group, while there was no difference between the groups in terms of other parameters of respiratory mechanics. The incidence of SAD malrotation was higher in the i-gel group.

Uppal and colleagues compared the i-gel airway with the cuffed tracheal tube in elective patients under conditions of pressure-controlled ventilation (PCV) [31]. In this cross-over study, the authors recruited 25 patients scheduled for abdominal hysterectomies or laparoscopic cholecystectomies. Following standardized induction to general anesthesia, an i-gel airway was initially inserted, leak volumes and fractions were measured, and then i-gel was replaced by a cuffed endotracheal tube.

The authors did not find any difference in leak volumes or leak pressures between the i-gel and endotracheal tube during PCV at 15 or 20 cmH_2O. There was significant difference when using higher pressures (25 cmH_2O, difference in leak fractions was 0.02 – $p = 0.014$; difference in leak volume was 26.5 ml – $p = 0.006$). The conclusion of this study was that i-gel may replace tracheal tube during procedures with PCV but only when peak pressures do not exceed 20-25 cmH_2O.

Singh studied the clinical performance of the i-gel in elective surgical procedures, including laparoscopic surgery, and compared it with the LMA ProSeal [32].

In total 13 patients in this study underwent laparoscopic cholecystectomy. The authors found the i-gel easier to insert. Insertion of a gastric tube was also easier in the i-gel group. The incidence of postoperative complaints was higher in the ProSeal LMA group.

Donaldson inserted an i-gel in a patient with a suspected subglottic stenosis scheduled for laparoscopic cholecystectomy. The procedure was performed without complications and without airway leaks, even during increased peak pressures associated with capnoperitoneum [9]. Some features of the i-gel important for laparoscopic procedures have been studied in both humans and cadavers. Nawaz et al. compared oropharyngeal seal pressures (OSP) of the i-gel before and after insertion of a silicone gastric tube in thirty patients undergoing elective surgical procedures [33]. They did not find any significant difference in the OSP before (23.3 ± 8.0 mmHg) and after the insertion (24.4 ± 8.4 mmHg) of a gastric tube. The results of this study implicate that insertion of a gastric tube through the gastric channel of the i-gel does not influence its seal pressure. Three different SADs (ProSeal LMA, cLMA, i-gel) were inserted into the unfixed cadaver model in another study [34].

The esophageus was then filled with water using two regimens – a slow increase in esophageal pressure and a fast increase in the pressure imitating active vomiting. The ProSeal LMA withstood high esophageal pressures up to 58 cmH_2O. The cLMA lost its esophageal seal at 37 cmH_2O and i-gel at an even lower level – at 13 cmH_2O. Both the ProSeal LMA and i-gel were able to drain esophageal fluid effectively through their additional lumens.

A recent study compared regurgitation of a dye indicator (indigo carmine green) in 73 patients scheduled for elective surgeries in the supine position [35]. Patients were randomized into two groups – in 36 of them an i-gel airway was used while the remaining 37 received a LMA Supreme. The authors did not note any regurgitation during controlled ventilation but two patients in the i-gel group (5.5%) had a small amount of dye detected inside the bowl during spontaneous ventilation. If the i-gel is to be used in laparoscopic surgery the gastric tube should be always inserted through the additional channel of device into stomach, its position confirmed and gastric contect actively suctioned (Figure 1).

The i-gel Airway in Lateral and Prone Position Surgeries

The majority of surgical procedures are performed with patients in the supine position. However some operations require lateral, or even prone positioning of the patient. Apart from thoracic surgery, lateral positions are used for removals of lipomas, fibromas and melanomas from the back, lateral chest and abdominal wall and for some operations on the buttock and lower extremities.

Table 3. Studies and case reports describing use of the i-gel in laparoscopic surgery. Legend: LC – laparoscopic cholecystectomy, GL – gynecological laparoscopy

Study, year	Number of patients	Procedures	Regurgitation/ Aspiration
Singh, 2009 [32]	6	LC	0/0
Donaldson, 2010 [9]	1	LC	0/0
Sharma, 2010 [30]	30	LC	0/0
Teoh, 2010 [28]	50	GL	0/0
Ibrahim, 2011 [29]	30	LC	0/0

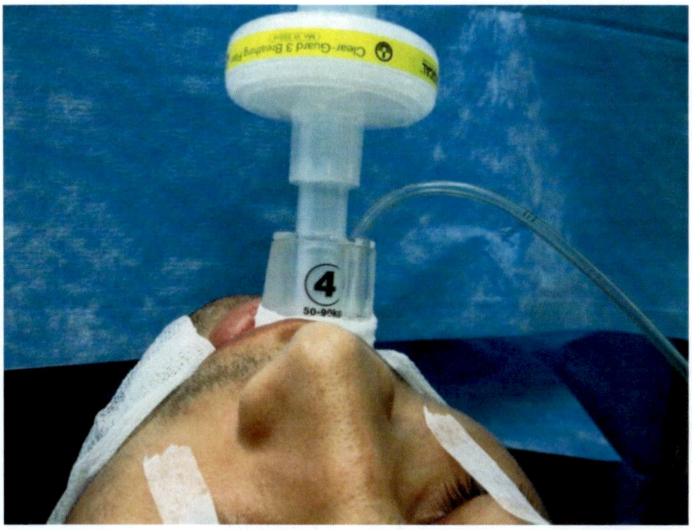

Figure 1. i-gel airway inserted for a laparoscopic procedure with a gastric tube inserted through the drainage channel.

Other minor operations in these locations such as drainage of abscesses, debridements or suturing of minor traumatic wounds may be also performed in the lateral position. The prone position is routinely employed for selected procedures on the back, perianal region and the posterior surface of the lower extremities.

For procedures in the lateral position, the i-gel may be inserted in supine position and patients may be turned over to the lateral position after fixation of the device or it may be inserted with the patient in the lateral position, using the same technique as for insertion in the supine position – "sniffing morning air" with jaw thrust applied by an assistant (Figure 2) [36]. Garcia et al. studied insertion of the i-gel airway in the lateral position [37]. The authors inserted an i-gel airway in 32 patients, 16 of them were operated in the lateral position, 16 in the supine position. The i-gel was inserted in patients already placed on their sides in the "lateral position" group. First attempt insertion success and insertion times were similar in both groups. Peak pressures and tidal volumes also did not differ between the groups. However, the low number of patients in the study meant that it was underpowered. In a retrospective evaluation of the i-gel airway in 300 patients, device was inserted in the lateral position in 55 of them. The authors did not report any complications associated with insertion in this position [7]. We routinely use the i-gel in female breast procedures – the device is inserted in the supine position, the patient is turned over to the lateral position for an application of paravertebral block and then turned back [38]. We have not experienced any significant malpositioning of device during this change of the patient´s position in more than 70 patients.

Use of the i-gel has been reported also for a prone position surgery (Figure 3) in two case reports. Taxak describes a case where the patient positioned himself in the prone position with his head turned laterally for induction. The device was inserted at the first attempt [39]. Another report describes insertion of the i-gel size 3 already in prone position [40].

Their patient was a 10-year old boy indicated for pyeloplasty. The authors favored i-gel over the laryngeal mask because of its semirigid non-inflatable cuff which should theoretically have lower potential for kinking.

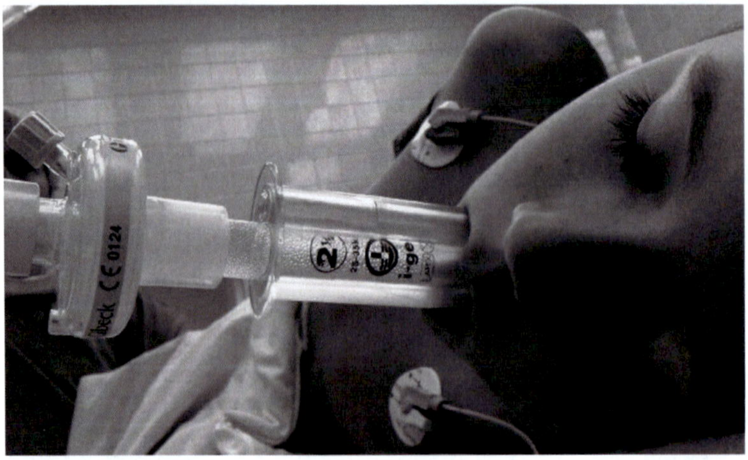

Figure 2. i-gel insertion in the lateral position.

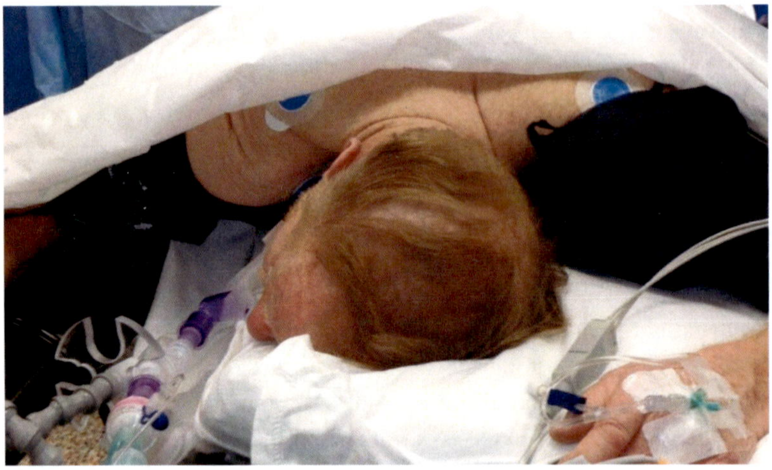

Figure 3. i-gel inserted for surgery in the prone position.

The main risks using SADs in the prone position include difficulty of insertion, airway obstruction or difficulties in readjusting the airway in case of malpositioning of the device [41].

Other Indications for Non-Conventional Use of the i-gel

The i-gel airway has also been used in thoracic anesthesia, in the magnetic resonance imaging suite and in intensive care settings.

i-gels were used as a conduit for a fiberscope-guided insertion of bronchial blocker in twenty-five patients scheduled for various thoracic operations (Figures 4a,b) [8]. All patients were scheduled for elective cases and did not have any risk factors for gastric content regurgitation. The majority of the procedures were video-assisted thoracic surgeries and lateral minithoracotomies.

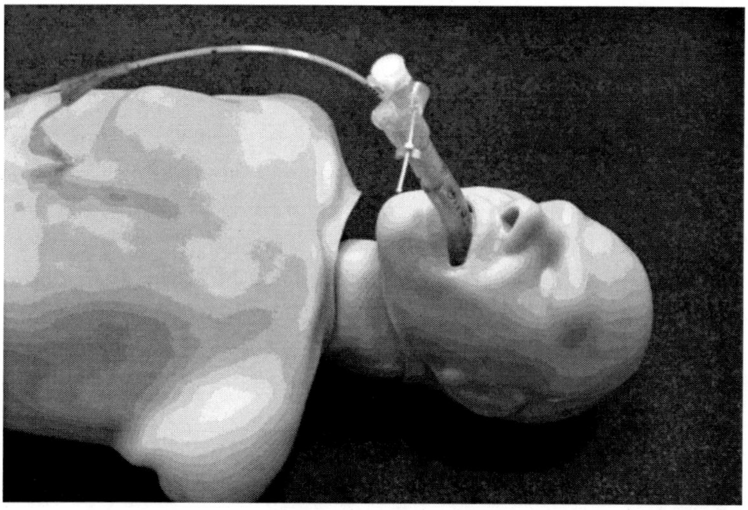

a)

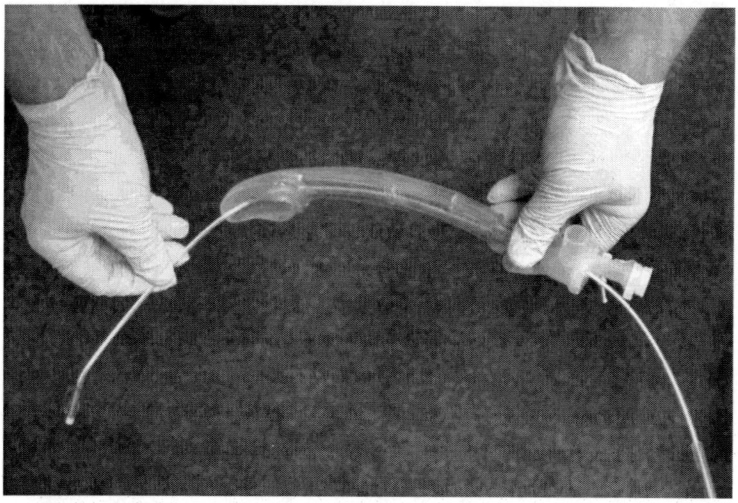

b)

Figure 4 a, b. A bronchial blocker inserted through the i-gel supraglottic airway (mannequin simulation).

An experienced thoracic anesthesiologist was able to insert a bronchial blocker under fiberoptic guidance into the selected main bronchus (Figure 5), No major leak or any other complications occurred in this study.

Sanuki et al. used a modified i-gel for the procedures of oral and dental surgery [42]. They cut the stem of device and inserted a reinforced tracheal tube through its breathing channel.

Their reason for cutting i-gel was to avoid interference of the airway device with the surgical field. However, this modification is not approved by the manufacturer.

Other non-conventional indications for i-gel insertion outside the operating suite are described in detail in Chapter 11.

PATIENTS WITH TRACHEAL STENOSIS AND I-GEL

Management of the airway in patients with tracheal stenosis is frequently challenging. The most commonly employed technique in this clinical scenario is insertion of a narrow-diameter tracheal tube to pass the stenotic segment. However, this technique may cause tracheal trauma with bleeding, mucosal edema and worsening of obstruction or perforation of the trachea. The vocal cords are usually visualized without any difficulty but passing the tracheal tube through the stenotic part of trachea may be very difficult or impossible. Repeated intubation attempts may lead to further narrowing of stenotic segment due to edema and may eventually lead to hypoxia. Even in cases of minor mucosal edema, patients may experience difficulties during and after extubation – stridor, acute respiratory insufficency or negative pressure pulmonary edema.

The use of supraglottic airways in tracheal stenosis has been advocated by some clinicians.

Asai published his experience with a classical laryngeal mask airway in children with stenosis of the trachea. The use of various supraglottic airways has been reported in the literature including laryngeal masks and EasyTube (EasyTube®, Rüsch-Teleflex, Limerick, PA, US) airway device [43-46]. These devices have been employed with both spontaneous and controlled ventilation. We used an i-gel supraglottic airway in one female patient with a subglottic stenosis of non-cancer origin [9]. This woman was scheduled for a laparoscopic cholecystectomy and had reported previous difficulties with insertion of an endotracheal tube for routine elective gynecological surgery. The i-gel was used for the examination of trachea (Figure 6) and airway maintenance during her laparoscopic cholecystectomy.

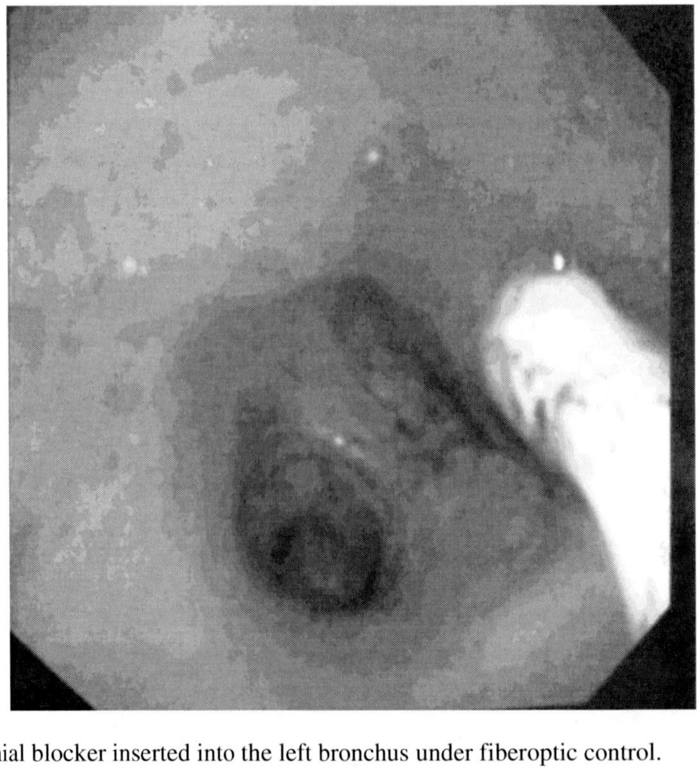

Figure 5. Bronchial blocker inserted into the left bronchus under fiberoptic control.

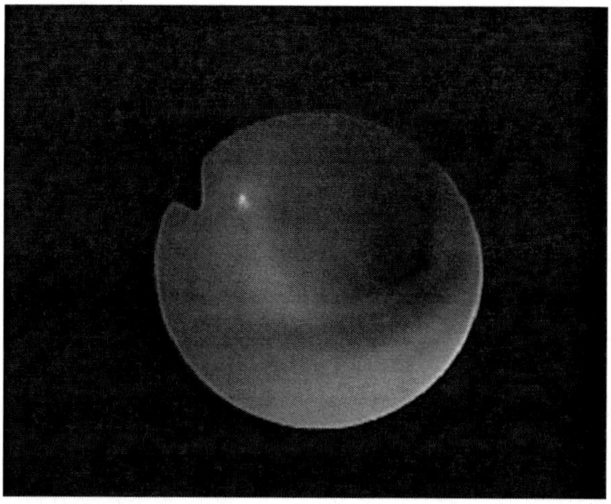

Figure 6. Subglottic tracheal stenosis examined through the i-gel airway.

The device was inserted after induction of general anesthesia without any difficulties, providing effective ventilation and a good seal (seal pressure over 25 mmHg). The 12-French gastric tube was then inserted through the suction channel of device and the stomach was decompressed.

Fiberoptic examination of the airway revealed normal vocal cords and a narrowing in the subglottic segment of trachea caused probably by a prominent cricoid cartilage. The surgical procedure, removal of the i-gel device and postoperative course were uneventful.

CONCLUSION

The i-gel airway is 2nd generation SAD and its main mechanism of seal is by anatomical matching of the cuff design with the perilaryngeal structures [47]. As with other 2nd generation SADs, the i-gel has been used for indications other than routine elective superficial surgeries in the supine position.

Improved airway seal pressures in comparison with the 1st generation SADs allow the use of i-gel in laparoscopic procedures. The i-gel seems to be an alternative to endotracheal tube for this indication; there have been no complications recorded in 117 patients in total but larger studies are needed to confirm its safety.

Regarding regurgitation and aspiration of gastric content: careful evaluation of the patient´s risk factors is probably more important than selection of airway device [48]. Aspiration of gastric contents may occur even with 2nd generation SADs, mainly due to malpositioning, poor seal or during massive vomiting [49, 50].

The use of i-gel in the lateral position has been described in the literature [7, 37]. According to published data, this technique may be recommended for lateral position surgery as well as for turning the patient from supine to lateral position for regional anesthesia procedures (caudal anesthesia, paravertebral block).

i-gel insertion and use in the prone position is also possible, however it may be associated with potentially serious problems due to loss of the airway and delay in re-establishment of its patency.

References

[1] T. M. Cook and B. Howes, Supraglottic airway devices: recent advances, *Cont. Educ. Anaesth. Crit. Care Pain* 2, 56-61 (2011).

[2] J. R. Brimacombe and A. Berry, The incidence of aspiration associated with the laryngeal mask airway: a meta-analysis of published literature, *J. Clin. Anesth.* 7, 297-305 (1995).

[3] C. Keller, J. Brimacombe, J. Bittersohl, P. Lirk and A. von Goedecke, Aspiration and the laryngeal mask airway: three cases and the review of the literature. *Br. J. Anaesth.* 93, 579-82 (2004).

[4] Bernardini and G. Natalini, Risk of pulmonary aspiration with laryngeal mask airway and tracheal tube: analysis on 65 712 procedure with positive pressure ventilation, *Anaesthesia* 64, 1289-94 (2009).

[5] D. M. Miller, A proposed classification and scoring system for supraglottic sealing airways: a brief review, *Anesth. Analg.* 99, 1553-9 (2004).

[6] I. J. Brain, C. Verghese and P. J. Strube, The LMA "ProSeal": a laryngeal mask with an oesophageal vent, *Br. J. Anaesth.* 84, 650-4 (2000).

[7] O. A. Bamgbade, W. R. Macnab and W. M. Khalaf, Evaluation of the i-gel airway in 300 patients, *Eur. J. Anaesthesiol.* 25, 865-6 (2008).

[8] J. Arevalo Ludena, J. J. Arcas Bellas, V. Lopez Perez, A. Cuarental Garcia and R. Alvarez-Rementeria Carbonell, Placement of a bronchial blocker through the i-gel supraglottic airway device for single-lung ventilation, *Rev. Esp. Anestesiol. Reanim.* 57, 532-5 (2010). [Article in Spanish with English abstract]

[9] W. Donaldson and P. Michalek, The use of an i-gel supraglottic airway for the airway management of a patient with subglottic stenosis: a case report, *Minerva Anestesiol.* 76, 369-72 (2010).

[10] T. A. Stellato, History of laparoscopic surgery, *Surg. Clin. North Am.* 72, 997-1002 (1992).

[11] F. J. Gerges, G. E. Kanazi and S. I. Jabbour-Khoury, Anesthesia for laparoscopy: a review, *J. Clin. Anesth.* 18, 67-78 (2006).

[12] A. Kaba and J. Joris, Anaesthesia for laparoscopic surgery, *Curr. Anaesth. Int. Care* 12, 159-65 (2001).

[13] C. P. Henny and J. Hofland, Laparoscopic surgery: pitfalls due to anesthesia, positioning, and pneumoperitoneum, *Surg. Endosc.* 19, 1163-71 (2005).

[14] C. N. Gutt, T. Oniu, A. Mehrabi, P. Schemmer, A. Kashfi, T. Kraus and M. W. Büchler, Circulatory and respiratory complications of carbon dioxide insufflation, *Dig. Surg.* 21, 95-105 (2004).

[15] Russo, E. Marana, D. Viviani, L. Polidori, S. Colicci, M. Mettimano, R. Proietti and E. Di Stasio, Diastolic function: the influence of pneumoperitoneum and Trendelendurg positioning during laparoscopic hysterectomy. *Eur. J. Anaesthesiol.* 26, 923-7 (2009).

[16] K. Thörn, S. E. Thörn and M. Wattwil, The effects on the lower oesophageal sphincter of sevoflurane induction and increased intra-abdominal pressure during laparoscopy, *Acta Anaesthesiol. Scand.* 50, 978-81 (2006).

[17] B. L. Duffy, Regurgitation during pelvic laparoscopy, *Br. J. Anaesth.* 51, 1089-90 (1979).

[18] P. P. Bapat, C. Verghese, Laryngeal mask airway and the incidence of regurgitation during gynecological laparoscopies, *Anesth. Analg.* 85, 139-43 (1997).

[19] Y. Lim, S. Goel and J. R. Brimacombe, The ProSeal laryngeal mask airway is an effective alternative to laryngoscope-guided tracheal intubation for gynaecological laparoscopy, *Anaesth. Intensive Care* 35, 52-6 (2007).

[20] J. R. Maltby, M. T. Beriault, N. C. Watson, D. J. Liepert and G. H. Fick, LMA-Classic and LMA-ProSeal are effective alternatives to endotracheal intubation for gynecologic laparoscopy, *Can. J. Anaesth.* 50, 71-7 (2003).

[21] G. Natalini, G. Lanza, A. Rosano, P. Dell´Agnolo and A. Bernardini, Standard laryngeal mask airway and LMA-Proseal during laparoscopic surgery, *J. Clin. Anesth.* 15, 428-32 (2003).

[22] J. R. Maltby, M. T. Beriault, N. C. Watson, D. Liepert and G. H. Fick, The LMA-ProSeal is an effective alternative to tracheal intubation for laparoscopic cholecystectomy, *Can. J. Anaesth.* 49, 857-62 (2002).

[23] J. M. Belena, J. L. Gracia, J. L. Ayala, M. Nunez, J. A. Lorenzo, A. de los Reyes, J. L. Perez and J. Yuste, The laryngeal mask airway Supreme for positive pressure ventilation during laparoscopic cholecystectomy, *J. Clin. Anesth.* 23, 456-60 (2011).

[24] W. Abdi, R. Amathieu, A. Adhoum, C. Poncelet, V. Slavov, W. Kamoun, X. Combes and G. Dhonneur, Sparing the larynx during gynecological laparoscopy: a randomized trial comparing the LMA Supreme and the ETT, *Acta Anaesthesiol. Scand.* 54, 141-6 (2010).

[25] D. Viira and P. S. Myles, The use of the laryngeal mask in gynaecological laparoscopy, *Anaesth. Intensive Care* 32, 560-3 (2004).

[26] R. Greif and L. Theiler, The use of supraglottic airway devices in pediatric laparoscopic surgery, *Minerva Anestesiol.* 76, 575-6 (2010).

[27] B. Richez, L. Saltel, F. Banchereau, R. Torielli and A. M. Cros, A new single use supragottic airway device with a noninflatable cuff and an esophageal vent: an observational study of the i-gel, *Anesth. Analg.* 106, 1137-9 (2008).

[28] W. H. Teoh, K. M. Lee, T. Suhitharan, Z. Yahaya, M. M. Teo and A. T. Sia, Comparison of the LMA Supreme vs the i-gel in paralysed patients undergoing gynaecological laparoscopic surgery with controlled ventilation, *Anaesthesia* 65, 1173-9 (2010).

[29] M. Ibrahim, A. Ragab and H. ElShamaa, i-gel vs cuffed tracheal tube during volume controlled ventilation in elective laparoscopic cholecystectomy, *Egypt. J. Anaesth.* 27, 7-11 (2011).

[30] B. Sharma, R. Sekhal, C. Sahai and J. Sood, PLMA vs. i-gel: a comparative evaluation of respiratory mechanics in laparoscopic cholecystectomy, *J. Anaesthesiol. Clin. Pharmacol.* 26, 451-7 (2010).

[31] V. Uppal, G. Fletcher and J. Kinsella, Comparison of the i-gel with the cuffed tracheal tube during pressure-controlled ventilation, *Br. J. Anaesth.* 102, 264-8 (2009).

[32] Singh, M. Gupta and M. Tandon, Comparison of clinical performance of i-gel^{TM} with LMA-Proseal^{TM} in elective surgeries, *Ind. J. Anaesth.* 53, 302-5 (2009).

[33] S. Nawazi, A. A. Butter, A. Taqi and A. Shafique, A comparison of seal pressure of i-gel before and after insertion of a gastric tube, *J. Univ. Med. Dental Coll. (JUMDC)* 3, 12-5 (2012).

[34] W. Schmidbauer, S. Bercker, T. Volk, G. Bogusch, G. Maher and T. Kerner, Oesophageal seal of the novel supralaryngeal airway device i-gel^{TM} in comparison with the laryngeal mask airways Classic^{TM} and ProSeal^{TM} using a cadaver model, *Br. J. Anaesth.* 102, 135-9 (2009).

[35] S. G. Russo, S. Cremer, U. Muhlhauser, C. Eich, M. Quintel and M. Bauer, Investigating the fluid seal of supraglottic airway devices in humans using indicator dye via the drainage tube: a potential roadmap for future studies, *Open J. Anesthesiol.* 2, 18-22 (2012).

[36] User guide, i-gel® single use supraglottic airway, available on: www.i-gel.com.

[37] C. A. Garcia, A. J. Ludena, A. J. Bellas and A. R. Alvarez, Insertion of the supraglottic airway device i-gel in the lateral position: preliminary results, *Eur. J. Anaesthesiol.* 27, 252 (2010) [abstract].

[38] W. Donaldson, A. Abraham, M. Deighan and P. Michalek, i-gel^{TM} vs. AuraOnce^{TM} laryngeal mask for general anaesthesia with controlled ventilation in paralyzed patients, *Biomed. Pap.* 155, 155-63 (2011).

[39] S. Taxak and A. Gopinath, Insertion of the i-gel airway in prone position, *Minerva Anestesiol.* 76, 381 (2010).

[40] M. Senthil Kumar, R. Pandey and P. Khanna, Successful use of i-gel airway in prone position surgery, *Paediatr. Anaesth.* 19, 176-7 (2009).

[41] A. M. Lopez and R. Valero, Use of supraglottic airway devices in patients positioned other than supine, *Trends Anaesth. Crit. Care* 2, 65-70 (2012).

[42] T. Sanuki, S. Sugioka and J. Kotani, Modified i-gel airway for oral surgery, *Anesth. Prog.* 58, 124-5 (2011).

[43] H. Ischii, H. Fujihara, T. Ataka, H. Baba, T. Yamakura, T. Tobita, K. Taga, and K. Shimoji, Successful use of laryngeal mask airway for a patient with tracheal stenosis with tracheobronchopathia osteochondroplastica, *Anesth. Analg.* 95, 781-2 (2002).

[44] T. Asai, K. Fujise, and M. Uchida, Laryngeal mask and tracheal stenosis, *Anaesthesia* 48, 81 (1993).

[45] W. T. Hung, S. M. Liao and J. M. Su, Laryngeal mask airway in patients with tracheal stents who are undergoing non-airway related interventions: report of three cases, *J. Clin. Anesth.* 16, 214-6 (2004).

[46] M. Urtubia and P. Leyton, Successful use of the EasyTube for facial surgery in a patient with glottic and subglottic stenosis, *J. Clin. Anesth.* 19, 77-8 (2007).

[47] R. M. Levitan and W. C. Kinkle, Initial anatomic investigation of the i-gel airway: a novel supraglottic airway without inflatable cuff, *Anaesthesia* 60, 1022-6 (2005).

[48] T. Asai, Who is at increased risk of pulmonary aspiration? *Br. J. Anaesth.* 93, 497-50 (2004).

[49] J. Brimacombe and C. Keller, Aspiration of gastric contents during use of a ProSeal™ laryngeal mask airway secondary to unidentified foldover malposition, *Anesth. Analg.* 97, 1192-4 (2003).

[50] B. Gibbison, T. M. Cook and C. Seller, Case series: protection from aspiration and failure of protection from aspiration with the i-gel airway, *Br. J. Anaesth.* 100, 415-7 (2008).

Conflict of interest: Prof. Pavel Michalek has lectured for several companies manufacturing supraglottic airway devices inluding Intersurgical Ltd., AMBU Ltd. and Intavent Orthofix Ltd.

In: The i-gel Supraglottic Airway
Editors: Pavel Michalek and William Donaldson
ISBN: 978-1-62417-897-9

Chapter 7

CLINICAL EVIDENCE FOR THE USE OF THE I-GEL IN PEDIATRIC ANESTHESIA

Lorenz Theiler* and Robert Greif
University Department of Anaesthesiology and Pain Therapy,
Inselspital, Bern University Hospital and University of Bern, Switzerland

ABSTRACT

The pediatric i-gel is a promising 2nd generation supraglottic airway device. It is available in sizes 1, 1.5, 2, 2.5 and 3. The smallest size ventilates children over 2kg of weight. Overall insertion success rates in randomized controlled studies range from 93-100%; airway leak pressures are 22-26 cm H_2O. Although experience in small children is scarce, the available evidence suggests that the i-gel performs well in children weighing more than 15-20 kg but it tends to slide upwards and out of the mouth in smaller children. Apart from airway maintenance during elective procedures under general anesthesia, it may be also used as a "rescue airway device" in pediatric difficult laryngoscopy scenarios.

INTRODUCTION

The pediatric airway and pediatric respiratory physiology are considerably different from those of the adult. The larynx is shifted cranially, the tongue is comparatively large and the epiglottis is relatively longer and more u-shaped [1]. Additionally, airway narrowing occurs in relation to depth of anesthesia, especially in children who snore at night [2]. Increased airway narrowing during anesthesia occurs throughout the entire upper airway and is most pronounced in the hypopharynx at the level of the epiglottis [2]. These anatomical and functional airway problems and the increased oxygen consumption in children increase the risk of de-oxygenation and airway disaster, especially if the anesthesiologist in charge is not very experienced in pediatric anesthesia [3]. Episodes of laryngospasm and bronchospasm are

* Corresponding author: Lorenz Theiler. E-mail address: lorenz.theiler@insel.ch.

frequent. Another functional airway problem encountered with facemask ventilation is gastric air insufflation; this can occur despite using a proper technique and correct positioning. Increased gastric air reduces ease of ventilation and thereby facilitates further gastric air insufflation [1]. Therefore, gastric suctioning is highly recommended following mask ventilation, mainly in infants [1]. Because of this fact, some experts argue that "the 'impaired' normal pediatric airway may be handled by anesthesiologists experienced with children, whereas the expected difficult pediatric airway requires dedicated pediatric anesthesia specialist care and should only be managed in specialized centers" as mentioned recently by Engelhardt and Weiss [4].

The introduction of the first supraglottic airway device (SAD), the Laryngeal Mask Airway™ in 1983 opened a new door in pediatric airway management. Supraglottic airway devices are recommended in many difficult airway algorithms and during lifesaving procedures [5, 6]. Compared with difficulties that may be encountered during facemask ventilation, SADs are easy to insert in children. They generally provide sufficiently high airway seal pressures for controlled mechanical ventilation [7] freeing up the provider's hands for other tasks. SADs are less invasive than tracheal tubes, and their use is associated with fewer complications compared with tracheal tubes [8-10].

The classic LMA and its derivatives are still in use in many pediatric anesthesia departments. Their use is clearly limited regarding airway seal pressures and lack of gastric access with inability to suction gastric air. The more advanced second generation of SADs overcome some of these limitations and offer potential benefits [11]. These 2nd generation supraglottic airway devices include the ProSeal LMA™, the Supreme LMA™ and the i-gel™.

Whereas the first pediatric ProSeal became available in 2003, other 2nd generation pediatric supraglottic airway devices have only recently become commercially available and clinical experience with them is therefore limited. In studying pediatric supraglottic airway devices, we face two problems:

1 No agreement has been reached so far about what the "gold standard" is for pediatric supraglottic airway devices.
2 It is not wise to deduce the performance of devices in children from data in adults because of the previously described differences in airway anatomy and function. However, clinicians need to know which device will perform and with what success in order to base their decisions about the use of these devices on solid knowledge.

This chapter aims to provide an overview of the performance of the pediatric sizes of the i-gel, based on available evidence.

THE PEDIATRIC I-GEL

The i-gel for pediatric patients is available in sizes 1-3 (Figure 1). The manufacturer recommends selecting the size of the i-gel according to the patient's body weight (http://www.i-gel.com/igel-for-anaesthesia):

size 1: 2-5 kg

size 1.5: 5-12 kg
size 2.0: 10-25 kg
size 2.5: 25-35 kg
size 3: 30-60 kg

That might be translated to age as (see Table 1): [12]

size 1: 0-1.7 years
size 1.5: 1.7-2 years
size 2: 1.3-8 years
size 2.5: 8-11 years
size 3: 9.5-16 years

There is certainly some overlap between sizes. Some authors argue that, when in doubt, you should choose a larger size with the aim of providing a better seal. As with other SADs, the shape of the pediatric i-gel is maintained, and not adapted to the pediatric airway.

The devices are simply smaller in size than adult devices. With the exception of the size 1, a nasogastric tube can be advanced through all sizes of the i-gel. A size 10 (FG) nasogastric tube fits through a size 1.5 i-gel and larger i-gel sizes allow for passage of a size 12. From our clinical experience we recommend following the manufacturer's guidelines for insertion: not to rotate the device in the mouth [13], to use water-based lubrication without lignocaine [14] and secure the device in place with taping "maxilla to maxilla"

Table 1. i-gel sizes and the corresponding weight, age, nasogastric tubes and recommended endotracheal tubes [12]

i-gel size	Weight (kg)	Age (years)	Nasogastric tube size (FG)	Recommended endotracheal tube mm ID (Microcuff™)
1	2-5	0-1.7	--	3.0
1.5	5-12	1.7-2	10	3.0-3.5
2	10-25	1.3-8	12	3.5-5.0
2.5	25-35	8-11	12	5.5-6.0
3	30-60	9.5-16	12	5.5-7.0

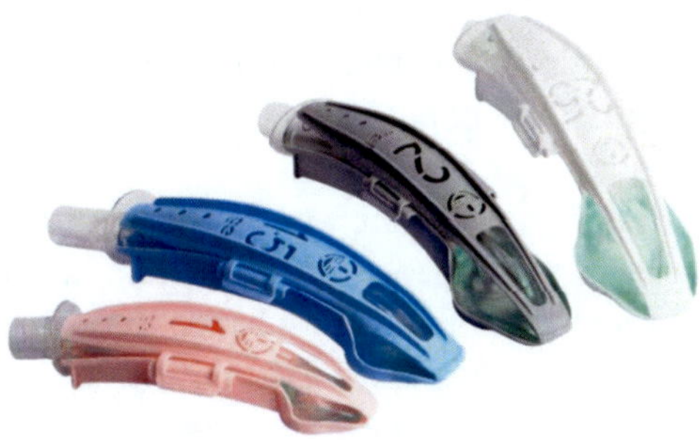

Figure 1. Pediatric sizes of the i-gel supraglottic airway.

The choice of induction technique does not seem to influence results [15]. In common with other SADs, adequate depth of anesthesia (unresponsiveness to jaw thrust) needs to be maintained at insertion to avoid coughing, bucking, and laryngospasm.

Spontaneous Vs. Controlled Ventilation (Using Intermittent Positive Pressure Ventilation)

Some authors prefer not using controlled ventilation in children less than 20 kg of weight when the airway is maintained with a supraglottic airway device; because airway leak pressures tend to be lower and the risk of gastric air insufflation is increased [1].

The use of controlled ventilation with a 2nd generation supraglottic airway devices has potential advantages such as improved ventilation because of the ability to control tidal volume, end-tidal CO_2, and PEEP [7]. In general, under spontaneous ventilation, the anesthesia provider needs to strike a balance between the depth of anesthesia level with the risk of high end-tidal CO_2 or apnea under deep anesthesia, and too light a plane of anesthesia with the risks of laryngospasm or bronchospasm and awareness. This may be overcome by using 2nd generation SADs, which are characterized by higher airway seal pressures and their ability to allow pressure controlled mechanical ventilation with the use of PEEP.

It might be prudent to check the airway leak pressure of every supraglottic airway device inserted. This is accomplished, according to Keller's suggestions [16], by connecting the airway circuit to the ventilator and closing the airway valve with a gas flow of 3 liters per minute. This raises the airway pressure to the point when audible air is leaking and an "equilibrium is reached" [17].

Because the new generation of SADs seals nearly perfectly in some cases, we do not allow the pressure to rise above 30 cmH_2O when performing this test to avoid possible barotrauma of the lungs, but we are aware that others allow airway pressures of up to 40 cmH_2O [18, 19]. This knowledge of the airway leak pressure should guide the clinician's decision about the preferred mode of controlled ventilation. Knowing this fact, administering pressure controlled ventilation (while limiting the upper pressure limit) can safely be used, even in children under 20 kg, as long as the supraglottic airway device does not leak and a minimum tidal volume of 5-8 ml/kg body weight can be delivered.

The ability to drain gastric air with the newer SADs is an advantage in those rare cases when gastric insufflation occurs despite following the precautions mentioned above.

The use of non-depolarizing neuromuscular blocking drugs is not contraindicated when using supraglottic airways for airway maintenance [18] but it is rarely necessary. Intubation through the i-gel is possible, both with cuffed and uncuffed tracheal tubes, but no study has investigated this in a pediatric patient population.

The relatively large breathing tube of the i-gel allows easy insertion of age-adjusted tube sizes (see Table 1). From the experiences published in adult studies, we would also recommend the use of a fiberoptic scope when intubating through a pediatric i-gel.

Because removal of the SAD after tube insertion can easily lead to dislocation of the tracheal tube, we also strongly support the use of an airway exchange catheter to secure access to the pediatric airway throughout the entire procedure [20]. In short cases, the SAD may be left in place.

RANDOMIZED CONTROLLED CLINICAL STUDIES

A few recent studies have looked at the performance of the i-gel in pediatric patients. Lee and colleagues [18] compared the pediatric i-gel with the classic LMA (cLMA) and included 99 patients, aged 1 month – 9 years. No patients could be enrolled for the size 1 i-gel; the groups for sizes 1.5 -2.5 were equally proportioned for each device.

The first-time attempt success rates were 96% and 92% for the i-gel and cLMA, respectively. All devices could be inserted within two attempts, and in all cases, sufficient ventilation could be established - defined as proper chest movement and square-shaped capnography readings. All patients received neuromuscular blocking agents. The median insertion time was shorter for the i-gel, 17 vs. 21 seconds ($p=0.002$).

Median airway leak pressures were comparable: 22 cmH_2O for the i-gel vs. 20 cmH_2O for the cLMA ($p=0.117$). The maximum pressure allowed was 40 cmH_2O. The fiberoptic view of the glottis was better for the i-gel, providing a full view in 16% vs. 8% ($p<0.001$).

One strength of this study was that a relatively large number of smaller children (5-9 kg) were enrolled. Unfortunately, the authors only reported the overall performance; they did not report the performance of the different i-gel sizes.

Goyal and colleagues performed a prospective randomized trial, comparing the size 2 i-gel with the ProSeal and the cLMA in a total of 120 children (40 per group) aged 2–5 years, weighing 10–20 kg [19]. No difference in performance was found:

Their overall insertion success rate was 100% in all three groups. Insertion attempts (1/2/3 attempts, n=40) were 38/2/0 for the i-gel, 36/3/1 for the ProSeal, and 36/3/1 for the classic LMA with no differences between the groups ($p > 0.05$). The ease of insertion was similar for all three devices.

The mean airway leak pressure was higher for the i-gel compared with the other devices, but it was comparable between ProSeal and classic LMA: 26 ± 2.6 cmH_2O for the i-gel, 23 ± 1.2 cmH_2O for the ProSeal, and 22 ± 2.3 cmH_2O for the cLMA ($p<0.01$). The maximum pressure allowed was 40 cmH_2O.

No cases of sore throat were reported, blood staining occurred in 2, 4 and 3 cases for the i-gel, ProSeal, and cLMA, respectively. There were no hemodynamic differences between the devices before, during or after insertion.

In this study, only children from 10-20 kg were enrolled. The comparison of three different devices (ProSeal, cLMA, and i-gel) is its major strength.

Our own group (Theiler and colleagues) investigated the performance of the pediatric i-gel with the pediatric sizes of the Ambu Aura Once in 208 patients with a mean age of 6 years (range 0.75-12 years) [15]. The i-gel size 1 was not studied because these patients (< 5kg) were all intubated according to the standard operating procedures at our institution.

The first attempt success rate was 91% in the i-gel group and 93% in the Ambu group. Overall success rates were 93% and 98% for the i-gel and Ambu, respectively ($p=0.10$). All failures were because of inadequate ventilation; defined as an absence of symmetric chest movements, stable oxygen saturation, stable square wave capnography, no audible oropharyngeal leak, and a tidal volume of at least 6 ml per kg body weight.

The airway leak pressure was higher in the i-gel group: 22 ±5 cmH_2O vs. 19 ±3 cmH_2O ($p<0.01$).

A full fiberoptic view of the glottis was achieved in 87% (i-gel) and 89% (Ambu). Insertion of a gastric tube was possible in 99% of all i-gel cases. Interestingly, gastric content was suctioned in 76% of these cases despite all of the children being fasted [21].

There were more minor airway interventions necessary in the i-gel group (49 vs. 8%, $p<0.01$). The successfully inserted i-gels needed to be secured by taping in place to ensure a seal in 44% (0% with the Ambu, $p<0.01$). Overall, the smaller i-gel had a tendency to slip out but this was easy to overcome by taping down the smaller i-gel sizes (size 2 and below).

We speculated that this happens because the i-gel is a smaller copy of the adult version, but as mentioned above the airway anatomy, especially in smaller kids, is considerably different. Therefore, some adjustments in the design of the i-gel tube might be needed to overcome the sliding-out of the smaller sizes of the i-gel.

Insertion was faster with the Ambu (24±8 vs. 27±11 seconds, $p=0.02$). Because of the different weight groups, a subgroup analysis according to weight was performed with four subgroups consisting of 1) 5–9.9 kg, 2) 10–19.9 kg, 3) 20–29.9 kg, and 4) 30–50 kg. The mean airway leak pressures for the 4 groups were 27, 20, 22, and 23 cmH_2O ($p=0.05$). Of note, only 3 children for each SAD were in the smallest group. In general, younger children required more airway interventions.

This study analyzed a fairly large patient population. The evidence obtained is limited in children using the size 1.5 i-gel; only 3 children could be enrolled.

Observational Studies, Case Reports and Case Series

Beylacq and colleagues evaluated the size 3 i-gel in 50 children over 30 kg. The first-attempt insertion success rate was 100% [22]. The mean airway leak pressure was 24.9 cmH_2O. The maximum pressure allowed was 35 cmH_2O. Insertion of a gastric catheter was easy in 98%, with difficulty in one case.

Because only children over 30 kg were evaluated, the evidence for smaller children is somewhat limited.

A cohort study by Beringerand and colleagues looked at 120 uses of the pediatric i-gel in children from 0.4-13 years (median: 5 years) with a body weight of 7-35 kg (mean: 20 kg) [23]. They found a first attempt insertion success rate of 92%, with 98% being successful within two attempts. A sufficient tidal volume (defined as 7 ml/kg) was established in 96%.

Median airway leak pressures were 26, 20 and 20 cmH_2O for i-gel sizes 1.5 (n=13), 2.0 (n=70) and 2.5 (n=37), respectively. The maximum pressure allowed was 30 cmH_2O. Side effects such as sore throat were reported in 4% immediately after surgery and 8% after 24hours. Blood on the device was noted in 3% of cases.

Another cohort study by Hughes and colleagues in 154 children with a median age of 5 years (interquartile range 2-7) showed a first attempt success rate of 93.5%, and an overall success rate of 99.3% [24]. Median airway leak pressures were in size 1 (n=3): 20 cmH_2O, in size 1.5: 19 cmH_2O, in size 2: 20 cmH_2O, in size 2.5: 22 cmH_2O, and overall: 20 cmH_2O. The maximum pressure allowed was 30 cmH_2O.

Overall, the i-gel was used successfully in 96%. In seven cases, an alternative device had to be used. Failure rates were 12% (3 out of 26) for size 1.5, 5% (4 out of 77) for size 2 and 0% for size 1 and size 2.5. Blood on the device was noted in 7%.

In a prospective observational study, our group studied the performance of the i-gel in 2049 patients [25]. In this multicenter study, patients aged 6-91 years have been analyzed.

Of the 2049 cases, 127 patients were <18 years old. In this subgroup, the mean age was 13 years and the overall success rate of the i-gel supraglottic airway device was 96%. The mean airway leak pressure was 25.6 ± 8cmH_2O. There were no significant complications reported in this subgroup of patients.

CONCLUSION

Based on the evidence available, the pediatric i-gel is a promising 2nd generation SAD. It offers gastric access and has reasonably high success rates of 93-98% and airway leak pressures of 20-26 cmH_2O. The leak pressures should not be analyzed out of context. Whilst airway leak pressures are widely used as a marker of performance, the methods used are not uniform, e.g. the maximum airway pressure will influence the mean pressure, and the age of the child being studied is important. Similarly, the value of success rates needs to be seen in the context of the definition of success, and preferably in comparison with another SAD. But as observed for other SADs, the success rate for the i-gel tends to be lower in smaller children. How low is too low? According some authors, the lowest observed overall success rate of 93% for the i-gel is too low and a rate of 95% is preferred [26]. The anesthetic community should seek a success rate of at least 95%, which means that 1 in 20 devices does not work. Obviously, a 90% success rate is unacceptable for such devices, because that means only 9 out of 10 devices are working. Success rates in clinical studies may be lower because they depend on definitions of success that are stricter than what would be acceptable clinically. However, randomized controlled trials offer the benefit of comparing success rates and airway leak pressure with other devices. The airway leak pressures reported for the i-gel are generally higher than those reported for the pediatric classic LMA (< 20 cmH_2O), and at least as high as those reported for the pediatric Supreme-LMA [27], but lower than reported for the pediatric ProSeal (up to 31cmH_2O) [28, 29]. Taking all of the above into consideration, it seems to be too early to recommend the pediatric i-gel in prone positions or even for laparoscopic surgeries [30]. The airway leak pressures in children are also lower than those reported for the adult i-gel (24–30 cmH_2O) [31, 32].

As mentioned previously, the pediatric i-gel has the tendency to displace upwards out of the mouth [15, 23] and needs to be taped securely to avoid this, especially in smaller children. The reason for this may be that the shape of the pediatric i-gel is the same as the adult device and not specifically designed for small children.

In smaller children, the angle towards the glottic inlet is rather large when compared with other supraglottic airway devices (Figure 1). This may not match the relatively anterior and cranial position of the pediatric larynx [1]. Adjustments of this angle to match the pediatric laryngeal position may be necessary to overcome this problem and should further enhance the performance of the pediatric i-gel supraglottic airway device.

After summarizing the available results from i-gel studies available, it is clear that some research questions are still open and should be addressed in rigorously executed and properly powered randomized controlled trials. These research questions might be:

- The primary outcome should be overall insertion success rate. We need sufficiently powered studies that enroll smaller children. So far, there is not sufficient evidence to answer the question, what is the success rate of the pediatric i-gel in children below 10 kg of weight?
- Secondary outcomes should focus on safety. There are no data about side effects in children after the use of the i-gel. It is difficult to assess subjective side effects such as sore throat, and a large study population is necessary to find rare side effects.
- There are no data about mucosal pressures exerted by the i-gel in children.
- There is no evidence about how and if the airway leak pressure changes over time.
- Ideally, a randomized controlled study should be performed involving several anesthesia departments in order to generate sufficient power and include high numbers of small children as well.

The following two unpublished clinical studies are registered at the clinical trials or at the ISRCTN database as of July 2012, and we eagerly await their results:

- In 2011, C. Keller launched a study in Switzerland and Austria to compare the i-gel with the ProSeal in children 18 months – 6 years old
- J.R. Lee from Korea is evaluating the i-gel in comparison with the cLMA in neonates and infants up to 1 year old.

REFERENCES

[1] R. J. Holm-Knudsen and L. S. Rasmussen, Paediatric airway management: basic aspects, *Acta Anaesthesiol. Scand.* 53, 1-9 (2009).

[2] R. G. Evans, M. W. Crawford, M. D. Noseworthy and S. J. Yoo, Effect of increasing depth of propofol anesthesia on upper airway configuration in children, *Anesthesiology* 99, 596-602 (2003).

[3] Murat, I. Constant and H. Maud'huy, Perioperative anaesthetic morbidity in children: a database of 24,165 anaesthetics over a 30-month period, *Paediatr. Anaesth.* 14, 158-66 (2004).

[4] T. Engelhardt and M. Weiss. A child with a difficult airway: what do I do next? *Curr. Opin. Anaesthesiol.* 25, 326-32 (2012).

[5] M. Weiss and T. Engelhardt, Proposal for the management of the unexpected difficult pediatric airway, *Paediatr. Anaesth.* 20, 454-64 (2010).

[6] Practice guidelines for management of the difficult airway: an updated report by the American Society of Anesthesiologists Task Force on Management of the Difficult Airway, *Anesthesiology* 98, 1269-77 (2003).

[7] K. Goldmann, C. Roettger and H. Wulf, Use of the ProSeal laryngeal mask airway for pressure-controlled ventilation with and without positive end-expiratory pressure in paediatric patients: a randomized, controlled study, *Br. J. Anaesth.* 95, 831-4 (2005).

[8] S. H. Yu and O. R. Beirne, Laryngeal mask airways have a lower risk of airway complications compared with endotracheal intubation: a systematic review, *J. Oral Maxillofac. Surg.* 68, 2359-76 (2010).

[9] R. Tait, U. A. Pandit, T. Voepel-Lewis, H. M. Munro and S. Malviya, Use of the laryngeal mask airway in children with upper respiratory tract infections: a comparison with endotracheal intubation, *Anesth. Analg.* 86, 706-11 (1998).

[10] K. Goldmann, Recent developments in airway management of the paediatric patient, *Curr. Opin. Anaesthesiol.* 19, 278-84 (2006).

[11] M. C. White, T. M. Cook and P. A. Stoddart, A critique of elective pediatric supraglottic airway devices. *Paediatr. Anaesth.* 19, S55-65 (2009).

[12] J. Mauch, T. Haas and M. Weiss, Distance from the laryngeal mask grip to endotracheal tube tip. A crucial point during fiberoptic intubation in children, *Anaesthesist* 61, 123-8 (2012). [Article in German, English abstract]

[13] B. Ghai, J. K. Makkar, N. Bhardwaj and J. Wig, Laryngeal mask airway insertion in children: comparison between rotational, lateral and standard technique, *Paediatr. Anaesth.* 18, 308-12 (2008).

[14] C. Keller, H. J. Sparr and J. R. Brimacombe, Laryngeal mask lubrication. A comparative study of saline versus 2% lignocaine gel with cuff pressure control, *Anaesthesia* 52, 592-7 (1997).

[15] L. G. Theiler, M. Kleine-Brueggeney, B. Luepold, F. Stucki, S. Seiler, N. Urwyler and R. Greif, Performance of the pediatric-sized i-gel compared with the Ambu AuraOnce laryngeal mask in anesthetized and ventilated children, *Anesthesiology* 115, 102-10 (2011).

[16] C. Keller, J. R. Brimacombe, K. Keller and R. Morris, Comparison of four methods for assessing airway sealing pressure with the laryngeal mask airway in adult patients, *Br. J. Anaesth.* 82, 286-7 (1999).

[17] J. Brimacombe, C. Keller, S. Kurian and J. Myles, Reliability of epigastric auscultation to detect gastric insufflation, *Br. J. Anaesth.* 88, 127-9 (2002).

[18] J. R. Lee, M. S. Kim, J. T. Kim JT, H. J. Byon, Y. H. Park, H. S. Kim and C. S. Kim, A randomised trial comparing the i-gel (TM) with the LMA Classic (TM) in children, *Anaesthesia* 67, 606-11 (2012).

[19] R. Goyal, R. N. Shukla, and G. Kumar, Comparison of size 2 i-gel supraglottic airway with LMA-ProSeal and LMA-Classic in spontaneously breathing children undergoing elective surgery, *Paediatr. Anaesth.* 22, 355-9 (2012).

[20] M. Weiss, J. Mauch, K. Becke, J. Schmidt, and M. Johr, Fibre optic-assisted endotracheal intubation through the laryngeal mask in children, *Anaesthesist* 58, 716-21 (2009). [Article in German, English abstract]

[21] Practice guidelines for preoperative fasting and the use of pharmacologic agents to reduce the risk of pulmonary aspiration: application to healthy patients undergoing elective procedures: an updated report by the American Society of Anesthesiologists Committee on Standards and Practice Parameters, *Anesthesiology* 114, 495-511 (2011).

[22] L. Beylacq, M. Bordes, F. Semjen and A. M. Cros, The i-gel, a single-use supraglottic airway device with a non-inflatable cuff and an esophageal vent: an observational study in children. *Acta Anaesthesiol. Scand.* 53, 376-9 (2009).

[23] R. M. Beringer, F. Kelly, T. M. Cook, J. Nolan, R. Hardy, T. Simpson and M. C. White, A cohort evaluation of the paediatric i-gel() airway during anaesthesia in 120 children, *Anaesthesia* 66, 1121-6 (2011).

[24] C. Hughes, K. Place, S. Berg and D. Mason, A clinical evaluation of the i-gel(TM) supraglottic airway device in children, *Paediatr. Anaesth.* 22 765-71 (2012).

[25] L. Theiler, M. Gutzmann, M. Kleine-Brueggeney, N. Urwyler, B. Kaempfen and R. Greif, i-gel™ supraglottic airway in clinical practice: a prospective observational multicentre study, *Br. J. Anaesth.* (2012), Epub ahead of print.

[26] J. J. Pandit, If it hasn't failed, does it work? On 'the worst we can expect' from observational trial results, with reference to airway management devices, *Anaesthesia* 67, 578-83 (2012).

[27] N. Jagannathan, L. E. Sohn, A. Sawardekar, J. Gordon, K. E. Langen and K. Anderson, A randomised comparison of the LMA Supreme™ and LMA ProSeal™ in children, *Anaesthesia* 67, 632-9 (2012).

[28] K. Goldmann and C. Jakob, A randomized crossover comparison of the size $2^{1/2}$ laryngeal mask airway ProSeal versus laryngeal mask airway-Classic in pediatric patients, *Anesth. Analg.* 100, 1605-10 (2005).

[29] M. Lopez-Gil and J. R. Brimacombe,The ProSeal laryngeal mask airway in children, *Paediatr. Anaesth.* 15, 229-34 (2005).

[30] R. Greif and L. Theiler L, The use of supraglottic airway devices in pediatric laparoscopic surgery, *Minerva Anestesiol.* 76, 575-6 (2010).

[31] B. Richez, L. Saltel, F. Banchereau, R. Torrielli and A. M. Cros, A new single use supraglottic airway device with a noninflatable cuff and an esophageal vent: an observational study of the i-gel, *Anesth. Analg.* 106, 1137-9 (2008).

[32] L. G. Theiler, M. Kleine-Brueggeney, D. Kaiser, N. Urwyler, C, Luyet, A. Vogt, R. Greif and M. M. Unibe, Crossover comparison of the laryngeal mask supreme and the i-gel in simulated difficult airway scenario in anesthetized patients, *Anesthesiology* 111, 55-62 (2009).

Conflict of interest: Dr. Lorenz Theiler and Prof. Dr. Robert Greif, MME, FERC do not have any conflict of interest and did not receive any financial support from SAD providers. The authors received supraglottic airway devices from various manufacturers free of charge for research purposes. All their studies were carried out based on departmental grants or peer reviewed grants from anesthesia societies.

In: The i-gel Supraglottic Airway
Editors: Pavel Michalek and William Donaldson
ISBN: 978-1-62417-897-9

Chapter 8

EVALUATION OF THE I-GEL AIRWAY IN CHILDREN

Yukako Abukawa,[1] Koichi Hiroki[1] and Makoto Ozaki[1,*]

[1]Department of Anesthesiology, Tokyo Women´s Medical University, Tokyo, Japan

ABSTRACT

The pediatric version of the i-gel airway is designated for the airway maintenance of wide range of pediatric patients undergoing elective surgeries. Th smallest sizes may be used in neonates while the size 3 is suitable for adolescents and small females.

We present our first clinical evaluation of the i-gel device in pediatric patients. Low success rates and higher rates of complications have been recorded in the smaller sizes, mainly with the size 1.5. The main complications noted have been: device malpositioning, laryngospasm and temporary dysphonia. Fiberoptic views through the device have also been evaluated – with the larger sizes showing a significantly higher proportion of vocal cord covering than smaller sizes. The size 1.5 i-gel should be used with caution because it covers pediatric patients aged from 2 months to 2 years, whose airway anatomy may be entirely different.

INTRODUCTION

The pediatric airway and respiratory physiology are considerably different from those of the adult. Pediatric anesthetic practice made significant advances with the invention of the laryngeal mask airway (LMA). Several other useful supraglottic airway devices (SADs) have been developed since but, however, there are still some difficulties associated with device insertion in pediatric patients. Anesthesiologists using SADs in pediatric patients must look out for several differences unique to this population: higher position of the larynx inside the

* Corresponding author: Makoto Ozaki. E-mail address: mozaki@anes.twmu.ac.jp.

throat (C2-3), a larynx that is more angled over the glottis, a cone-shaped larynx, long epiglottis and hypertrophy of the adenoids. All these factors may contribute to problems with device insertion. The Pro-Seal LMA® was a very important invention that enabled the effective drainage of gastric contents. However, in some cases, insertion of the Pro-Seal LMA® requires a change in technique to the rotation method, gum elastic bougie (GEB)-guided technique or digital technique [1-3]. In addition, difficulty inserting the gastric tube and achieving adequate seal pressures have been associated with the use of the Pro-Seal LMA in pediatric anesthesia [4, 5].

The i-gel™ supraglottic airway (Intersurgical Ltd., Wokingham, United Kingdom) is a 2nd generation, single-use, supraglottic airway device, available for pediatric patients since 2010. Four pediatric sizes of i-gel airway allow its use in a wide range of pediatric patients from neonates to large children. This chapter will focus on clinical experience with the i-gel airway in pediatric patients.

Anatomy of the Upper Airway in Children

There are various anatomical differences between the airways of neonates, infants, small children and adolescents. For a full understanding of the upper airway function, it is vital to understand the main stages of human dvelopment. Postnatally, the growth of the airways follows the growth of the skeleton of the head, neck and thorax [6]. Growth is accelerated during the first 2 years of life; thereafter, it linearly follows the growth of the body [6]. The tongue is relatively large and causes obstruction at the level of pharynx during and after anesthesia. Mathru et al. [7] demonstrated that the minimum antero-posterior diameter of the pharynx at the level of the soft palate decreased from 6.6±2.2 mm (Mean±SD) in the fully conscious state to 2.7±1.5 mm during propofol anesthesia and showed that it increased to 8.4±2.5 mm after application of nasal CPAP. Using magnetic resonance imaging, Litmanet al. [8] confirmed that the upper airway of a sedated, spontaneously breathing child is wider in the lateral position (total airway volume 8.7 ml) than in the supine position (total airway volume 6.0 ml). Furthermore, Arai et al. [9] showed that lateral positioning combined with airway maneuvers improved airway patency more than airway maneuvers applied alone in patients positioned supine. After anesthesia, jaw thrust combined with lateral positioning allows easy maintenace of airway patency in children.

Choosing the Appropriate Size of the i-gel Airway Device

The i-gel supraglottic airway device has a non-inflatable cuff that is made from a soft, gel-like material (Figure 1). There are four sizes of i-gel airway designated for pediatric patients. All sizes apart from the smallest one possess an additional gastric channel (Figure 2).

The appropriate size is mainly determined according to the patient's body weight. Either a size 1.5 or a size 2.0 can be used for patients weighing between 10-12 kg, whilst remembering the variety of laryngeal sizes in this age group. It may be quite difficult to select an appropriate size for patients with body weight within this range but age can be used as a second factor, including for low birth weight infants. However, further evaluation is often required, such as checking the size of larynx with the ultrasound.

THE DEPTH OF DEVICE INSERTION

The pediatric sizes of the i-gel airway device do possess a marking on the integral bite block to help determine the correct position. The optimal position varies between individuals and is hard to predict. According to our experience, anesthesia trainees/residents tend to insert the i-gel deeper, until it cannot progress any further.

Specialists/consultants in anesthesia avoid inserting the i-gel too deep by measuring the distance from the connector wing to the teeth: the average distance for the i-gel airways from size 1.5 to 2.5 is 5.6 cm.

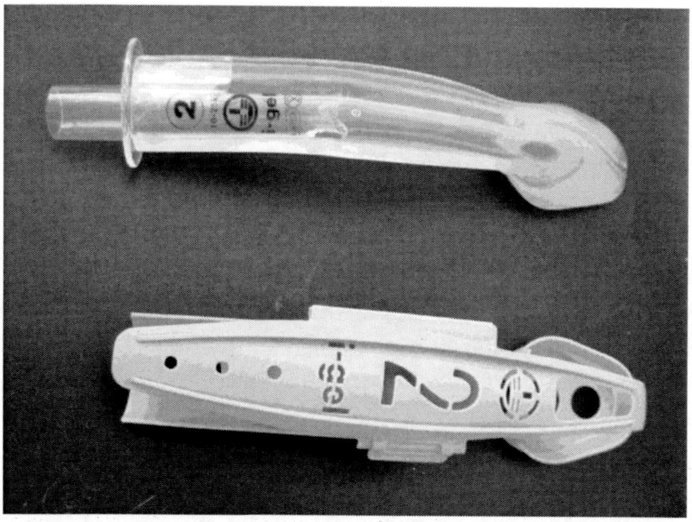

Figure 1. Size 2 i-gel with its protective cradle.

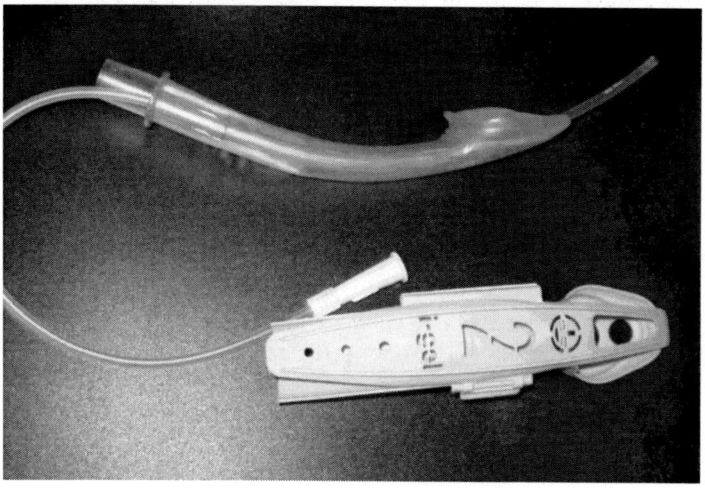

Figure 2. Size 2 i-gel with a gastric tube inserted.

Our institution uses three criteria to determine if the i-gel airway has been successfully inserted:

a Appropriate chest expansion
b Visible $etCO_2$ (square shape) waveform on capnography
c No leak heard at a tidal volume of 6-10 ml/kg.

OUR EXPERIENCE WITH I-GEL IN PEDIATRIC PATIENTS

In following paragraphs, we would like to report our initial clinical experience with the i-gel in pediatric patients. The i-gel airway was used in 70 children for various elective surgical procedures.

Induction of General Anesthesia

There is no difference in the success rate, ease of i-gel insertion, leak pressure or complications rate between propofol induction and sevoflurane induction as demonstrated in our study [10]. In patients without an intravenous cannula, general anesthesia was induced by inhalation of 8% sevoflurane in a mixture of nitrous oxide with oxygen. Fentanyl (at a dose of 2 $mcg.kg^{-1}$) was administered after securing intravenous access. Patients who arrived at the operating room with an intravenous cannula in situ received 2 $mcg.kg^{-1}$ of fentanyl followed by 2-3 $mg.kg^{-1}$ of propofol. Anesthesia was maintained by inhalation of 5% sevoflurane in 100% oxygen until the insertion of the i-gel airway. The i-gel airway was inserted once the patient had reached a sufficient depth of anesthesia, based on the absence of an eyelash reflex, presence of mandibular relaxation, and the absence of limb movements. General anesthesia was then maintained with 2–3% sevoflurane in a mixture of oxygen and air (FiO_2 = 0.35). Neuromuscular blocking agents were not routinely used.

Insertion of the i-gel Airway

The smooth inner surface of the i-gel airway, including the distal end of the gastric channel, should be lubricated before insertion using a water-based lubricant. In contrast to some SADs, insertion of the i-gel under adequate general anesthesia is very easy. When the i-gel is being inserted by residents they are always supervised by experienced pediatric anesthesiologists. A study of the perceived ease of insertion of the i-gel airway device reported that inexperienced residents under supervision found insertion to be 'easy' on 98% of occasions [10]. The overall success rate of insertion of the i-gel airway was 99%, and the first attempt insertion success rate was 94% [10]. Insertion of a gastric tube was easily achieved by residents in all cases. If three attempts at the insertion of i-gel failed, tracheal intubation was performed.

The square shape of the capnographic trace, audibility of air leak, and leak pressure were measured once adequate chest movements indicated the proper positioning of the i-gel airway. The fresh gas flow was set at 3 ml/min, and the pressure adjustment valve was set at 70 cmH_2O. Leak pressure recorded when residents detected leakage by a stethoscope at the patient's neck was 23 ± 5 cmH_2O (21 ± 4, 24 ± 5, 20 ± 3 cmH_2O for i-gel airway size 1.5, 2.0 and 2.5 respectively). The overall tidal volume divided by body weight at the leak pressure was 24 ± 10 ml/kg (17 ± 6, 27 ± 10, 22 ± 10 ml/kg for i-gel airway size 1.5, 2.0 and 2.5 respectively. The expiration valve was opened when the leak pressure reached 30 cmH_2O.

Fiberoptic Scores

A fiberscope with 3.1 mm of internal diameter (Olympus LP-TP) or 2.8 mm diameter (Karl-Storz, Tuttlingen, Germany) was placed 1 cm inside the soft non-inflatable cuff of the i-gel airway device. The aperture view was assessed when the fiberscope was in a natural position and was scored according to the Inagawa grading scale (Table 1) [11]. Vocal cord visibility was 67% for i-gel airway size 1.5, 75% for i-gel airway size 2.0, and 100% for i-gel airway size 2.5 (Figure 3).

There was no reduction in tidal volumes, even if only the epiglottis was visible via the fiberscope. It was often quite difficult to visualize the vocal cords because of epiglottic down-folding with the smaller sized i-gel airway (size 1.5). An Inagawa grade 1 was seen in 8% of cases and grade 2 in 25% of cases (Table 2).

Table 2. Inagawa grading scale for assessment of fiberoptic views through the SADs [11]

Grading	Description
Grade 1	the aperture view is completely covered by the anterior surface of epiglottis, but the airway remains open
Grade 2	the anterior epiglottis is seen for more than two-thirds of the diameter of the aperture view
Grade 3	the anterior epiglottis is seen for more than one-third, but less than two-thirds, of the diameter of the aperture view
Grade 4	the anterior epiglottis is seen for less than one-third of the diameter of the aperture view

Table 3. Fiberoptic assessement through the i-gel airway

	Size 1.5 (n=12)	Size 2 (n=43)	Size 2.5 (n=14)
Fiberoptic score			
Grade 4	5 (42%)	19 (46%)	13 (93%)
Grade 3	3 (25%)	12 (29%)	1 (7%)
Grade 2	3 (25%)	8 (20%)	0
Grade 1	1 (8%)	2 (5%)	0
Missing data	0	2 (5%)	0

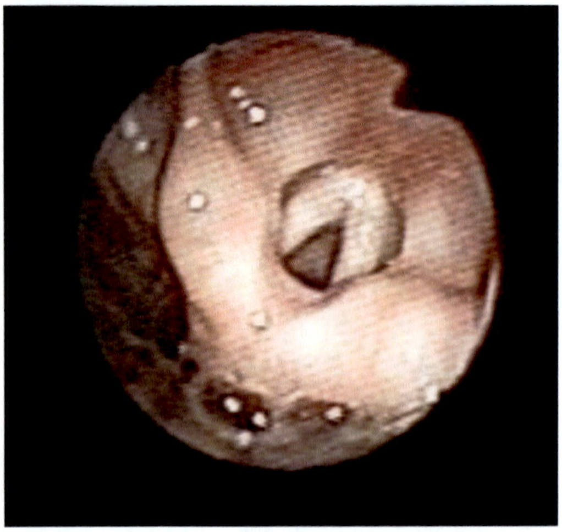

Figure 3. Fibreoptic view through the pediatric i-gel showing the vocal cords.

Clinically, all observed patients had unobstructed airways. Von Ungern-Sternberg et al. [12] reported that complete down-folding of the epiglottis over the laryngeal inlet occurred in 11% of children, and partial down-folding occurred in 32% of patients using a size 1.5 cLMA. Hughes et al. reported that the vocal cords were visible on fiberoptic examination in 97% of patients [13]. Epiglottic down-folding was observed in 2% of patients, but with clinically unobstructed airways [13].

Removal of the i-gel

The tidal volumes were checked after patients started to breathe spontaneously and the i-gel airway was removed if an adequate tidal volume (>6 ml/kg) was recorded and a normal respiratory rate was present. No patients bit onto the i-gel airway device, and it could be easily removed in all cases.

Complications

Only one patient (1.4%) experienced a brief episode of hypoxia. The i-gel airway became displaced in two patients (2.8%). One patient, a 9-month-old male (body weight, 9.4 kg) who received a size 1.5 i-gel device (leak pressure 25 cmH_2O and tidal volume 99 ml) experienced airway obstruction just before the operation started. The i-gel was immediately removed, the patient was ventilated via face mask and then tracheal intubation was performed. Another patient, a 10-month-old male (body weight, 8.4 kg) who received a size 1.5 i-gel device (leak pressure 16 cmH_2O and tidal volume 80 ml) could not be ventilated through the i-gel airway device after his position was changed from supine to lateral. Displacement of the i-gel airway was diagnosed and the patient was given 100% oxygen. The patient was turned back to the supine position, where he could be successfully ventilated via the i-gel airway device; subsequently, a tracheal tube was inserted. Dysphonia was observed in one patient who received a size 1.5 i-gel device. This patient, a 6-month-old female (body weight, 6.8 kg), could breathe well after the i-gel airway was removed, but her voice changed. She was observed in the recovery room, and her dysphonia disappeared within 10 min without any treatment. There were no cases of blood on the device upon removal, and no cases of coughing (Table 3).

Comparison with Other Studies

Kelly et al. [14] showed in their study a first-attempt success rate of 100%, median leak pressure of 23 cmH_2O, an airway obstruction rate of 10% and a laryngospasm rate of 5% with the size 1.5 ProSeal LMA. In our study, the first-attempt success rate with the i-gel airway device size 1.5 was 92% (12/13), median leak pressure was 21 cmH_2O, and device displacement rate was 15% (2/13).

The incidence of temporary dysphonia was 8% (1/12), and laryngospasm was observed in 8% (1/12). This incidence of laryngospasm is relatively high. However, laryngospasm is more common in young patients that in adults, because it is more common for children to have an upper respiratory infection (URI) before the operation. Bagshaw reported a rate of complications with a size 1.5 LMA as high as 42% [15]. Recently, Theiler et al. demonstrated that the efficacy of the pediatric i-gel airway device and the Ambu AuraOnce™ for the ventilation of anesthetized children was comparable to the ProSeal LMA and LMA Classic™. They concluded that the i-gel might be advantageous because of its easy gastric access. Their overall success rate with devices of size 1.5 (n=3), 2.0 (n=38), 2.5 (n=34) was 93%, leak pressure was 22 ± 5cmH_2O, the incidence of laryngospasm was 4%, and the blood on device was seen in 1% of patients. This is similar to the results obtained in our study.

WHY CHOOSE THE I-GEL AIRWAY FOR PEDIATRIC PATIENTS?

The average time to perform minor pediatric surgery is short and most patients do not require neuromuscular blockade. Insertion of the i-gel airway device is easy without using neuromuscular blocking agents. Furthermore, the insertion of a gastric tube is also easy. The reflex stimulation associated with tracheal intubation is significantly greater than that during i-gel insertion. Irritation of tracheal mucosa occuring with tracheal intubation should be avoided in patients with bronchial asthma. The i-gel airway device therefore provides several advantages in terms of its ease of insertion, its ability to achieve adequate ventilation and its easy gastric tube insertion by residents in pediatric patients.

Table 3. Complications associated with pediatric i-gels

Complications	Size 1.5 (n=13)	Size 2 (n=43)	Size 2.5 (n=14)
Overall	4 (31%)	0	0
Displacement	2 (15%)	0	0
Hypoxia	1 (8%)	0	0
Changed voice	1 (8%)	0	0

Is It Safe to Use i-gel in Children with Upper Respiratory Tract Infection?

Anesthesia for the child who presents for surgery with a URI presents a challenge to the anesthesiologist. Tait et al. demonstrated that there was no difference in the incidence of laryngospasm and bronchospasm in children with active URI, recent URI (within 4 weeks) and asymptomatic children [17]. However, children with active and recent URI had more episodes of breath holding, major desaturation events (oxygen saturation < 90%) and a greater incidence of overall adverse respiratory events than children with no URI [17]. Independent risk factors for adverse respiratory events in children with active URI included use of an endotracheal tube (less than 5 years of age), history of prematurity, history of reactive airway disease, paternal smoking, surgery involving the airway, presence of copious secretions and nasal congestion [17]. Flicket al. demonstrated that the incidence of laryngospasm increased in patients with URI or airway abnormalities, even if their airway was managed using a LMA. Von Ungern-Sternberg and colleagues reported that the incidence of laryngospasm after the use of an LMA was higher in children with a recent URI than in healthy children [19]. In our hospital, not only the presence of copious secretions but also the breathing pattern when anesthesia is induced, is used to judge whether to choose a SAD or tracheal tube in a child who has had a recent URI. If we observe breathing pattern with strenuous respirations, we always choose tracheal intubation.

Conclusion

The i-gel airway is a promising novel pediatric supraglottic airway device but its position in pediatric airway management will only be confirmed by future major observational and randomized controlled trials. The i-gel airway device can be used easily and quickly to protect the airway not only in elective situations. The role of the LMA in difficult airway management is well recognized. For pediatric patients, it should be fitted in the best position possible for patients of all ages and abnormities. The i-gel airway has the potential to be a life-saving device in pediatric patients in both difficult airway management and cardio-pulmonary resuscitation.

The size 1.5 i-gel airway device should be used with extreme care because this size covers a wide rage in body weight, from 5 to 12 kg, that corresponds to children from 2-months to 2-years old. It would be advantageous if this size were to be divided into two separate sizes in the future.

References

[1] Y. T. Jeon, H. S. Na, S. H. Park, A. Y. Oh, H. P. Park, M. J. Yun, J. H. Kim and J. W. Hwang, Insertion of the ProSeal laryngeal mask airway is more successful with the 90 degrees rotation technique, *Can. J. Anaesth.* 57, 211-5 (2010).

[2] M. Lopez-Gil, J. Brimacombe, L. Barragan and C. Keller, Bougie-guided insertion of the ProSeal laryngeal mask airway has higher first attempt success rate than the digital technique in children, *Br. J. Anaesth.* 96, 238-41 (2006).

[3] C. Y. Teoh and F. S. Lim, The Proseal laryngeal mask airway in children: a comparison between two insertion techniques, *Paediatr. Anaesth.* 18, 119-24 (2008).

[4] M. Lopez-Gil, J. Brimacombe and G. Garcia, A randomized non-crossover study comparing the ProSeal and Classic laryngeal mask airway in anaesthetized children, *Br. J. Anaesth.* 95, 827-30 (2005).

[5] H. Shimbori, K. Ono, T. Miwa, N. Morimura, M. Noguchi and K. Hiroki, Comparison of the LMA-ProSeal and LMA-Classic in children, *Br. J. Anaesth.* 93, 528-31 (2004).

[6] P. Pohunek, Development, structure and function of the upper airways, *Paediatr. Resp. Reviews.* 5, 2-8 (2004).

[7] M. Mathru, O. Esch, J. Lang, M. E. Herbert, G. Chaljub, B. Goodacre and E. van Sonnenberg, Magnetic resonance imaging of the upper airway. Effects of propofol anesthesia and nasal continuous positive airway pressure in human, *Anesthesiology* 84, 273-9 (1996).

[8] R. S. Litman, N. Wake, L. M. Chan, J. M. McDonough, S. Sin, S. Mahboubi and R. Arens, Effect of lateral positioning on upper airway size and morphology in sedated children, *Anesthesiology* 103, 484-8 (2005).

[9] Y. C. Arai, K. Fukunaga, S. Hirota and S. Fujimoto, The effects of chin lift and jaw thrust while in the lateral position on stridor score in anesthetized children with adenotonsillar hypertrophy, *Anesth. Analg.* 99, 1638-41 (2004).

[10] Y. Abukawa, K. Hiroki and M.Ozaki, Initial experience of the i-gel supraglottic airway by the residents in pediatric patients, *J. Anesth.* 26, 357-61 (2012).

[11] G. Inagawa, K. Okuda, T. Miwa and K. Hiroki, Higher airway seal does not imply adequate positioning of laryngeal mask airways in paediatric patients, *Paediatr. Anaesth.* 12, 322-6 (2002).

[12] B. S. Von Ungern-Sternberg, C. J. Wallace, S. Sticks, T. O. Erb and N. A. Chambers, Fibreoptic assessment of paediatric sized laryngeal mask airways, *Anaesth. Intensive Care* 38, 50-4 (2010).

[13] C. Hughes, K. Place, S. Berg and D. Mason, A clinical evaluation of the i-gel(TM) supraglottic airway device in children, *Paediatr. Anaesth.* 22, 765-71 (2012).

[14] F. Kelly, S. Sale, G. Bayley, T. Cook, P. Stoddart and M. White, A cohort evaluation of the pediatric ProSeal laryngeal mask airway in 100 children, *Paediatr. Anaesth.* 18: 947-51 (2008).

[15] O. Bagshaw, The size 1.5 laryngeal mask airway (LMA) in paediatric anaesthetic practice, *Paediatr. Anaesth.* 12, 420-3 (2002).

[16] L. G. Theiler, M. Kleine-Brueggeney, B. Luepold, F. Stucki, S. Seiler, N. Urwyler and R. Greif, Performance of the pediatric-sized i-gel compared with the Ambu AuraOnce laryngeal mask in anesthetized and ventilated children, *Anesthesiology* 115, 102-10 (2011).

[17] R. Tait, S. Malviya, T. Voepel-Lewis, H. M. Munro, M. Seiwert and U. A. Pandit, Risk factors for perioperative adverse respiratory events in children with upper respiratory tract infections, *Anesthesiology* 95, 299-306 (2001).

[18] R. P. Flick, R. T. Wilder, S. F. Pieper, K. van Koeverden, K. M. Ellison, M. E. Marienau, A. C. Hanson, D. R. Schroeder and J. Sprung, Risk factors for laryngospasm in children during general anesthesia, *Paediatr. Anaesth.* 18, 289-96 (2008).

[19] B. S. von Ungern-Sternberg, K. Boda, C. Schwab, C. Sims, C. Johnson and W. Habre, Laryngeal mask airway is associated with an increased incidence of adverse respiratory events in children with recent upper respiratory tract infections, *Anesthesiology* 107, 714-9 (2007).

Conflict of interest: The authors declare no conflict of interest.

In: The i-gel Supraglottic Airway
Editors: Pavel Michalek and William Donaldson

ISBN: 978-1-62417-897-9

Chapter 9

THE ROLE OF THE I-GEL IN THE MANAGEMENT OF THE DIFFICULT AIRWAY

Pavel Michalek[1,2,*]

[1]Department of Anesthesia and Intensive Medicine,
First Medical Faculty of the Charles University and
General University Hospital, Prague, Czech Republic
[2]Department of Anaesthesia, Antrim Area
Hospital, Antrim, UK

ABSTRACT

Tracheal intubation is usually performed using direct laryngoscopy. In some situations, laryngoscopy cannot visualize the vocal cords and alternative methods have to be used in order to achieve oxygenation and ventilation. Supraglottic airway devices (SAD) including the i-gel may be used in these scenarios. The use of an SAD as a "Plan B" in unexpected difficult intubation is supported by various guidelines.

The i-gel supraglottic airway may be used for both blind and fiberscope-guided tracheal intubation. Its use for these indications is supported by a number of case reports, case series and by four randomized trials. The i-gel supraglottic airway provides very good coverage of the laryngeal inlet even in patients with abnormal anatomy of the perilaryngeal structures.

According to several published trials, the i-gel is as successful as the Intubating Laryngeal Mask Airway (ILMA) when used as a conduit for fiberoptic tracheal intubation but has a lower success rate than the ILMA for blind tracheal intubation without fiberoptic guidance.

The recent availability of pediatric sizes may reveal the i-gel to be a potential conduit for tracheal intubation in neonates, infants and older children with predicted or unexpected difficult laryngoscopy.

* Corresponding author: Pavel Michalek. E-mail address: pafkamich@yahoo.co.uk.

INTRODUCTION

Supraglottic airway devices (SADs) play a very important role in difficult airway management. In this role they belong to the group of "dedicated airways" – devices that are defined as: "Any upper airway device dedicated to the maintenance of a patent airway while other major airway interventions (mainly tracheal intubation) are anticipated or performed" [1]. For more than two decades, SADs have been used in difficult airway situations providing adequate oxygenation and ventilation in clinical situations where direct laryngoscopy was not successful. In addition, some SADs also have the potential as conduits for blind or fiberscope-guided insertion of an endotracheal tube [2, 3].

The ability of these devices to perform this function is determined by their positioning over the glottic opening. The most commonly used conduits for tracheal intubation have been the Intubating Laryngeal Mask Airway (ILMA, Fastrach, Laryngeal Mask Company, Mahe, Seychelles) and the CTrach Laryngeal Mask (CTrach, Laryngeal Mask Company, Mahe, Seychelles) [4-7]. Techniques using fiberscope generally have higher success rates and potentially lower incidence of complications than blind techniques [8].

The first evaluation of the i-gel performed in cadavers showed that the device provided very good coverage of the glottis after insertion – the authors reported that in all 65 cadavers, a Percentage of Glottic Opening (POGO) score of greater than 50% was achieved and in two thirds a full view of the glottic opening was achieved [9].

This feature should theoretically allow adequate ventilation and provide direct access to the trachea in difficult airway situations. The i-gel airway has been used in difficult airway management for two indications – as an airway device for temporary airway maintenance in difficult laryngoscopy [10, 11] and as a conduit for tracheal intubation [12-14].

SUPRAGLOTTIC AIRWAY DEVICES IN DIFFICULT INTUBATION SCENARIOS

The use of SADs is incorporated into various guidelines and recommendations in difficult intubation scenarios. SADs may be classified according to their sealing mechanism, presence of an additional channel for drainage of gastric content and other features [15]. For the purpose of difficult airway management they are further subclassified into devices allowing passage of an appropriate size of the endotracheal tube and other SADs which require insertion of an introducer due to their narrow lumen (Table 1) [2]. Various SADs may be used as conduits for tracheal intubation (Table 2) [2, 3].

The American Society of Anesthesiologists (ASA) recommends use of a classic laryngeal mask airway (cLMA) if initial intubation attempts have failed and facemask ventilation is inadequate. The cLMA may be used as a conduit for tracheal intubation either with or without fiberoptic guidance [16, 17].

The Difficult Airway Society (UK) supports use of the ILMA or cLMA with fiberscope-guided insertion of an endotracheal tube through these devices as their "Plan B" (back-up plan) if the first four attempts at tracheal intubation using direct laryngoscopy fail. This algorithm is relevant for elective cases in patients with a low risk of gastric content aspiration [18].

Insertion of the cLMA or ProSeal LMA is also recommended as a "plan B" following failed direct laryngoscopy in patients undergoing rapid sequence induction (RSI) and as a back-up plan for "cannot intubate, cannot ventilate" (CICV) situations (www.das.uk.com).

First generation SADs (cLMA, ILMA) are also components of German and French guidelines for the management of difficult airways. Of note, Canadian and Italian guidelines do not support the use of SADs in these scenarios. The i-gel supraglottic airway is only mentioned as an alternative airway device in the ERC guidelines [19]. Other guidelines and algorithms do not include the i-gel, despite the fact that this device seems to be very promising in situations of difficult or failed laryngoscopy.

DEVELOPMENT OF TECHNIQUE

In their cadaveric study, Levitan and Kinkle were the first to demonstrate the very good covering of the glottis by the i-gel. Their study also showed a low incidence of downfolding of the epiglottis [9].

These findings led Sharma et al. to the idea of using the i-gel as a conduit for tracheal intubation in an unexpected difficult airway scenario [13]. They anesthetized an adolescent patient scheduled for a closure of ileostomy and found a Cormack and Lehane grade IV view on laryngoscopy using a classical MacIntosh laryngoscopic blade. Subsequent insertion of size 4 laryngeal mask Classic™ provided sufficient ventilation but fiberoptic intubation through the device did not succeed. The operators decided to use a size 4 i-gel supraglottic airway which provided good ventilation. They could clearly see the vocal cords through the device using a 4.1 mm bronchoscope and, after removal of the fiberscope, they blindly inserted endotracheal tube into the trachea [13].

This case report encouraged our team to practise fiberoptic intubation through the i-gel on mannequins (Figure 1, Figure 2). Due to the ease of this technique and our high success rate in the airway skills laboratory, we decided to use this approach in the management of expected difficult intubation in patients for whom awake fiberoptic intubation was not feasible.

Table 1. Classification of supraglottic airways in relation to their use in difficult airway management (modified according to Miller) [15]

<table>
<tr><td rowspan="2">Direct insertion of tracheal tube through the SAD</td><td colspan="2">1st generation</td><td colspan="2">2nd generation (esophageal vent/sealing cuff)</td></tr>
<tr><td>Reusable</td><td>Disposable</td><td>Reusable</td><td>Disposable</td></tr>
<tr><td>YES</td><td>ILMA
Air-Q ILA
CTrach</td><td>ILMA
Air-Q ILA
Aura-i LM</td><td></td><td>i-gel</td></tr>
<tr><td>NO</td><td>cLMA</td><td>uLMA
AuraOnce</td><td>LMA ProSeal
Baska airway</td><td>LMA Supreme
SLIPA
LTS II
Baska airway</td></tr>
</table>

Table 2. Benefits and downfalls of most commonly used supraglottic airway devices in difficult intubation [2]

SAD	Direct TT placement	Channel for drainage of gastric content	Pediatric size	Disposable version
ILMA	+	-	-	+
CTrach LMA	+	-	-	-
i-gel	+	+	+	+
Aura-i	+	-	+	+
Air-Q	+	-	+	+

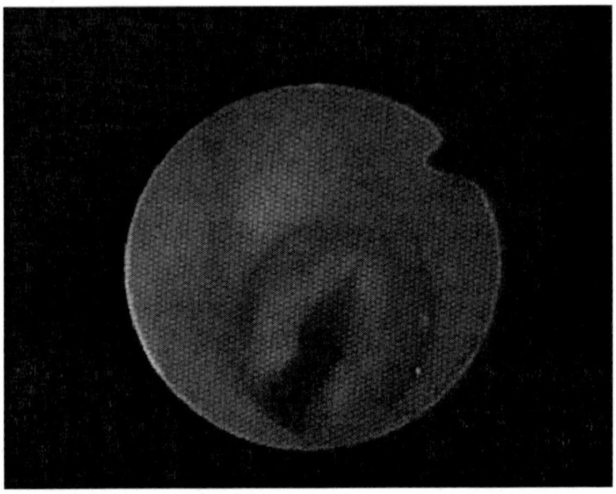

Figure 1. Fiberoptic view through the i-gel showing a clear view of the vocal cords.

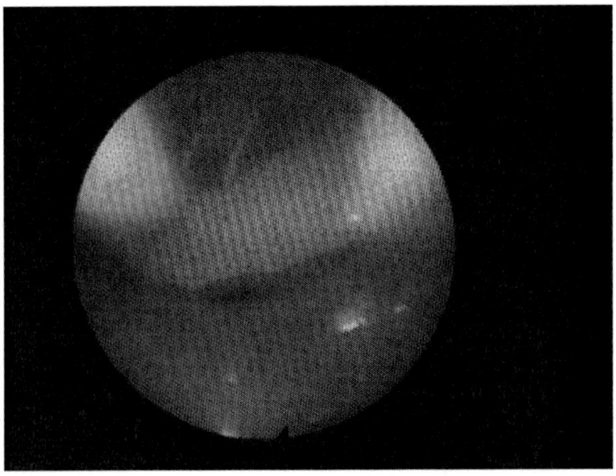

Figure 2. Fiberoptic view through the i-gel in a mannequin showing an incomplete view of the glottic opening and the Aintree intubating catheter caught on the arytenoids.

Two patients with genetic syndromes, (Hunter syndrome – mucopolysaccharidosis and Waardenburg syndrome) who presented with predicted difficult laryngoscopy at preoperative assessment, were scheduled for complex dental surgery under general anesthesia.

These patients were not suitable for an awake fiberoptic intubation due to a lack of cooperation and severe anxiety. Both patients were premedicated using buccal midazolam and then induced to general anesthesia. An i-gel was then inserted providing good ventilation and oxygenation, although there was an audible leak in the second patient.

The fiberoptic view through the SAD using a 3mm scope showed a clear view of the vocal cords (Figure 3, Figure 4) without the epiglottis downfolding and both patients were intubated without any difficulties.

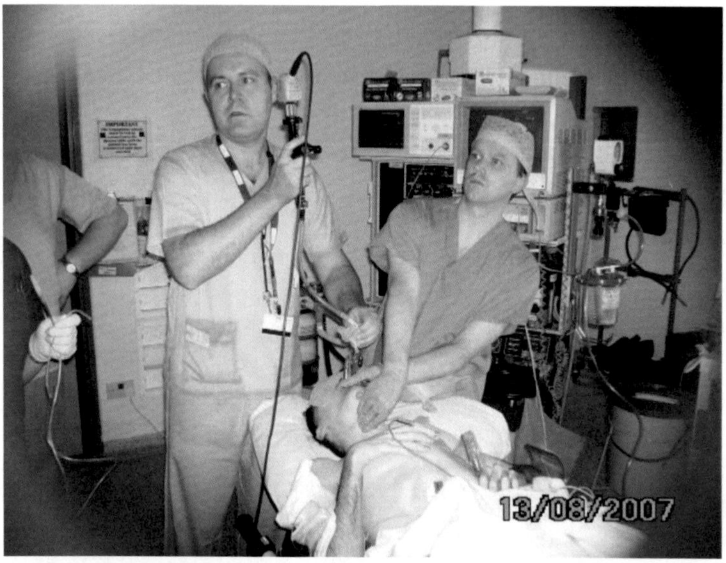

Figure 3. Tracheal intubation of a patient with mucopolysaccharidosis through the i-gel.

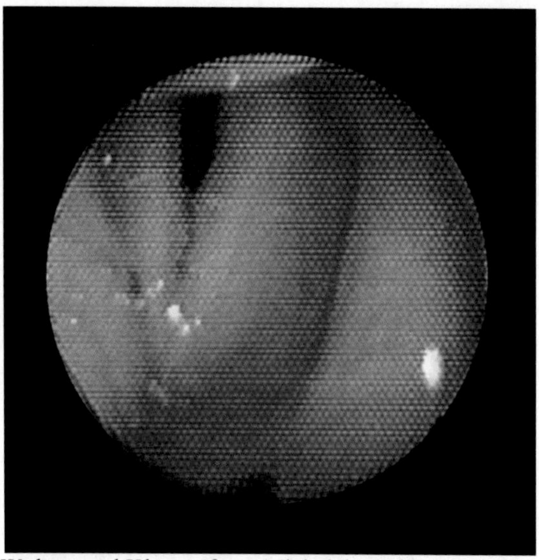

Reprinted with permission of Wolters and Kluwer from Michalek et al., Anesth. Analg. 2008;106: 1501-4.

Figure 4. Fiberoptic view through the i-gel showing a clear view of the anatomical changes to the vocal cords in a patient with mucopolysaccharidosis.

Equipment used for these cases included soft tracheal tubes size 6.0 (i-gel size 3) and 7.0 (i-gel size 4) and fiberoptic bronchoscope (Figure 5). The i-gel was eventually removed using a silicone stabilizer ("pusher") (Figure 6). This removal technique was identical to that previously described with the ILMA [12]. The i-gel has since been used as a device for a rescue airway maintenance in cases of difficult laryngoscopy as well as a conduit for blind or fiberscope-guided insertion of an endotracheal tube.

Clinical Evidence Supporting the Use of i-gel in Difficult Intubation Scenarios

Randomized Controlled Trials (RCT)

There have been several studies published comparing the i-gel with other supraglottic airway devices as conduits for tracheal intubation. Some have used the i-gel as a conduit for blind intubation whereas two studies have compared the i-gel with other SADs as conduits for fiberoptic intubation.

Tracheal Intubation through i-gel without Fiberoptic Guidance

Wadhwa and colleagues compared the ILMA and i-gel in sixty ASA I and II patients without predicted difficult laryngoscopy who were scheduled for various elective operations requiring tracheal intubation [20].

Following insertion of the SADs, they inserted a lubricated endotracheal tube blindly through the devices. The position of the tube in the trachea was confirmed using auscultation and a capnography track analysis. The authors found that insertion of the i-gel was faster than insertion of the ILMA but that the time taken for tracheal intubation through the devices was shorter in the ILMA group.

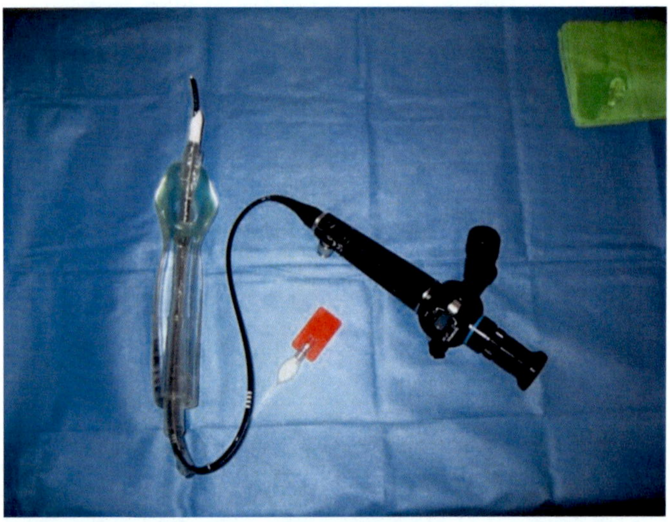

Figure 5. Equipment used for difficult intubation through the i-gel – a soft tracheal tube loaded on the intubating fiberscope.

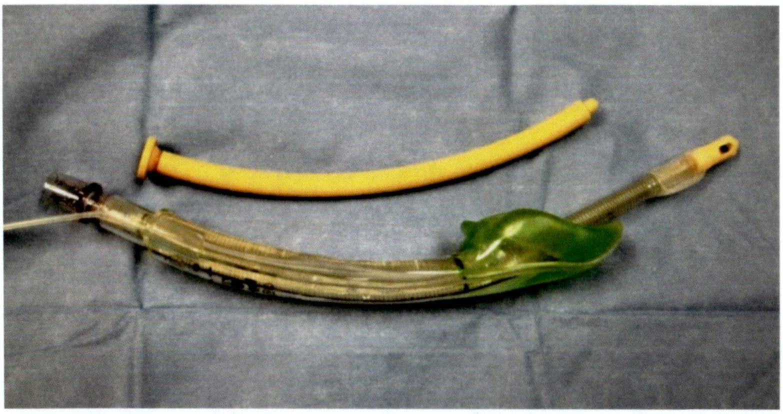

Figure 6. Removal technique of the i-gel using a silicone stabilizer.

Table 3. Independent risk factors for difficult airways [21]

Independent risk factors for difficult airways
1. Documented difficult intubation in the history
2. Obesity (BMI over 30 $kg.m^{-2}$)
3. Thyromental distance less than 6 cm
4. Inability to protrude lower jaw or retrognathia
5. Abnormal neck anatomy
6. Malampati score more than II or mouth opening less than 3.5 cm

Regarding hemodynamic parameters, there was no significant difference between the groups – in terms of heart rate and mean arterial pressure (MAP). Theiler et al. studied tracheal intubation without fiberoptic guidance in eighty patients with at least one independent predictor of difficult laryngoscopy (Table 3).

Blind intubation through the ILMA (69%) was significantly more successful than through the i-gel (15%). Due to the very low success rate the authors do not recommend using the i-gel as a conduit for blind tracheal intubation.

No difference between the devices was found with regards to insertion success rate, insertion time, airway leak pressures or tidal volumes. There was also no significant difference in the removal time of the SADs following successful insertion of the tube into trachea [21]. The authors also studied hemodynamic parameters during insertion of the SADs and during endotracheal tube placement.

Differences in MAP or heart rate did not achieve statistical significance between the groups. Intraoperative complications and postoperative complaints were generally low and did not differ between the ILMA and i-gel.

Halwagi et al. studied the success rate of blind tracheal intubation through i-gel in 160 patients without predicted difficult airways [22]. Eighty patients had an i-gel inserted while the remaining half was intubated through the ILMA. The authors found a similar first time success rate of tracheal intubation (69% in the i-gel group and 74% in the ILMA group) but a significantly higher total intubation success rate in the ILMA group.

Another trial compared the adequacy of ventilation through the i-gel versus the ILMA and success rate of blind intubation through the devices in 80 patients. Both supraglottic airway devices showed similar efficacy in providing effective ventilation but significantly higher success rate for blind tracheal intubation through the SADs was achieved with the ILMA (70% vs. 40% in the i-gel group, $p = 0.013$) [23].

Fiberscope-Guided Tracheal Intubation through the i-gel

Two randomized clinical trials have been completed that studied the i-gel as a conduit for fiberscope-guided tracheal intubation. Kleine-Brueggeney et al. studied 160 ASA I-IV patients indicated for elective procedures under general anesthesia. The conduits used in the study were the i-gel airway and single-use ILMA (sILMA). The participants had at least one independent risk factor for difficult airways (Table 3). The first attempt intubation success rate was 96% with the i-gel and 90% with the sILMA ($p = 0.21$). Airway leak pressure was significantly higher in the sILMA group. There was no difference in SAD insertion times, intubation times or in the incidence of postoperative complaints [24]. This study is analyzed in Chapter 10. Our team compared three different SADs as conduits for fiberscope-guided tracheal intubation. One hundred and twenty patients scheduled for elective surgery requiring tracheal intubation were randomized into three groups. All patients had at least one predictor of difficult laryngoscopy. Three SADs as conduits for fiberoptic tracheal intubation were used – ILMA, i-gel supraglottic airway and CTrach laryngeal mask. Before insertion of the SAD, direct laryngoscopy was performed by a different person to the operator. Tracheal intubation was performed under direct vision in all three groups – using a fiberscope in the ILMA and i-gel groups and using the built-in camera in the CTrach group. The SADs were removed following confirmation of the correct tube position in the trachea (etCO_2, breathing excursions, expiratory volumes).

The primary outcome was the total success rate of tracheal intubation through the devices, whilst the secondary outcomes were: speed of tracheal intubation, time for the SAD insertion, fiberoptic views through the SADs and the incidence of postoperative complications. Total success rates were similar in all three groups and varied between 95-100%. The i-gel showed the shortest insertion and intubation times and provided better coverage of the vocal cords than other two devices [25].

Theiler et al. compared the i-gel with the LMA-Supreme in a simulated difficult airway scenario under general anesthesia. They applied a neck collar to the anesthetized patients, limiting their mouth opening and neck movements and then inserted the SADs. Both devices showed similar insertion success rates. The i-gel caused less epiglottic downfolding and showed better fiberoptic views. On the other hand, insertion times for the LMA-Supreme were shorter [26].

Case Reports and Case Series

There have been several other case reports published (following the initial two case reports) describing the use of an i-igel as a conduit for tracheal intubation, Emmerich and Dummler described the use of a size 4 i-gel in a patient with previously reported difficult direct laryngoscopy (Cormack and Lehane grade III with a McCoy laryngoscopic blade) [27]. This patient was scheduled for re-laparotomy and evacuation of retroperitoneal hematoma. A modified "rapid sequence induction – RSI" using 0.45 $mg.kg^{-1}$ of rocuronium was used.

Conventional maneuvers to facilitate direct laryngoscopy such as use of the McCoy blade, optimization of head position and BURP ("backward, upward and rightward external pressure on the larynx) failed. An i-gel airway was inserted which provided good ventilation and allowed a clear direct view to the cords with a 4-mm flexible bronchoscope. A size 6.0 cuffed tube was subsequently placed into the trachea under fiberoptic guidance.

Asai used i-gels in three patients with difficult laryngoscopy and difficult bag-mask ventilation [28]. The i-gel airway provided satisfactory ventilation in all three patients. Two of them were intubated through the device using an intubating fiberscope and the third patient was eventually intubated using the Airtraq laryngoscope.

Another case report described use of the i-gel in an Intensive Care Unit setting [14]. An extremely obese male (BMI 44) with COPD and obstructive sleep apnea was admitted to the ICU with respiratory failure secondary to pneumonia. Shortly after admission he developed acute respiratory distress with hypoxemia and became confused and aggressive. Awake fiberoptic intubation was not feasible under these conditions and RSI was performed. Direct laryngoscopy revealed a grade 4 view (Cormack and Lehane) and the patient´s oxygen saturation decreased rapidly.

Insertion of a cLMA did not provide sufficient ventilation and it was eventually removed. At this point bag-mask ventilation became increasingly difficult. A size 4 i-gel was inserted and immmediatelly provided effective ventilation and oxygenation. A size 7.0 cuffed endotracheal tube was inserted with the aid of an intubating fiberscope five minutes later when the oxygen saturation had improved from 78% to 91%.

Tiesmeier and Emmerich used an i-gel airway as a conduit for blind tracheal intubation in the pre-hospital setting [29]. Their patient was found collapsed outside the physiotherapy department 11 days following a cardiac operation.

The cause of his cardiac arrest was ventricular fibrillation. A size 4 i-gel was inserted immediatelly without any interruption in the chest compressions and provided ventilation without any leak. A size 7.0 cuffed endotracheal tube was inserted blindly through the i-gel into trachea at the first attempt. The i-gel was left in place, helping to stabilize the tracheal tube position.

Piraccini et al. used the i-gel in a patient with an arched palate in whom the insertion of endotracheal tube under direct laryngoscopy was technically difficult. The size 3 i-gel airway allowed ventilation, oxygenation and blind insertion of an endotracheal tube into the trachea [30].

The same authors have also described tracheal intubation through an i-gel in cardio-pulmonary resuscitation without interruption of chest compressions [31] and use of an i-gel in failed intubation in a partiturient [32].

The i-gel has been successfully inserted in a difficult laryngoscopy scenario during induction of thoracic case. The authors used a size 4 i-gel as a conduit for placement of a size 6.5 Univent tube. The Univent tube was railroaded over the pediatric fiberscope and a bronchial blocker inserted into the right bronchus without difficulty [33].

Corso et al. described the i-gel use in a case scenario of "cannot intubate, cannot ventilate – CICV" [11]. Their patient arrived in the operating room for a revision after uvulopalato-pharyngoplasty and tonsillectomy. Both direct laryngoscopy and bag-mask ventilation were unsuccessful and a cLMA did not provide satisfactory ventilation. An i-gel was inserted as a last resort choice before attempting a surgical airway. The i-gel allowed good quality ventilation and facilitated fiberoptic intubation.

Mannequin Studies

The i-gel as a conduit for tracheal intubation has been also trialed in two mannequin studies.

DeLloyd et al. compared the i-gel and cLMA as conduits for fiberscope-guided intubation in mannequin settings [34]. Insertion of the tracheal tube through the i-gel was faster and participants generally preferred the i-gel over the cLMA [88].

We compared the i-gel with the ILMA for both blind and fiberoptic intubation in three different airway trainers. Blind insertion of the gum elastic bougie, Aintree intubating catheter, soft tracheal tube and fiberscope were evaluated. We found that both conduits performed well a without difference using a fiberscope, but for blind intubation the ILMA was significantly more successful [35]. Both studies are analyzed in detail in Chapter 10.

The i-gel in Pediatric Difficult Airway Management

Until recently, SADs that allow for direct tracheal tube placement were not available in pediatric sizes. Laryngeal masks were inserted in difficult laryngoscopy to establish oxygenation and ventilation.

There have been three SADs introduced recently which permit uncomplicated tracheal tube insertion through them. The Ambu-i laryngeal mask is available in pediatric sizes 1, 1.5, 2 and 2.5. The inner diameter of the Aura-i allows placement of 3.5-5.5 tracheal tubes [36]. The air-Q ILA is available in four pediatric sizes from newborns, (size 1) to bigger children (size 2.5, 30-50 kg). A soft tracheal tube may be placed into the trachea through the air-Q even without fiberoptic guidance [37].

The i-gel supraglottic airway also allows direct placement of a tracheal tube. The available pediatric sizes are 1 (neonates, 2-5 kg), 1.5 (infants, 5-12 kg), 2 (small children, 10-25 kg), 2.5 (large children, 25-35 kg) [38]. Theoretically, size 1 i-gel permits insertion of 3.5 tracheal tube, size 2 placement of 4.5 tube and size 2.5 insertion of 5.5-mm tracheal tube (Figure 7).

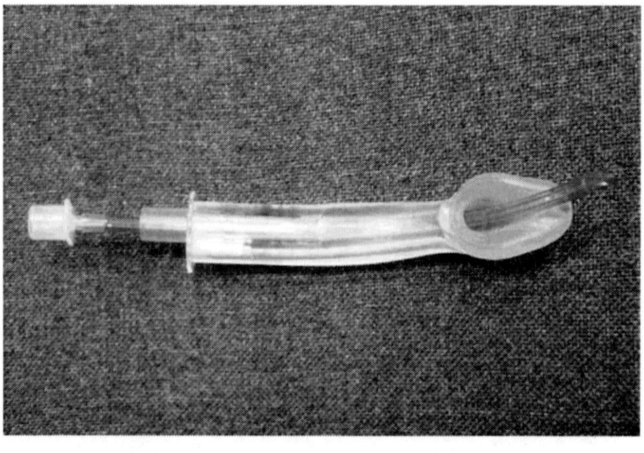

Figure 7. A 4.5 mm uncuffed tracheal tube inserted through a size 2 i-gel.

Despite the potential of this device for a pediatric difficult airway management, there is only one case report describing the use of an i-gel in a pediatric setting; it was used as a conduit for a fiberscope-guided tracheal intubation in a 9-year-old child with neck contractures following burns. A 5.5-mm uncuffed tracheal tube railroaded onto a pediatric flexible bronchoscope was easily inserted through the size 2.5 i-gel [39].

CONCLUSION

SADs are very useful tools in failed laryngoscopy scenarios and other difficult airway situations. The ILMA is still recommended as a "first choice" conduit for tracheal intubation in adult patients with unpredicted difficult airways. The i-gel may provide an efficient and cheap alternative to the ILMA based on published studies and case reports. Furthermore, this device is easier to insert than the ILMA and anesthesiologists may prefer it over ILMA because they are familiar with the i-gel from their routine anesthetic practice. Fiberoptic guidance for a placement of the tracheal tube through i-gel should improve the success rate of tracheal intubation through the device.

REFERENCES

[1] P. Charters and E. O´Sullivan, The "dedicated airway": a review of the concept and an update of current practice, *Anaesthesia* 54, 778-86 (1999).

[2] P. Michalek, W. Donaldson and F. McAleavey, The role of supraglottic airway devices in difficult intubation scenarios, In: P. E. Doebrich and C. R. Antunes, *Intubation: Preparation, Procedures and Complications,* Nova Biomedicals, New York 1-37 (2012).

[3] A. Timmermann, Supraglottic airways in difficult airway management: successes, failures, use and misuse, *Anaesthesia* 66, S45-S56 (2011).

[4] N. S. Gerstein, D. A. Braude, O. Hung, J. C. Sanders and M. F. Murphy, The Fastrach™ intubating laryngeal mask airway: an overview and update, *Can. J. Anesth.* 57, 588-601 (2010).

[5] D. Z. Ferson, W. H. Rosenblatt, M. J. Johansen, I. Osborn, and A. Ovassapian, Use of the intubating LMA-Fastrach in 254 patients with difficult-to-manage airways, *Anesthesiology* 95, 1175-81 (2001).

[6] P. J. F. Baskett, M. J. A. Parr and J. P. Nolan, The intubating laryngeal mask. Results of a multicentre trial with experience of 500 cases, *Anaesthesia* 53, 1174-7 (1998).

[7] E. H. Liu, R. Wender and A. J. Goldman, The LMA CTrach in patients with difficult airways. *Anesthesiology* 110, 941-3 (2009).

[8] H. S. Joo and D. K. Rose, The intubating laryngeal mask airway with and without fiberoptic guidance, *Anesth. Analg.* 88, 662-6 (1999).

[9] R. M. Levitan and W. C. Kinkle, Initial anatomic investigation of the i-gel airway: a novel supraglottic airway without inflatable cuff, *Anaesthesia* 60, 1022-6 (2005).

[10] N. A. Joshi, M. Baird and T. M. Cook, Use of an i-gel for airway rescue, *Anaesthesia* 63, 1020-1 (2008).

[11] R. M. Corso, E. Piraccini, V. Agnoletti and G. Gambale, Use of an i-gel in a "can´t intubate/can´t ventilate" situation, *Anaesth. Intensive Care* 38, 212 (2010).

[12] P. Michalek, P. Hodgkinson and W. Donaldson, Fiberoptic intubation through an i-gel supraglottic airway in two patients with predicted difficult airway and intellectual disability, *Anesth. Analg.* 106, 1501-4 (2008).

[13] S. Sharma, S. Scott, R. Rogers and M. Popat, The i-gel airway for ventilation and rescue intubation, *Anaesthesia* 62, 419-20 (2007).

[14] J. Campbell, P. Michalek and M. Deighan, i-gel supraglottic airway for rescue airway management and as a conduit for tracheal intubation in a patient with acute respiratory failure, *Resuscitation* 80, 963 (2009).

[15] D. M. Miller, A proposed classification and scoring system for supraglottic sealing airways: a brief review, *Anesth. Analg.* 99, 1553-9 (2004).

[16] J. L. Benumof, Laryngeal mask airway and the ASA difficult airway algorithm, *Anesthesiology* 84, 686-99 (1996).

[17] American Society of Anesthesiologists Task Force on the Management of Difficult Airway, Practice guidelines for management of the difficult airway: an updated report by the American Society of Anesthesiologists Task Force on the Management of Difficult Airway, *Anesthesiology* 98, 1269-77 (2003).

[18] J. J. Henderson, M. T. Popat, I. P. Latto and A. C. Pierce, Difficult Airway Society guidelines for management of the unanticipated difficult intubation, *Anaesthesia* 59, 675-94 (2004).

[19] J. P. Nolan, J. Soar, D. A. Zideman, D. Biarent, L. L. Bossaert, C. Deakin, R. W. Koster, J. Wyllie, B. Böttiger, European Resuscitation Council Guidelines for Resuscitation 2010, *Resuscitation* 1219-1451 (2010).

[20] R. Wadhwa and S. Kalra, Comparison of hemodynamic changes and ease of endotracheal intubation through i-gel vs. ILMA, *J. Anaesth. Clin. Pharmacol.* 26, 379-82 (2010).

[21] L. Theiler, M. Kleine-Brueggeney, N. Urwyler, T. Graf, C. Luyet, and R. Greif, Randomized clinical trial of the i-gel™ and Magill tracheal tube or single-use ILMA™ and ILMA™ tracheal tube for blind intubation in anaesthetized patients with a predicted difficult airway. *Br. J. Anaesth.* 107, 243-50 (2011).

[22] E. Halwagi, N. Massicotte, A. Lallo, A. Gauthier, D. Boudreault, M. Ruel and F. Girard, Tracheal intubation through the i-gel™ supraglottic airway versus the LMA Fastrach™: a randomized controlled trial, *Anesth. Analg.* 114, 152-6 (2012).

[23] J. A. Sastre, T. Lopez, J. C. Garzon, Blind tracheal intubation through two supraglottic devices: i-gel versus Fastrach intubating laryngeal mask airway, *Rev. Esp. Anestesiol. Reanim.* 59, 71-76 (2012). [Article in Spanish, English abstract]

[24] M. Kleine-Brueggeney, L. Theiler, N. Urwyler, A. Vogt and R. Greif, Randomized trial comparing the i-gel™ and Magill tracheal tube with the single-use ILMA™ and ILMA™ tracheal tube for fibreoptic-guided intubation in anaesthetized patients with a predicted difficult airway, *Br. J. Anaesth.* 107, 251-7 (2011).

[25] A. Abraham, P. Michalek, F. McAleavey, W. Donaldson, C. Telford and R. Mathers, Comparison of CTrach, intubating laryngeal mask (ILMA) and i-gel for tracheal intubation. NWAC 2011 Abstract CD-ROM.

[26] L. G. Theiler, M. Kleine-Brueggeney, D. Kaiser, N. Urwyler, C. Luyet, A. Vogt, R. Greif and M. M. Unibe, Crossover comparison of the laryngeal mask supreme and the i-

gel in simulated difficult airway scenario in anesthetized patients, *Anesthesiology* 111, 55-62 (2009).

[27] M. Emmerich, R. Dummler, Use of the i-gel laryngeal mask for management of a difficult airway, *Anaesthetist* 57, 779-81 (2008). [Article in German, English abstract]

[28] T. Asai, Successful use of i-gel in three patients with difficult intubation and difficult ventilation, *Masui* 60, 850-2 (2011). [Article in Japanese, English abstract]

[29] J. Tiesmeier, M. Emmerich, Successful use of the i-gel supraglottic airway as a conduit for blind pre-hospital intubation during resuscitation, *Resuscitation* 82, 1358-9 (2011).

[30] E. Piraccini, A. Bartolini, V. Agnoletti, R. Corso, G. Gambale and C. Vicini, The use of the i-gel in a developing country, *Am. J. Emerg. Med.* 28, 840-1 (2010).

[31] E. Piraccini, R. M. Corso, V. Agnoletti, S. Maitan and G. Gambale, Use of the i-gel for tracheal intubation without the interruption of chest compressions, *J. Emerg. Med.* 43, e67-8 (2012).

[32] M. Berger, R. M. Corso, E. Piraccini, V. Agnoletti, E. Valtancoli, and G. Gambale, The i-gel in failed obstetric intubation, *Anaesth. Intensive Care* 39, 136-7 (2011).

[33] T. Lopez, J. A. Sastre, and C. Muriel, Use of i-gel airway in an intermediate step toward intubating difficult airway for thoracic surgery, *Rev. Esp. Anestesiol. Reanim.* 63, 1020-1 (2008).[Article in Spanish, English abstract]

[34] L. de Lloyd, I. Hodzovic, S. Voisey, A. R. Wilkes and I. P. Latto, Comparison of fibrescope guided intubation via the classic laryngeal mask airway and i-gel in manikin, *Anaesthesia* 65, 36-43 (2010).

[35] P. Michalek, W. Donaldson, C. Graham and J. D. Hinds, A comparison of the i-gel supraglottic airway as a conduit for tracheal intubation with the intubating laryngeal mask airway: a manikin study, *Resuscitation* 81, 74-77 (2010).

[36] J. Mauch, T. Haas and M. Weiss, Distance from the laryngeal mask grip to endotracheal tube tip. A crucial point during fiberoptic intubation in children, *Anaesthetist* 61, 123-8 (2012).

[37] N. Jagannathan, A. G. Roth. L. E. Sohn, T. Y. Pak, S. Amin and S. Suresh, The new air-Q intubating laryngeal airway for tracheal intubation in children with anticipated difficult airway: a case series, *Paediatr. Anaesth.* 19, 618-22 (2009).

[38] L. Beylacq, M. Bordes, F. Semjen and A. M. Cros, The i-gel, a single-use supraglottic airway device with a non-inflatable cuff and an esophageal vent: an observational study in children, *Acta Anaesthesiol. Scand.* 53, 376-9 (2009).

[39] R. Gupta, R. Gupta, S. Wadhawan and P. Bhadoria, Tracheal intubation through i-gel conduit in a child with post-burn contracture, *J. Anaesthesiol. Clin. Pharmacol.* 28, 397-8 (2012).

Conflict of interest: Prof. Pavel Michalek has lectured for several companies manufacturing supraglottic airway devices inluding Intersurgical Ltd., AMBU Ltd. and Intavent Orthofix Ltd.

In: The i-gel Supraglottic Airway
Editors: Pavel Michalek and William Donaldson
ISBN: 978-1-62417-897-9

Chapter 10

THE I-GEL AS A CONDUIT FOR FIBEROPTIC TRACHEAL INTUBATION

Lorenz Theiler** and Robert Greif
University Department of Anaesthesiology and
Pain Therapy, Inselspital, Bern University Hospital
and University of Bern, Switzerland

ABSTRACT

The i-gel supraglottic airway device establishes a patent airway for ventilating the patient's lungs and also offers gastric access. It can also be used as a guide for tracheal intubation. Several randomized controlled trials confirm high success rates (of 96-100%) for first attempt fiberoptic intubation. Blind intubation through the i-gel fails in 25-85% and therefore cannot be recommended. There is only weak evidence that an intubation stylet or a gum elastic bougie would facilitate blind intubation through the i-gel, but a tracheal tube with a soft tip may be useful for both blind and fiberoptic intubation through the i-gel.

INTRODUCTION

The "cannot intubate cannot ventilate" (CICV) situation is a potential nightmare for every anesthesiologist. In a CICV situation, the most important step for the patient is to first establish oxygenation and then ventilation of the lungs [1]. This life-threatening situation has fortunately lost some of its mortal character with the introduction, in the last two decades, of supraglottic airway devices (SADs) into the anesthetic toolbox. In most of the cases a CICV situation can be converted in a "can ventilate" situation with the aid of an SAD, avoiding deoxygenation of the patient and further harm. In such an event a common strategy, that is a part of nearly all airway management guidelines, is to terminate anesthesia, wake the patient up and plan to perform an "awake fiberoptic" intubation at a later stage. It seems fine as part

* Corresponding author: Lorenz Theiler. E-mail address: lorenz.theiler@insel.ch.

of an algorithm, but after having secured the patient's oxygenation, the clinical anesthesialogist is often confronted with the fact that the surgical procedure or the diagnostic intervention mandates tracheal intubation because of the urgency of the situation or because of the intraoperative positioning of patients. A special challenge in such an airway emergency is the non-fasted patient or other patients who are at risk of pulmonary aspiration of gastrointestinal contents. Of all the many ways to secure an airway with a tracheal tube (e.g. direct laryngoscopy, video-laryngoscopy, flexible and rigid fiberoptic devices, blind intubation, retrograde intubation) intubation through a supraglottic airway used as a guide is a core topic of most of the rescue strategies if intubation is required. Therefore, in this chapter, we focus on clinical aspects and experimental results of the i-gel as a conduit for tracheal intubation.

Mannequin Trials

De Lloyd and colleagues presented a mannequin study evaluating fiberoptic intubation through the i-gel vs. the classic LMA (cLMA) [2]. A Laerdal Airway Management Trainer was used as an airway model and 32 anesthetists participated in the study. Each anesthetist inserted both supraglottic airway devices. Two rounds of fiberoptic intubation were performed in each device, each with and without the additional help of an Aintree Intubation Catheter (AIC). The i-gel provided faster intubation times, 22 seconds vs. 43 seconds without AIC ($p < 0.001$), and 37 vs. 46 seconds with AIC ($p < 0.001$). Interestingly, in 5 cases out of 64 in the cLMA group the esophagus was intubated without noticing. This did not happen with the use of an AIC and in the i-gel group.

Michalek and colleagues published a mannequin trial in 2010, evaluating both fiberoptic and blind intubation through the i-gel with and without the help of guidance catheters (bougie and AIC) [3]. Twenty-five participants intubated three different mannequins through the i-gel and the intubating laryngeal mask Fastrach (ILMA). Blind intubation proved to be more successful through the ILMA, regardless whether the tracheal tube was placed on its own or if a bougie or an AIC was used ($p < 0.001$ for all three scenarios). The success rates were:

- 88% (ILMA) vs. 64% (i-gel) using a bougie
- 80% (ILMA) vs. 47% (i-gel) using an AIC
- 88% (ILMA) vs. 51% (i-gel) for blind passage of the tracheal tube without any aid.

The fiberoptic views through both devices were equally good ($p=0.26$). Apparently, a good view through the SAD did not predict successful blind intubation. Fiberoptic intubation was equally successful in both devices; the fiberoptic intubation success rate in both devices was 98.6%.

In their mannequin study, Scutt et al. evaluated whether fiberscope-guided intubation through supraglottic airway devices would be faster than guidance with the single-use videoscope Ambu aScope™ [4]. They compared the i-gel with the cLMA and ILMA. Generally, intubation times were faster when using a supraglottic airway device as a conduit than without (between 16-31 seconds in the SAD groups vs. 54-87 seconds in the oral intubation groups, $p = 0.02$). There was no influence of the type of fiberoptic scope on intubation time ($p = 0.30$), but the i-gel provided faster intubation times: it was 12 seconds faster than the cLMA (31 seconds, no p-value provided) and 5 seconds faster than the ILMA (24 seconds, no p-value provided).

CLINICAL TRIALS

Kleine-Brueggeney and colleagues looked at the success rate of fiberoptic intubation through the i-gel in a predicted difficult airway scenario [5]. This randomized controlled study compared the success of fiberscope-guided tracheal intubation using a standard PVC tracheal tube through the i-gel with the intubation success of a soft ILMA tube through the single use ILMA.

The authors included 160 adult patients with predictors for a difficult airway, defined as any of the following: documented difficult intubation in patient history, obesity with BMI >30 kg/m^2, thyromental distance > 6 cm, inability to protrude the mandible or retrognathia, abnormal neck anatomy, modified Mallampati score > II, or mouth opening < 3.5 cm.

The first attempt insertion and ventilation success rate was 94% for both devices; overall ventilation success rate was 99%. The success rate of fiberoptically guided tracheal intubation was 96% using the i-gel with the PVC tracheal tube compared with 90% using the ILMA with its ILMA tracheal tube ($p=0.21$).

Intubation time was limited to 5 minutes and included correction maneuvers, such as anticlockwise rotation of the tracheal tube by 90°, adjusting the SAD by using 'Chandy' maneuvers [6], by the 'up-down' maneuver, or by changing the position of the patient's head. The mean time necessary for intubation was 72±42 seconds for the i-gel group and 65±37 seconds for the ILMA group ($p=0.34$). The time taken to intubate the trachea with the fiberoptic scope did not differ between the i-gel and ILMA, but the time to railroad the tube over the fiberscope into the trachea was longer with the i-gel: 28 vs. 18 seconds, ($p < 0.001$).

Sore throat was reported in 14% (i-gel) and 9% (ILMA), respectively ($p = 0.45$). After successful intubation, the SADs were removed with the help of the ILMA exchange rod.

The same group, Theiler and colleagues, also compared the success rate of first attempt blind intubation through the i-gel (using a PVC tube) with blind intubation through the single use ILMA (using a soft ILMA tracheal tube) in 80 patients with a predicted difficult airway [7].

The setting was similar to the study evaluating fiberoptic intubation success [5] except, this time, the fiberoptic scope was only advanced up to the tip of the tube (and not beyond). The fiberscope did not guide the tube into the trachea (manipulation during the blind insertion attempt was avoided) but it enabled visualization of the advancement of the tube to judge if the tube found its "blind" way into the trachea or not.

This procedure could be termed 'visualized blind technique' or 'tube first fiberoptic technique' (Figure 1). At the same time, the view through the fiberoptic scope assured that the advancement of the tube could be stopped without applying force as soon as the tube was seen not to freely enter the vocal cords.

Only the first attempt success rate was evaluated. The success rate of the i-gel was 15% compared with 69% in the ILMA group ($p < 0.001$).

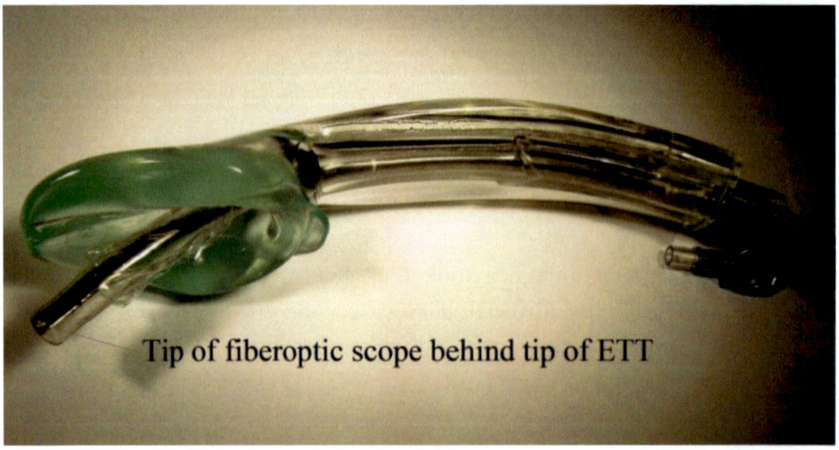

Figure 1."Tube first" fiberoptic technique.

The authors commented that when the tracheal tube exits the i-gel, it often gets caught in the arytenoid cartilage or other posterior structures of the larynx. In order to enter the trachea, fiberoptic scope and tracheal tube often needed to be pushed anteriorly to allow free passage into the trachea. This might be improved by reshaping the airway outlet of the i-gel to optimize the angle.

Halwagi and colleagues recently evaluated 160 patients without predictors of difficult airway for blind intubation success through the i-gel vs. through the ILMA [8].

In both groups, a PVC tracheal tube was used for intubation and up to three attempts including airway maneuvers were allowed. First and overall SAD device insertion success rates were 84% and 96% for the i-gel and 80% and 100% for the ILMA (p=0.68 and p=0.25).

First attempt blind intubation success rate was 69% (i-gel) vs. 74% (ILMA), p=0.60. Overall intubation success rate was 73% (i-gel) vs. 91% (ILMA), p=0.0035.

Overall intubation time was 22±13 seconds (i-gel) vs. 30±31seconds (ILMA), p=0.04. The authors mention that they observed a low first attempt intubation success rate through the i-gel of 23% in an unpublished preliminary study, but that they increased the success rate by 50% when the tracheal tube was rotated 90° counterclockwise before its insertion into the i-gel. This maneuver should prevent impingement of the tip of the tracheal tube on the right arytenoid cartilage during insertion.

Francksen et al. demonstrated, in a small randomized controlled study on 56 patients, how the use of a soft silicone tracheal tube may improve the blind intubation success rate compared with the (usually) stiffer PVC tube [9]. Both tracheal tubes were advanced through the i-gel. The success rate was 74% (17 out of 23) compared with 30% (10 out of 33) in the PVC group (p=0.003). The influence of tube type on intubation success rates was also investigated, in an additional analysis, in the above-mentioned study by Theiler and colleagues [7]. In a subgroup of 40 patients from the accompanying study [5], the alternative tracheal tube was used in a blind intubation attempt (soft ILMA tube for i-gel and stiff PVC tube for ILMA). The results were compared with the 80 patients from the blind intubation trial [7]. The following 2x2 table compares i-gel vs. ILMA and the soft ILMA tracheal tube vs. the stiffer PVC tracheal tube and reports the intubation success rate (and percentage). Intubation success did not depend on the used tube but highly significantly depended on the SAD used (Table 1).

Table 1. The relationship between type of tracheal tube and SADs [7]

Tracheal tube	Supraglottic airway device			
		i-gel (n=58)	ILMA n = 59	p-value
	PVC tube (n=59)	6 (15%)	12 (60%)	<0.01
	ILMA tube (n= 58)	4 (21%)	27 (69%)	<0.01
	p-value	0.59	0.48	

Case Reports and Case Series

In 2008, Michalek and colleagues reported, for the first time, two successful fiberoptic intubations through an i-gel SAD [10].

Campbell and colleagues described a successful fiberoptic intubation through the i-gel in an obese patient admitted to the ICU and who presented with a grade 4 laryngoscopic view, difficult bag-mask ventilation and failure of a cLMA as a rescue airway [11].

Emmerich and colleagues described fiberoptic intubation through i-gel in the operating room [12]. In other cases, blind intubations through the devices during resuscitation were described [13,14].

These case reports are described in detail in Chapter 9.

Comments Based on the Results of Clinical Studies

According the available evidence, the success rate of fiberoptic intubation through the i-gel is at least as high as through the ILMA, and better when compared with the classic LMA.

When the i-gel is used as a conduit for tracheal intubation, the use of a conventional fiberoptic scope, a single-use scope such as the Ambu aScope [4] or a fiberoptic stylet is strongly recommended. Blind intubation success rates are generally lower than 50%, which is unacceptable for elective airway procedures.

In an emergency scenario, we would attempt one single blind attempt, preferably using a tracheal tube with a soft, rounded tip such as the Parker™ tracheal tube (Figure 2, third from left). There is some evidence that a tracheal tube with a soft tip may be easier to insert blindly into the glottic opening [9], and it also seems to be easier to railroad a tracheal tube with a soft tip over the fiberoptic scope [15].

There is no evidence that a 2-step blind intubation – with either an AIC or another exchange catheter with passage of the tracheal tube over the catheter – would improve blind intubation. In one mannequin study, the use of a bougie was slightly favorable, but the evidence is far too weak to formulate any clinical recommendations.

A hollow bougie is favorable. After blind passage of a hollow bougie or tube exchange catheter into the trachea through an SAD, the correct tracheal placement of the catheter in the trachea can be confirmed by measuring end-tidal carbon dioxide concentration ($etCO_2$).

After confirmation of correct positioning, the SAD may be removed and the tracheal tube railroaded over the bougie into the correct position in the trachea [16].

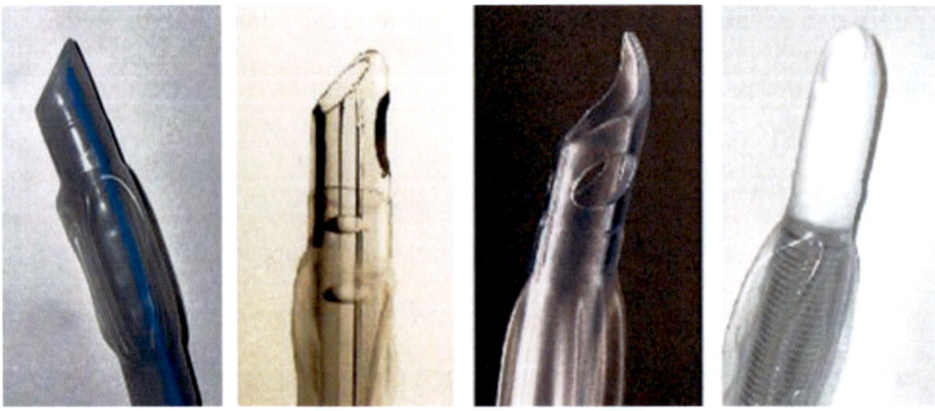

Figure 2. Different designs of tracheal tubes used for guided intubation through the SADs.

Significant differences in blind intubation success rates between the studies performed by Halwagi et al. [8] and by Theiler and colleagues [7] warrant further discussion, and it is not easy to explain them. Theiler et al. describe the alignment of the tip of the tube differently, but just as in the study by Halwagi et al, the tube was inserted with the concave side facing the arytenoid cartilage. The low intubation success rates by Theiler et al. might be explained by differences in the patient populations in the two studies: in the Theiler study patients had predictors of difficult airway management whereas in the Halwagi study patients with normal airways were investigated. Another possible explanation of the contradictory results is the methodical difference between the two studies in respect of the blind (Halwagi) vs. the "visualized blind" intubation (Theiler). With the visualized blind intubation method, the intubation attempt was immediately terminated when the tracheal tube was seen not to be entering the trachea. In a true blind intubation attempt, the anesthetist is more likely to accept a small degree of resistance of the tracheal tube as it passes the entry to the glottis, which then may lead to a higher success rate.

In order to minimize the risk of airway injury during intubation when using the i-gel as a conduit, fiberoptic guidance is strongly recommended because it enables direct visualization of the passage of the tracheal tube. Use of this method allows the clinician to observe and negotiate possible obstacles, whether they are at the glottic level or below.

If a blind intubation attempt is performed, the use of a tracheal tube with a soft tip may be beneficial and attempts to measure and verify the end-tidal CO_2 (via a bougie, exchange catheter or tracheal tube) throughout the procedure are highly recommended to ensure the tube finds its way into the trachea.

After successful intubation through the i-gel, there are multiple choices of how to manage the now redundant supraglottic airway device. For short procedures, the i-gel can be left in place [12], and removed following tracheal tube removal at the end of surgery. Initial reports found that the pressures exerted by the i-gel on the pharyngeal mucosa are comparable to those exerted by the cLMA [17].

Leaving the i-gel in place can provide for smooth emergence because the tube may be removed during deep anesthesia, minimizing coughing with the i-gel in place at emergence of anesthesia [18]. Alternatively, an airway exchange catheter can allow for the safe removal of the SAD [13]. Finally, either a specially designed silicone stabilizer ('pusher') may be used [3], or a smaller-sized tracheal tube as well as a narrow, but long clamp will suffice.

So far there is only one case report published regarding fiberoptic or blind intubation through the i-gel in pediatric patients. Considering the good fiberoptic view through the pediatric i-gel [19], a high fiberoptic intubation success rate would be expected, but we doubt that blind intubation will have an acceptably high success rate. Careful considerations have to be made, especially in children, concerning the removal of the i-gel after successful intubation. In short cases, the device may be left in place; otherwise an exchange catheter should be used [20].

OPEN QUESTIONS AND FURTHER DIRECTIONS OF CLINICAL STUDIES

At the time of this review, only two studies were registered either at ISRCTN (www.controlled-trials.com) or at the Clinical Trials website (www.clinicaltrials.gov). A randomized controlled trial from Antrim Area Hospital, UK, compared the success rates and intubation times of three SADs used as conduits for fiberscope-guided tracheal intubation. The i-gel airway, ILMA and CTrach laryngeal mask airway were inserted in 120 patients. The study was completed in September 2010 and presented at the NWAC Congress in Rome (May 2011). All three conduits performed well with fiberoptic guidance, with the i-gel being quickest to insert and to intubate through.

Another study performed at the University in Houston, Texas, looked at the difference in intubation success rate between the i-gel and LMA Unique. This study was completed in March 2011. We await the results of these trials with great interest.

In summarizing the results of the studies published on the i-gel as a conduit for tracheal intubation, we face the following research questions:

- First of all, there are a number of good mannequin-based studies but we need more high-quality patient studies. High quality means sufficiently high-powered studies with sample sizes that may convince clinicians to change their clinical practice. Few would change their clinical routine if results of such trials were not based on adequately powered studies with sufficient numbers of patients.
- As intubation through the i-gel will mainly be used as a rescue method, studies should be performed in patients with either established or known difficult airways, or at least in patients with predictors of difficult airway management.
- Because the pediatric airway is anatomically different from that of adults we need studies in children as well as in adults, for both fiberoptic guided intubation and for blind intubation, to either definitively abolish the blind technique or to recommend how to manage blind intubation safely and successfully for the pediatric patient.
- The primary outcome has to be intubation success. The main secondary outcomes should be safety and side effects. We know very little about these factors. The Innsbruck group, together with Keller and Brimacombe [17], should be acknowledged for their pioneering study on possible pressure damage to the pharyngeal mucosa. Large observational studies should provide data about such relatively rare side effects. Time to intubate the trachea as a secondary outcome is of lower importance because as long as oxygenation is maintained, intubation success is

the goal and a few seconds more or less for the intubation have little clinical meaning.

- Because the ILMA is still considered as the "gold standard" in guided intubation, studies should compare the i-gel with the ILMA; the classic LMA is almost outdated for this indication. With newer SADs developed specifically for intubation emerging, we need studies to provide evidence; such studies should compare the i-gel against other SADs designed for intubation (e.g. the Ambu Aura-i, CTrach LMA and the Air Q)
- Because the results related to blind intubation through the i-gel in adults are not favorable, we need more high-quality data about how this might be improved by either changing the approach to blind intubation or the design of the i-gel.
- The results relating to the use of exchange catheters or the AIC are mostly from mannequin studies. We lack the knowledge about this approach in real patients. We need to clarify if these intubation aids are really of use in emergency scenarios to help to secure a patent's airway.

Conclusion

The i-gel is suitable and safe as a conduit for fiberoptic intubation in adults. Fiberoptic intubation through the i-gel is as successful as it is with the Intubation Laryngeal Mask Airway ILMA. Because the placement of the i-gel is easy and highly successful, the i-gel is suitable as a rescue device in the difficult airway situation to help secure patients' oxygenation. After ensuring oxygenation and ventilation with the i-gel as a rescue device, fiberoptic intubation is recommended in cases where a tracheal tube needs to be placed. The available data suggest not attempting blind intubation through the i-gel, except in a clinical study. There is lack of data concerning intubation through the i-gel in children. No studies exist comparing the i-gel with newer SADs designed for intubation. Therefore we cannot comment on differences between these devices and the i-gel for the indications discussed in this chapter.

References

[1] J. J. Henderson, M. T. Popat, I. P. Latto and A. C. Pearce, Difficult Airway Society guidelines for management of the unanticipated difficult intubation, *Anaesthesia* 59, 675-94 (2004).

[2] L. de Lloyd, I. Hodzovic, S. Voisey, A. R. Wilkes and I. P. Latto, Comparison of fibrescope guided intubation via the classic laryngeal mask airway and i-gel in a manikin, *Anaesthesia* 65, 36-43 (2010).

[3] P. Michalek, W. Donaldson, C. Graham and J. D. Hinds, A comparison of the i-gel supraglottic airway as a conduit for tracheal intubation with the intubating laryngeal mask airway: a manikin study, *Resuscitation* 81, 74-7 (2010).

[4] S. Scutt, N. Clark, T. M. Cook, C. Smith, T. Christmas, L. Coppel and K. Crewdson, Evaluation of a single-use intubating videoscope (Ambu aScope™) in three airway

training manikins for oral intubation, nasal intubation and intubation via three supraglottic airway devices, *Anaesthesia* 66, 293-9 (2011).

[5] M. Kleine-Brueggeney, L. Theiler, N. Urwyler, A. Vogt and R. Greif, Randomized trial comparing the i-gel and Magill tracheal tube with the single-use ILMA and ILMA tracheal tube for fibreoptic-guided intubation in anaesthetized patients with a predicted difficult airway, *Br. J. Anaesth.* 107, 251-7 (2011).

[6] H. S. Joo and D. K. Rose, The intubating laryngeal mask airway with and without fiberoptic guidance, *Anesth. Analg.* 88, 662-6 (1999).

[7] L. Theiler, M. Kleine-Brueggeney, N. Urwyler, T. Graf, C. Luyet and R. Greif, Randomized clinical trial of the i-gel and Magill tracheal tube or single-use ILMA and ILMA tracheal tube for blind intubation in anaesthetized patients with a predicted difficult airway. *Br. J. Anaesth.* 107, 243-50 (2011).

[8] E. Halwagi, N. Massicotte, A. Lallo, A. Gauthier, D. Boudreault, M. Ruel and F. Girard, Tracheal intubation through the i-gel supraglottic airway versus the LMA Fastrach: a randomized controlled trial, *Anesth. Analg.* 114, 152-6 (2012).

[9] H. Francksen, J. Renner and J. Scholz, A comparison of two endotracheal tubes for intubation via new i-gel laryngeal mask, *Eur. J. Anaesthesiol.* 26, S45 (2009).

[10] P. Michalek, P. Hodgkinson and W. Donaldson, Fiberoptic intubation through an i-gel supraglottic airway in two patients with predicted difficult airway and intellectual disability, *Anesth. Analg.* 106, 1501-4 (2008).

[11] J. Campbell, P. Michalek and M. Deighan, i-gel supraglottic airway for rescue airway management and as a conduit for tracheal intubation in a patient with acute respiratory failure, *Resuscitation* 80, 963 (2009).

[12] M. Emmerich and J. Tiesmeier, The i-gel supraglottic airway - a useful tool in case of difficult fiberoptic intubation, *Minerva Anestesiol.* 2012.

[13] J. Tiesmeier and M. Emmerich, Successful use of the i-gel supraglottic airway as a conduit for blind pre-hospital intubation during resuscitation, *Resuscitation* 82, 1358-9 (2011).

[14] E. Piraccini, R. M. Corso, V. Agnoletti, S. Maitan and G. Gambale, Use of the i-gel for tracheal intubation without the interruption of chest compressions, *J. Emerg. Med.* 43, e67-8 (2012).

[15] M. S. Kristensen, The Parker Flex-Tip tube versus a standard tube for fiberoptic orotracheal intubation: a randomized double-blind study, *Anesthesiology* 98, 354-8 (2003).

[16] M. R. Hernandez, P. A. Klock Jr. and A. Ovassapian, Evolution of the extraglottic airway: a review of its history, applications, and practical tips for success, *Anesth. Analg.* 114, 349-68 (2012).

[17] S. Eschertzhuber, J. Brimacombe, M. Kaufmann, C. Keller and W. Tiefenthaler, Directly measured mucosal pressures produced by the i-gel(TM) and laryngeal mask airway Supreme(TM) in paralysed anaesthetised patients, *Anaesthesia* 67, 407-10 (2012).

[18] D. P. Dob, C. N. Shannon and P. M. Bailey, Efficacy and safety of the laryngeal mask airway vs Guedel airway following tracheal extubation. *Can. J. Anaesth.* 46, 179-81 (1999).

[19] L. G. Theiler, M. Kleine-Brueggeney, B. Luepold, F. Stucki, S. Seiler, N. Urwyler and R. Greif, Performance of the pediatric-sized i-gel compared with the Ambu AuraOnce laryngeal mask in anesthetized and ventilated children, *Anesthesiology* 115, 102-10 (2011).

[20] M. Weiss, J. Mauch, K. Becke, J. Schmidt and M. Johr, Fibre optic-assisted endotracheal intubation through the laryngeal mask in children, *Anaesthesist* 58, 716-21 (2009). [Article in German, English abstract]

Conflict of interest: Dr. Lorenz Theiler and Prof. Dr. Robert Greif, MME, FERC do not have any conflict of interest and did not receive any financial support from SAD providers. The authors received supraglottic airway devices from various manufacturers free of charge for research purposes. All their studies were carried out based on departmental grants or peer reviewed grants from anesthesia societies.

In: The i-gel Supraglottic Airway
Editors: Pavel Michalek and William Donaldson
ISBN: 978-1-62417-897-9

Chapter 11

USE OF THE I-GEL OUTSIDE OF THE OPERATING ROOM, BY PREHOSPITAL TEAMS AND IN MILITARY MEDICINE

Pavel Michalek[1,2,*] ***and Tomas Henlin***[3]

[1]Department of Anesthesia and Intensive Medicine, First Medical Faculty of the Charles University and General University Hospital, Prague, Czech Republic
[2]Department of Anaesthesia, Antrim Area Hospital, Antrim, UK
[3]Department of Anesthesia and Intensive Care, University Military Hospital, Prague, Czech Republic

ABSTRACT

Although the majority of indications for i-gel insertion are for airway maintenance during general anesthesia in elective operations, the i-gel possesses good features also for use as an airway device for procedures outside the operating room, in Intensive Care Unit settings and in pre-hospital emergency care. The i-gel may be used for airway management during Magnetic Resonance Imaging because it does not create any artifacts during scanning. In the Intensive Care Unit, use of the i-gel has been described in difficult intubation scenarios and also as an airway device during percutaneous dilational tracheostomy. The i-gel has been inserted also in pre-hospital care of trauma patients, by ambulance services as an alternative to tracheal intubation and may have potential for use in combat medicine.

* Corresponding author: E-mail address: pafkamich@yahoo.co.uk.

INTRODUCTION

The fact that supraglottic airway devices (SADs) perform very well in the operating room under conditions of general anesthesia is supported by many randomized controlled trials and other clinical studies [1, 2]. Conditions in the operating theatre are close to ideal: patients are under deep anesthesia and often administered neuromuscular blocking drugs, they are fasted and their airway reflexes are abolished.

Devices are usually inserted by experienced personnel, with well-instructed assistants and without any pressure. Under these circumstances, insertion of the SADs is highly successful, fast and the complication rate associated with them is extremely low.

On the other hand, the situation outside the operating room is entirely different: most patients have full stomachs in emergency and pre-hospital settings and the risk of regurgitation, vomiting and gastric content aspiration increases significantly. While the risk of gastric content aspiration in elective surgical procedures is less than 2:10,000 [3], in major trauma patients may be between 6-54% [4].

The "gold standard" for airway management outside the operating room has been, and will probably continue to be, tracheal intubation. This technique separates the respiratory and gastrointestinal tracts, protecting reasonably well against aspiration of gastric contents, and allows for positive pressure lung ventilation.

Its success rate is high when performed by experienced operators; however the degree of success decreases significantly in the hands of paramedics and other non-medical staff involved in emergency care [5].

Insertion of a supraglottic airway device may be the method of choice outside the operating room for diagnostic procedures under general anesthesia in elective patients such as MRI, CT scanning, PET-CT etc. Regarding resuscitation, trauma and emergency pre-hospital care, SADs including the i-gel may be inserted in patients with difficult and failed laryngoscopy or if the operator is not experienced enough in tracheal intubation [6, 7].

THE I-GEL AIRWAY IN MAGNETIC RESONANCE IMAGING SUITE

The i-gel may potentially be a very useful device for general anesthesia inside the Magnetic Resonance Imaging (MRI) suite. SADs are often chosen as airway devices for these conditions [8]. However, some SADs such as laryngeal masks contain small parts of ferromagnetic material. A special type of laryngeal mask airway was developed for use in the MRI suite (MRI-safe LMA). This device contains a silicone spring in the pilot balloon.

Zaballos et al. studied imaging artefacts caused by six different SADs under experimental conditions [9]. The Classic LMA, LMA Unique, LMA ProSeal, LMA Supreme, AMBU laryngeal mask and i-gel were placed on top and inside the phantom simulator (which is used by MRI technicians to diagnose compatibility of the MRI scanner with foreign materials and implanted devices). Four devices created different artifacts on the MRI images - cLMA, LMA Unique and LMA Supreme showed similar artifacts caused by the ferromagnetic parts contained inside the valve of the pilot balloon (Figure 1).

Scanning of phantom with LMA ProSeal inside was associated with most artifacts. These artifacts consisted of two different circles created by the pilot balloon and by ferro-magnetic material located inside the breathing tube of the device. Neither the i-gel airway nor the AMBU single-use laryngeal mask created any artifacts.

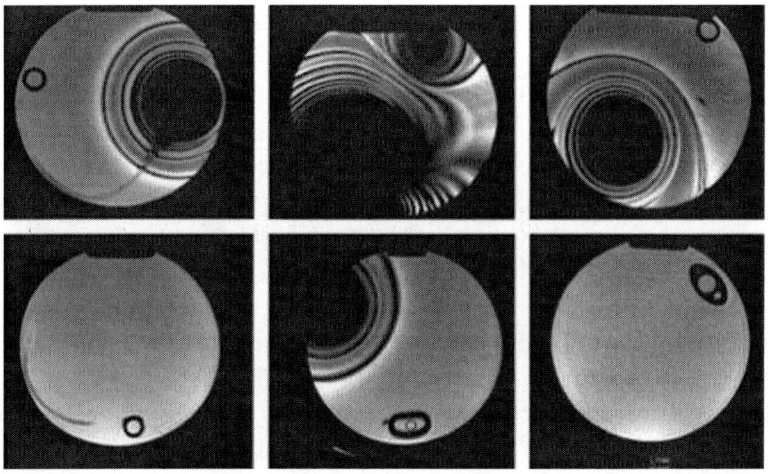

Reprinted with permission of John Wiley and sons from Zaballos et al., Anaesthesia 2010;65:569-72.

Figure 1. Axial magnetic resonance image showing artefacts as concentric circles produced by the metal spring of the pilot balloon in (a), (c) and (e) (corresponding to the Classic LMA, LMA Unique, and LMA Supreme); in (b), the two groups of concentric circles correspond to the metal in the pilot balloon and in the airway tube of the LMA ProSeal. In (d) (Ambu Disposable Laryngeal Mask) and (f) (i-gel supraglottic airway) there were no artefacts.

A recently published editorial highlighted the potential of the i-gel as a suitable device for procedures under general anesthesia in the MRI suite. The following benefits of the i-gel for this indication were discussed – its ease of insertion, good seal pressures, low morbidity, separation of respiratory and gastrointestinal tracts and lack of artifacts during imaging [10].

Taxak et al. described i-gel insertion in two small children (3-month-old and 3-years-old) for magnetic resonance imaging of the brain. The procedures were uneventful in both cases and no artifacts were created by the SAD [11].

Use of the i-gel Airway in the Intensive Care Setting

Although the standard methods of airway management in the ICU are tracheal intubation and tracheostomy, use of SADs including the i-gel airway has also been reported [12, 13].

The main problems associated with the long-term use of SADs in ICU patients are loss of the airway, risk of gastric content aspiration and risk of tissue and nerve trauma due to prolonged pressure exerted on the oropharyngeal structures.

SADs may be used in the ICU or Accident and Emergency Departments for airway maintenance in case of difficult laryngoscopy [12, 13]. The i-gel may have benefits over other SADs in terms of: easy and fast insertion, possibility of gastric content drainage and good access to the vocal cords through the breathing tube of the device with an intubating fiberscope. Campbell et al. used an i-gel as an airway rescue device in an ICU patient with respiratory failure [14]. This obese patient with a history of obstructive sleep apnea and pneumonia was initially managed using non-invasive ventilation but shortly after admission became uncooperative and required tracheal intubation. Having a predicted difficult laryngoscopy by Mallampati assessment and being unsuitable for awake fiberoptic intubation due to his uncooperativity, the patient was induced only with propofol. Laryngoscopy was tolerated well but failed to yield a view of the vocal cords (grade IV larynx). The cLMA was inserted as a rescue device but could not provide effective ventilation. The i-gel airway was available on the emergency airway cart and a size 4 was inserted. It provided good ventilation without leak and the patient´s oxygen saturation gradually improved. A size 7.0 mm endotracheal tube was then inserted through the i-gel with the aid of a 3-mm intubating fiberscope.

Another indication for SAD use in the ICU setting is fiberscope-controlled percutaneous dilational tracheotomy (PDTS) [15]. Two case studies have evaluated the i-gel airway as an airway maintenance device during PDTS. Dominguez Garcia et al. used an i-gel in PDTS in an ICU patient with respiratory insufficiency following an open repair of abdominal aortic aneurysm [16]. PDTS was indicated on day 14 because the patient could not be weaned from the ventilator. The authors replaced the orotracheal tube with a size 4 i-gel, inserted a gastric tube through the drainage channel of the device and performed PDTS under direct fiberoptic control. The vocal cords and trachea were easily examined through the device and the puncture needle, wire and insertion of tracheostomy cannula were fiberoptically observed in real-time. Corso and colleagues reported a case series of eight ICU patients who had PDTS performed with the i-gel as an airway device [17]. They were able to ventilate through the i-gel in seven patients, while the last patient had to be re-intubated due to difficulties during controlled ventilation with the i-gel. A fiberoptic bronchoscope was inserted through the i-gel until the level of the second tracheal ring (Figure 2) and PDTS (Blue Rhino™, Cook Critical Care, US) was perfomed under direct vision.

The authors highlighed some potential advantages of the i-gel over other airway devices. The i-gel offers an excellent fiberoptic view of the cords and subglottic area, allowing the identification of the upper tracheal rings and significantly decreases the risk of damage to the fiberscope. The i-gel may offer also some benefit over 1st generation SADs, providing a better view of the vocal cords, higher airway seal pressures and the possibility of stomach decompression using the i-gel's gastric channel.

The i-gel is considered as one of recommended airway management devices which should be available on all emergency airway trolleys in Intensive Care Units and Emergency Departments [18].

USE OF THE I-GEL IN EMERGENCY AND PRE-HOSPITAL CARE

There have been continuing debates whether paramedics should perform tracheal intubation without the direct supervision of a physician. Most countries do not have physicians in ambulances and paramedics have to deal with difficult airway situations in sub-optimal conditions (position of the patient, limited space, lack of light).

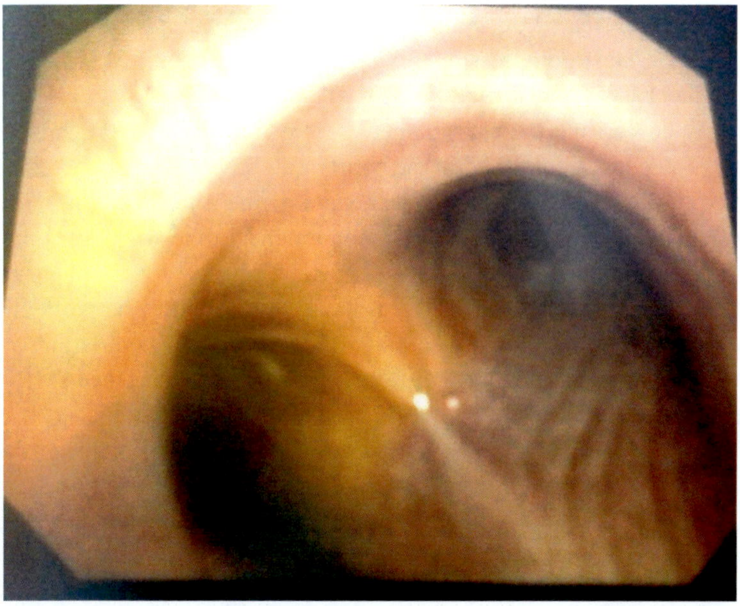

Figure 2. The i-gel in position and the endoscopic views of the trachea and its bifurcation during PDTS.

Some guidelines for airway management in the pre-hospital environment repeatedly suggest the insertion of SADs instead of tracheal intubation.

The i-gel airway can offer potential benefits over other SADs in emergency pre-hospital care. Its insertion is relatively easy and highly successful even for novices as shown by both human and manikin trials. Its cuff does not require inflation and the device can be used for ventilation and oxygenation of patients immediately following insertion. The integrated rigid bite block helps to protect device from kinking and airway obstruction caused by biting, whilst the gastric channel separates the respiratory and gastrointestinal tracts and may drain liquid gastric content. The i-gel airway tube has a wide bore which allows access to the trachea with a blindly inserted tracheal tube or fiberscope.

Based on findings from the operating room, Gabbott and Behringer pointed out the potential of i-gel use in resuscitation [19]. Soar reported very fast (10 sec) and effective insertion of i-gel airway in a patient with a cardiac arrest [20].

Thomas and Benger reported their relatively negative experience with the i-gel as an airway management device in patients following cardiac arrest [21]. In their report, the i-gel was inserted in 12 patients but did not provide effective ventilation in 7 of them (58%). The authors speculated that the lungs after cardiac arrest are less compliant and higher pressures for ventilation are required than the seal pressure of the i-gel can manage. One case report describes insertion of an i-gel airway in a young female patient with craniofacial trauma following a road traffic accident [22]. The patient´s Glasgow Coma Scale (GCS) suddenly decreased to 5 and the attending paramedic team expected difficulties in direct laryngoscopy due to the extent of craniofacial trauma. An i-gel size 4 was inserted and the stomach was decompressed with the insertion of a gastric tube. The patient was subsequently intubated through the i-gel (in the Emergency Department) with fiberoptic guidance.

Two other case reports have described use of the i-gel as a conduit for blind tracheal intubation in emergency situations outside the operating room. In one, an i-gel was inserted in an elderly patient who arrested on the medical ward. Placement of the device was very fast and did not interrupt chest compressions. A size 7.0 tracheal tube was inserted through the device into the trachea without difficulty [23]. Tiesmeier and Emmerich used an i-gel as an emergency airway device in a patient who had suffered a cardiac arrest caused by ventricular fibrillation [24]. The patient collapsed in the courtyard of a physiotherapy clinic. An i-gel was inserted because of poor light conditions at the site of the arrest and this provided effective ventilation and oxygenation immediately. An endotracheal tube was inserted blindly through the i-gel at the first attempt.

Two different supraglottic airway devices have been found to be ineffective in a patient who was resuscitated after drowning in seawater [25]. Bag-mask ventilation was difficult and caused significant gastric distension. The i-gel airway and, later, the AMBU AuraOnce™ laryngeal mask were inserted but could not provide efective ventilation.

The authors drew attention to the significantly decreased lung compliance and significantly increased pulmonary resistance in drowning victims. Peak pressures required for efficient lung ventilation are often higher than 40 cmH_2O and thus greatly exceed the typical seal pressures of SADs. The authors disputed the ERC guidelines from 2010 and do not recommend use of SADs for lung ventilation after drowning.

Military Medicine and Supraglottic Airway Devices

Battlefield trauma very often involves challenges in airway management. Victims may have extensive craniofacial or neck trauma, burns, thoracic injuries or traumatic upper airway obstruction [26].

Because of differing conditions and different types of victims, special guidelines for advanced life support are applied. Battlefield advance trauma life support (BATLS) guidelines comprise algorithms for the control of major hemorrhage, airway management including cervical spine stabilization, breathing assessment and ventilation, circulation control, disability and neurological deficit assessment, physical assessment of extremities, and evaluation of environmental and exposure factors (<C>ABCDE) [27].

Techniques of advanced airway management are crucial for the survival of victims. Basic airway management techniques involve bag-mask ventilation with or without an oral/nasal airway. Mask ventilation can be very difficult or even impossible in the injured patient with craniofacial or neck trauma. The airways of these victims have to be managed using either tracheal intubation or surgical cricothyrotomy [27-29].

Tracheal intubation in victims with trauma to the face or neck is very challenging even for very experienced anesthesiologists and it is not surprising that this method often fails in the hands of paramedics, combat medical technicians and corpsmen [30].

Adams et al. prospectively observed the techniques and success rates of airway management techniques in 6,875 combat casualties during Operation Iraqi Freedom [31]. They found that 86.6% of cases were intubated whilst 7.5% had a SAD inserted and 5.8% were managed using cricothyrotomy. Eleven endotracheal tubes (4.3%) were placed incorrectly (main bronchus, hypopharynx), however no esophageal intubation was detected. Mabry et al. evaluated a subgroup of 982 victims of combat trauma who died during operations in Iraq and Afghanistan (2003-2006 period) [32]. Eighteen people (1.8%) were found to have penetrating facial or neck injuries. Cricothyrothomy could have saved their lifes - it was attempted in five victims but without any success. Another paper analyzed the success and complication rates of pre-hospital cricothyrotomy in combat conditions [33]. Cricothyrotomy was successful in 68% of cases while in 26% of victims the corpsmen were unable to insert a cannula to the trachea. Performance of cricothyrotomy was not documented in 6% of victims who were found dead on arrival.

Von Goedecke and colleagues discussed the causes of field airway management disasters in an editorial [34]. Their article was focused mainly on unrecognized esophageal intubation. They pointed out that the equipment to verify correct placement of an endotracheal tube (such as capnography monitors) is often not available in pre-hospital emergency care. They recommend insertion of supraglottic airway devices rather than tracheal intubation if operators performing airway interventions are not sufficiently experienced in tracheal intubation. This editorial was challenged by Fraser and De Mello who, instead, recommended surgical cricothyrotomy as a plan A as opposed to tracheal intubation or the insertion of an SAD [35]. They argued that laryngoscopy or placement of a supraglottic airway device might irritate the hypopharynx and trigger vomiting.

There are very few papers supporting the use of SADs in military medicine. Navy corpsmen were instructed how to use Combitubes and laryngeal masks in an experimental study using videotapes and mannequin training [36]. Following this training, they were able to insert both devices with 100% success. Insertion of the LMA was faster than the endotracheal tube.

Sadler and de Mello presented an overview of the potential of the laryngeal mask airway (LMA) for use in battlefield medicine [37]. They pointed out the advantages of the LMA in combat scenarios – a shallow learning curve, quick insertion and infrequent failures.

The i-gel supraglottic airway may be considered as a rescue device in battlefield situations where direct laryngoscopy or surgical cricothyrotomy fail. It might also be used in stituations of upper airway obstruction where jaw thrust or triple maneuvers are not successful. In one mannequin study, the i-gel was the best performing device when inserted by corpsmen wearing chemical, biological, radiation, nuclear-personal protective equipment [38]. However, at the moment there is no evidence to support i-gel use in combat medicine.

CONCLUSION

A position of supraglottic airway devices in anesthesia is well supported by many randomized clinical trials. The classical laryngeal mask airway, ProSeal LMA, LMA Supreme and i-gel supraglottic airway are safe SADs allowing airway maintenance and controlled ventilation in elective surgical and diagnostic procedures. Use of SADs has been extended in last years to situations outside of the operating theatre [39, 40].

The i-gel might be an ideal airway management device for MRI procedures in the future due to its properties but further studies are needed. The use of the i-gel in ICU settings will be most likely limited to difficult intubation situations as a part of a Difficult airway trolley. The i-gel has also the potential to be included in Difficult airway algorithms for use by pre-hospital ambulance services and in military medicine.

REFERENCES

[1] J. R. Brimacombe, *Laryngeal mask anesthesia*, 2nd ed., W. B. Saunders, Philadelphia (2004).

[2] B. Bein and J. Scholz, Supraglottic airway devices, *Best Practice Res. Clin. Anaesthesiol.* 19, 581-93 (2005).

[3] A. Bernardini and G. Natalini, Risk of pulmonary aspiration with laryngeal mask airway and tracheal tube: analysis on 65 712 procedure with positive pressure ventilation, *Anaesthesia* 64, 1289-94 (2009).

[4] D. J. Lockey, T. Coats and M. J. Parr, Aspiration in severe trauma: a prospective study, *Anaesthesia* 54, 1097-98 (1999).

[5] M. J. Thomas and J. Benger, Prehospital intubation in cardiac arrest: the debate continues, *Resuscitation* 82, 367-8 (2011).

[6] F. X. Guyette, M. J. Greenwood, D. Neubecker, R. Roth and H. E. Wang, Alternative airways in the prehospital setting, *Prehospital Emerg. Care* 11, 56-60 (2007).

[7] E. Flavell and M. J. Boyle, Which is more effective for ventilation in the prehospital setting during cardiopulmonary resuscitation – the laryngeal mask airway or the bag-valve-mask? A review of the literature, *J. Emerg. Primary Health Care* 8, 990420 (2010).

[8] J. A. Langton, I. Wilson and D. Fell, Use of the laryngeal mask airway during magnetic resonance imaging, *Anaesthesia* 47, 532 (1992).

[9] M. Zaballos, E. Bastida, T. del Castillo, J. G. de Villoria and C. Jimenez, In vitro study of magnetic resonance imaging artefacts of six supraglottic airway devices, *Anaesthesia* 65, 569-72 (2010).

[10] K. N. Saxena, Airway management devices for general anesthesia for magnetic resonance imaging, *J. Anaesthesiol. Clin. Pharmacol.* 28, 153 (2012).

[11] S. Taxak, M. Bhardwaj and A. Gopinath, The i-gel™ – a promising airway device for magnetic resonance imaging suite, *J. Anaesthesiol. Clin. Pharmacol.* 28, 263-4 (2012).

[12] G. G. Lavery and B. V. McCloskey, The difficult airway in adult critical care, *Crit. Care Med.* 36, 2163-73 (2008).

[13] M. S. Lim and J. J. Hunt-Smith, Difficult airway management in the intensive care unit: alternative techniques, *Crit. Care Resuscitation* 5, 53-62 (2003).

[14] J. Campbell, P. Michalek and M. Deighan, i-gel supraglottic airway for rescue airway management and as a conduit for tracheal intubation in a patient with acute respiratory failure, *Resuscitation* 80, 963 (2009).

[15] U. Linstedt, M. Zenz, K. Krull, D. Hager and A. W. Prangel, Laryngeal mask airway or endotracheal tube for percutaneous dilatational tracheostomy: a comparison of visibility of intratracheal structures, *Anesth. Analg.,* 110, 1076-82 (2010).

[16] G. D. Dominguez, S. T. Leon, C. R. Tejera and D. E. Espinosa, Tracheotomy guided by fiberoptic bronchoscopy through an i-gel supraglottic airway device, *Rev. Esp. Anestesiol. Reanim.* 56, 643-5 (2009). [Article in Spanish, English abstract]

[17] R. M. Corso, E. Piraccini, V. Agnoletti, M. Baccanelli, A. Coffa and G. Gambale, The use of i-gel extraglottic airway during percutaneous dilatational tracheostomy: a case series, *Minerva Anestesiol.* 77, 852-3 (2011).

[18] P. Jeanrenaud, V. Girotra, T. Wharton, N. Main, R. Konuralp and G. Dempsey, Difficult airway trolleys for the critical care unit, *J. Intensive Care Soc.* 11, 98-103 (2010).

[19] D. A. Gabbott and R. Beringer, The iGEL supraglottic airway: a potential role for resuscitation? *Resuscitation* 73, 161-2 (2007).

[20] J. Soar, The i-gel supraglottic airway and resuscitation – some initial thoughts, *Resuscitation* 74, 197-9 (2007).

[21] M. Thomas and J. Benger, Pre-hospital resuscitation using the iGEL, *Resuscitation* 80, 1437 (2009).

[22] R. M. Corso, G. Giovannini, M. Berger, A. Fabbri and G. Gambale, The use of i-gel extraglottic airway in a trauma patient, *Am. J. Emerg. Med.* 30, 829-30 (2012).

[23] E. Piraccini, R. M. Corso, V. Agnoletti, S. Maitan and G. Gambale, Use of the i-gel for tracheal intubation without the interruption of chest compressions, *J. Emerg. Med.* 43, e67-8 (2012).

[24] J. Tiesmeier and M. Emmerich, Successful use of the i-gel supraglottic airway as a conduit for blind pre-hospital intubation during resuscitation, *Resuscitation* 82, 1358-9 (2011).

[25] P. A. Baker and J. B. Webber, Failure to ventilate with supraglottic airways after drowning, *Anaesth. Intensive Care* 39, 675-7 (2011).

[26] O. Langeron, A. Birenbaum and J. Amour, Airway management in trauma, *Minerva Anestesiol.* 75, 307-11 (2009).

[27] No authors listed, Battlefield advanced trauma life support: 1, *J. R. Army Med. Corps* 152, S5-72 (2006).

[28] J. Breeze and D. Bryant, Current concepts in the epidemiology and management of battlefield head, face and neck trauma, *J. R. Army Med. Corps.* 155, 274-8 (2009).

[29] K. C. Tang, J. W. Chiu and E. Low, Airway and ventilatory equipment in field anesthesia: what´s new? *Mil. Med.* 169, 342-8 (2004).

[30] R. L. Mabry and A. Frankfurt, Advanced airway management in combat casualties by medics at the point of injury: a sub-group analysis of the reach study, *J. Spec. Oper. Med.* 11, 16-9 (2011).

[31] B. D. Adams, P. A. Cuniowski, A. Muck and R. A. De Lorenzo, Registry of emergency airways arriving at combat hospitals, *J. Trauma* 64, 1548-54 (2008).

[32] R. L. Mabry, J. W. Edens, L. Pearse, J. F. Kelly and H. Harke, Fatal airway injuries during operation enduring freedom and operation Iraqi freedom, *Prehospital Emerg. Care* 14, 272-7 (2010).

[33] R. L. Mabry, An analysis of battlefield cricothyrotomy in Iraq and Afghanistan, *J. Spec. Oper. Med.* 12, 17-23 (2012).

[34] A. Von Goedecke, H. Herff, P. Paal, V. Dörges and V. Wenzel, Field airway management disasters, *Anesth. Analg.* 104, 481-3 (2007).

[35] N. H. Fraser and W. F. de Mello, Oxygenate rather than intubate, *Anesth. Analg.* 105, 1167-8 (2007).

[36] M. D. Calkins and T. D. Robinson, Combat trauma airway management: endotracheal intubation versus laryngeal mask airway versus combitube use by Navy SEAL and Reconnaissance combat corpsmen, *J. Trauma* 46, 927-32 (1999).

[37] P. J. Sadler and W. F. de Mello, The laryngeal mask airway (its potential for the military), *J. R. Army Med. Corps.* 142, 15-9 (1996).

[38] N. Castle, Y. Pillay and N. Spencer, Insertion of six different supraglottic airway devices whilst wearing chemical, biological, radiation, nuclear-personal protective equipment: a manikin study, *Anaesthesia* 66, 983-8 (2011).

[39] T. C. Mort, The supraglottic airway device in the emergency setting: its changing role outside the operating room, *Anesthesiology News* 37, 59-71 (2011).

[40] B. Young, The intubating laryngeal-mask airway may be an ideal device for airway control in the rural trauma patient, *Am. J. Emerg. Med.* 21, 80-5 (2003).

Conflict of interest: Prof. Pavel Michalek has lectured for several companies manufacturing supraglottic airway devices inluding Intersurgical Ltd., AMBU Ltd. and Intavent Orthofix Ltd.

In: The i-gel Supraglottic Airway
Editors: Pavel Michalek and William Donaldson

ISBN: 978-1-62417-897-9

Chapter 12

THE I-GEL AND CARDIOPULMONARY RESUSCITATION

Amy L. Williams,* Rebecca M. Anderson and Muhammed A. Nasir

Intersurgical Ltd, Wokingham, Berkshire, UK

ABSTRACT

The published evidence for i-gel® suggests the device has many attributes that make it a useful addition to the range of options available for airway management during resuscitation. After many reports of its easy and rapid insertion; relatively high seal pressures and ease of insertion by novices and a mechanism for managing regurgitant fluid, the indications for use were extended to include resuscitation in 2009. The potential of the i-gel in resuscitation has been acknowledged in the new 2010 ERC guidelines, where the device is described as 'easy to insert, requiring minimal training and seal pressures of 20-24cm H_2O can be achieved'.

The most recent development, the i-gel O_2 Resus Pack includes an i-gel with a supplementary oxygen port, a sachet of lubricant, a suction tube and an airway support strap for securing the device. The i-gel O_2 offers the opportunity of providing passive airway management (PAM) as an alternative to traditional ventilation techniques in the management of the witnessed cardiac arrest patient.

INTRODUCTION

In an editorial published in *Resuscitation* in 2009, entitled, 'Airway management for out-of-hospital cardiac arrest – more data required', Nolan and Lockey highlighted that virtually all data relating to the use of supraglottic airway devices (SADs) in cardiac arrest derive from low level studies [1]. They concluded that there is an urgent need for high-quality, randomised controlled trials of the use of SADs for cardiopulmonary resuscitation (CPR).

* Corresponding author: Amy L. Williams. E-mail address: awi@intersurgical.co.uk.

Whilst new airway devices appear frequently, they identified the i-gel® as one of three disposable SADs that should be studied for use during CPR.

Since tracheal intubation has long been considered the 'gold standard' for airway management during CPR, it would not be unreasonable to expect there to be high level data published confirming it improves patient outcome. However, Nolan and Lockey note that such data does not exist for tracheal intubation either. The European Resuscitation Council (ERC) also concludes that there is 'no data supporting the routine use of any specific approach to airway management during cardiac arrest' [2].

Until such data and evidence is published, decisions still have to be taken as to the most appropriate airway device to use during CPR, and it therefore seems logical to consider and review the evidence that is available, whilst acknowledging the potential limitations.

SUPRAGLOTTIC AIRWAY DEVICES AND RESUSCITATION

Classification of SADs might be helpful in deciding the safest and most appropriate type of device for use in a resuscitation scenario.

The simplest way of categorising SADs is into first and second-generation devices, as described in a review article published in *Pediatric Anesthesia* [3]. A 1st generation device was described as a 'simple airway tube', and 2nd generation as a device that 'incorporates specific design features to improve safety by protecting against regurgitation and aspiration'. In respect of resuscitation, this definition seems particularly relevant, as one concern over the use of SADs in this setting, has been the level of protection they may or may not offer against aspiration [4]. Since the i-gel incorporates a gastric channel, it has been designated as a 2nd generation device [3].

There are published studies on the use of the Combitube®, the LMA Classic® (cLMA), the Laryngeal Tube™ (LT) and the i-gel during CPR but none of these studies has included enough subjects to enable their impact on survival to be determined [2, 5]. However, the ease of use and rapid insertion of supraglottic airways without interrupting cardiac compression has prompted recommendations for their use during resuscitation [6].

CARDIOPULMONARY RESUSCITATION AND THE I-GEL AIRWAY

The i-gel was initially indicated for use in routine and emergency anesthesia. Following publication of studies reporting its easy and rapid insertion [7-10], relatively high seal pressures [8, 11, 12], a minimal training period for safe use [10] and ease of insertion by novices [7, 9] the indications for use were extended to include resuscitation. The first independently published report on the clinical use of the i-gel appeared as a correspondence [13]. A letter to the editor reported initial findings following clinical use in 100 patients for routine surgery.

The authors limited their use to size 4 devices only to assess whether there might be less dependence on size selection in adults with the i-gel than with other SADs, thus simplifying the process of airway selection in an emergency. Deakin et al. confirmed that a size 4 i-gel is suitable for a wide range of adults [14]. It is interesting to note the early identification of design features of the i-gel that might make it particularly suitable for use in a resuscitation scenario. Gabbott and Beringer reported that 98 of 100 devices were adequately positioned on the first or second attempt and peak airway pressures in excess of 30cm H_2O were possible in the vast majority of patients [13]. Airway trauma, demonstrated by visible blood on the device on removal, was only evident on one occasion [13].

Jasmeet Soar, chairman of both the Resuscitation Council UK Immediate Life Support committee and the ERC Immediate Life Support (ILS) working group, published a letter reporting use of the i-gel during a cardiac arrest [15]. The i-gel was inserted within 10 seconds of opening the packet and provided easy ventilation of the patient's lungs, which were ventilated asynchronously during chest compressions with no leak. Soar also confirmed that he was able to train five non-anesthetic trainee doctors in the intensive care unit to insert the i-gel and ventilate an anesthetized patient after minimal instruction. All of the trainees had received previous training on use of the laryngeal mask airway and rated the i-gel as being easier to insert [15].

Clinical Studies Related to Potential Use of the i-gel in CPR

Since these early reports, a number of clinical studies examining the use of the i-gel in anesthesia have been published, many of which have included data of significance to its potential use in CPR [5, 7-9, 16-18]. One study was specifically designed to evaluate its potential when used by non-anesthesiologists, such as medical students, non-anesthetic physicians and other allied healthcare professionals who were all unfamiliar with the i-gel [9]. In the manikin section of the study, 50 i-gels were inserted, with 88% of them placed at the first attempt in a mean insertion time of 14 seconds. In the patient section, i-gels were placed in 40 healthy anesthetized patients. The overall insertion success rate was 100%, with a median insertion time of 17.5 seconds. The authors confirmed that, 'Two recent studies of novice anesthetic trainees found the median insertion times for the LMA Classic to be 32 seconds (first-time success rate 80%, overall 95%) and the LMA-ProSeal 53 seconds (first-time success rate 73%, overall success rate 95%). Data from this study indicate the i-gel can be placed both faster (18 seconds) and with higher success rates (first time 83%, overall 100%) than reported in those studies' [9]. Ease of use by novices, was also confirmed in an audit report published in the European Journal of Anaesthesiology, which reported 90 successful insertions of the i-gel by first-time users such as medical students, firemen, nurses and paramedics [7]. In a particularly interesting study, designed to evaluate the speed with which different airway devices could be placed with and without interrupting chest compressions, Gatward et al. timed 40 doctors regularly involved in resuscitation inserting a tracheal tube, LMA Classic, LMA-ProSeal and i-gel into a manikin [10]. The i-gel was approximately 50% faster to insert than the other devices, and the authors concluded that 'The LMA ProSeal and i-gel (SADs with a gastric drain tube) were both faster to insert than the cLMA and offer additional benefits. They should be considered for use in CPR.'

A number of studies have confirmed the i-gel as being easy [7, 8] and rapid [7-9] to insert, and its seal pressure has been reported as higher than that with a standard laryngeal mask [11]. In fact, in two studies, mean seal pressures of 30cm H_2O or above have been reported [8, 12]. The ease of use and ability of the gastric channel to manage regurgitant fluid has also been studied, most notably by Schmidbauer et al., who inserted airway devices into unfixed cadavers with exposed esophaguses that had been connected to a water column producing both a slow and a fast esophageal pressure increase [17]. They concluded that both the LMA-ProSeal and i-gel quickly drained off gastrointestinal fluid through their esophageal lumen, 'Thus tracheal aspiration may be prevented with their use'. This combination of easy and rapid insertion, high seal pressures, steep learning curve for competent use and a mechanism for managing regurgitant fluid, suggest that the i-gel has many of the key attributes required for a device in resuscitation.

Earlier this year, the Royal College of Anaesthetists and the Difficult Airway Society published a prospective study of "Major complications of airway management in the UK" [19] during anesthesia, in the intensive care unit (ICU) and the emergency department. Whilst this seminal report did not examine use of airway devices in the out-of-hospital setting for cardiac arrest, it provided a wealth of information regarding the use of supraglottic airways that may have relevance in such scenarios, including the potential benefits of second generation devices such as the i-gel [19].

As already stated, there remains an urgent need for high quality, randomized controlled trials of the use of SADs for CPR before conclusions can be drawn about the suitability of one device compared with another. However, the potential of the i-gel in resuscitation has already been acknowledged in the new ERC guidelines [14, 20], where the device is described as 'very easy to insert, requiring only minimal training and laryngeal seal pressure of 20-24cm H_2O can be achieved. In two manikin studies, insertion of the i-gel was significantly faster than several other airway devices. The ease of insertion of the i-gel and its favourable leak pressure make it theoretically very attractive as a resuscitation airway device for those inexperienced in tracheal intubation. Use of the i-gel during cardiac arrest has been reported but more data on its use in this setting are awaited' [14, 20].

Successful use of the i-gel in cardiac arrest has been reported [15] but, as with virtually all other SADs, high-quality randomised controlled trials are still to be published. Tracheal intubation, long considered the gold standard, has many limitations in CPR, particularly in inexperienced hands [21, 22], and ERC guidelines state that there are 'no data supporting the routine use of any specific approach to airway management during cardiac arrest' [14, 20].

Resuscitation science continues to advance, and clinical guidelines are updated regularly reflecting these developments and to provide advice on best practice [20]. Nolan et al (2010) produced a report presenting the widely accepted view of how resuscitation should be undertaken both safely and effectively.

However, when new and revised treatment recommendations are produced it does not imply that current clinical care is ineffective or unsafe [20].

REPORTS ON THE USE OF THE I-GEL IN CPR

There have been several case reports published reporting the use of i-gel in cardiopulmonary resuscitation scenarios. As already mentioned in previous paragraphs, Soar first reported insertion of the i-gel in cardiac arrest in 2007 [15].

Two letters to the editor reported an insertion of the i-gel during cardiopulmory resuscitation and its subsequent use as a conduit for blind tracheal intubation. The first described the case of an elderly patient who suffered cardiac arrest on a medical ward. An i-gel airway was immediately available and placed within seconds whilst a second operator performed chest compressions. A tracheal tube was inserted through the device into trachea at the first attempt [21]. Tiesmeier and Emmerich used an i-gel in a man who collapsed outside a rehabilitation clinic. Ventricular fibrillation was diagnosed on the ECG, defibrillation and CPR commenced, and the airway was managed using the i-gel airway. A tracheal tube was later inserted through the i-gel without difficulty [22].

Larkin et al. published their experience with the i-gel as an airway device during CPR inside the hospital [23]. This has been the most extensive report on the i-gel use in resuscitation so far. The authors reported i-gel insertion in 100 cases of in-hospital emergency situations where either tracheal intubation was impossible or the member of staff managing the airway was not competent to intubate the trachea.

Only size 4 devices were inserted because that size covers a wide range of the adult population (40-100 kg). Devices were inserted by nurses in 49%, by junior doctors in 47% and by resuscitation officers in the remaining 4% of cases. The results are summarized in Table 1.

There have also been two reports published discussing the potential limitations of the i-gel airway (and also other SADs) in cardiopulmonary resuscitation.

Table 1. Results of i-gel insertion during cardiopulmonary resuscitation in 100 patients [23]

Insertion parameters	Success rate
Overall success rate	99/100 (99%)
– 1st attempt	82/100 (82%)
– 2nd attempt	17/100 (17%)
– Failure	1/100 (1%)
Ease of insertion	
Easy insertion	83/100 (83%)
Moderate insertion	15/100 (15%)
Difficult insertion	2/100 (2%)
Insertion before bag-mask ventilation	16/100 (16%)
Insertion after bag-mask ventilation	46/100 (46%)
Data not available	38/100 (38%)
Audible leak (assessed in 61 patients during synchronous ventilation and chest compressions)	
No leak	36/61 (59%)
Audible leak, but visible chest movement	24/61 (39%)
Ventilation during asynchronous ventilation and chest compressions (assessed in 31 patients)	23/31 (74%)

Thomas and Benger used i-gels in 12 patients who suffered cardiac arrest and were resuscitated by the ambulance crew. Ventilation using the i-gel was not effective in 5 persons (42%). This might have be caused by laryngospasm or higher inspiratory pressures for lung ventilation due to the decreased lung compliance following cardiac arrest [24]. Two different SADs (Ambu® AuraOnce™ and i-gel) have been found to be ineffective in a victim who arrested following drowning in seawater.

Peak inspiratory pressures required for effective lung ventilation in the case were 40 cmH_2O - which significantly exceeds the seal pressures of both SADs [6].

Simulated Cardiopulmonary Resuscitation

The importance of early, uninterrupted chest compressions is emphasised throughout the ERC guidelines [14, 20] to minimize No-Flow Time (NFT) [20], as prolonged NFT compromises tissue perfusion [25]. In a study by Ruetzler et al., 40 voluntary emergency medical technicians - none of whom had advanced airway management experience - performed airway management with 6 devices during on-going chest compressions on a manikin. The hands-off time was 15.9s for the i-gel compared to 48 seconds for an endotracheal tube. The authors concluded that supraglottic devices appear to be a reasonable emergency airway management strategy, even for inexperienced personnel [25].

Wiese et al. compared the LTS-D and i-gel in a manikin-based cardiac arrest scenario. They state that 'An ideal supraglottic airway should be inserted rapidly with minimal training and it should enable controlled ventilation' [26]. During the study, the i-gel met these criteria during resuscitation performed on a manikin and NFT was kept as low as possible, consistent with ERC guidelines [26].

Concept of Passive Oxygenation during CPR

Cardiocerebral resuscitation (CCR) or compression-only CPR might be equivalent or superior to conventional CPR in patients with out of hospital cardiac arrest in both survival rate and neurological benefits [27]. The American Heart Association (AHA) in 2005 stated "Laypersons should be encouraged to do compression-only CPR if they are unable or unwilling to provide rescue breaths" [27, 28]. However, compression-only CPR may only be sufficient for the first few minutes post arrest, and is not as effective for an arrest of non-cardiac origin, such as the victim of drowning or asphyxiation [30].

Another approach to oxygenation during cardiac arrest is continuous oxygen insufflation. Positive pressure ventilation during cardiac arrest increases intrathoracic pressure, reducing cardiac output [31]. The consequences of this can be exacerbated by the well-documented tendency of some health care professionals to deliver excessive ventilations during cardiac arrest [31].

Steen et al. demonstrated that continuous insufflation of oxygen into the trachea of swine resulted in an improved 2hr post-resuscitation survival compared to the use of positive pressure ventilation [31, 32].

Hayes and associates showed that, in a swine model, continuous high flow oxygen insufflation resulted in 24-h neurologically intact survival similar to that achieved with the positive pressure ventilation advocated by the ASA Guidelines [33]. The authors state the advantages of insufflation by saying it is 'faster and simpler to initiate and easier to manage than positive pressure ventilation techniques. All that is required is placement of an oropharyngeal airway, a non-rebreathing mask, and a high flow source of oxygen. Once applied, this allows an EMS provider to undertake other duties, such as obtaining intravenous access, or helping with continuous chest compressions. Insufflation technique avoids the possible adverse hemodynamic effects from increased intrathoracic pressures during intermittent positive pressure ventilation' [31]. It also prevents the tendency to hyperventilate the cardiac arrest victim [31]. Chen-lu et al. agree that CCR is easier to manage and may bring about more neurological benefits, making it an increasingly popular choice for the management of the out-of-hospital cardiac arrest patient [28].

A study by Bobrow et al. also confirms that, 'among adult, witnessed, VF/Ventricular tachycardia, out-of-hospital cardiac arrest resuscitated with minimally interrupted cardiac resuscitation, adjusted neurologically intact survival to hospital discharge was higher for individuals receiving initial passive ventilation than those receiving initial bag-valve-mask ventilation' [34].

According to several previous studies the neurological outcome of patients who suffer out-of-hospital cardiac arrest (OHCA) mainly depends on the blood flow to the brain during resuscitation. Chen-lu et al. state that 'chest compressions create blood flow to the brain by compressing the chest and increasing intrathoracic pressure and, thus, deliver a small but critical amount of oxygen and substrate to the brain. This critical cerebral perfusion is lost when the rescuer stops chest compressions for mouth-to-mouth ventilation' [28].

Whilst passive oxygenation, as a component of CCR, for management of the cardiac arrest patient looks promising, the current ERC guidelines for resuscitation conclude that, 'There is insufficient evidence to support or refute the use of passive oxygen delivery during CPR to improve outcome when compared with oxygen delivery by positive pressure ventilation. Until further data are available, passive delivery without ventilation is not recommended for routine use during CPR'[14,20]. The AHA guidelines make a similar statement: 'At this time there is insufficient evidence to support the removal of ventilations from CPR performed by ACLS providers' [33].

Development of the i-gel 0_2 Resus Pack

As management of the cardiac arrest patient continues to evolve with these radical new concepts of compression-only resuscitation and passive oxygenation, the i-gel® itself has evolved. Following the extension of the indications for use of the i-gel to include resuscitation, the indications have been extended still further to include use as a conduit for intubation with fiberoptic guidance. The latter may have a role in the resuscitation setting and use of the device for this technique is discussed further in the chapter on the role of i-gel in the management of the difficult airway (Chapter 9).

The most recent development is the 'i-gel O_2 Resus Pack' (Figure 1). This includes an i-gel with a supplementary oxygen port (Figure 2) (Figure 3), a sachet of lubricant, a suction tube and an airway support strap for securing the device (Figure 4). The i-gel O_2 offers the opportunity of providing passive airway management (PAM) as an alternative to traditional ventilation techniques in the management of the witnessed cardiac arrest patient.

CONCLUSION

For the i-gel, the evidence available suggests that this device has many attributes (easy and rapid insertion, high seal pressures, steep learning curve for competent use and a mechanism for managing regurgitant fluid) that make it a useful addition to the range of options available for airway management during resuscitation. As with all other airway devices, there remains a need for high quality randomised controlled trials of its use in the resuscitation setting.

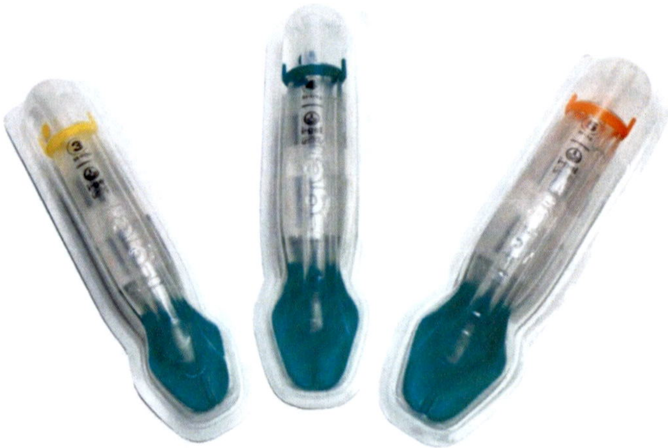

Figure 1. i-gel O_2 Resus Packs® sizes 3, 4 and 5, designated for adults (courtesy of Intersurgical® Ltd., UK).

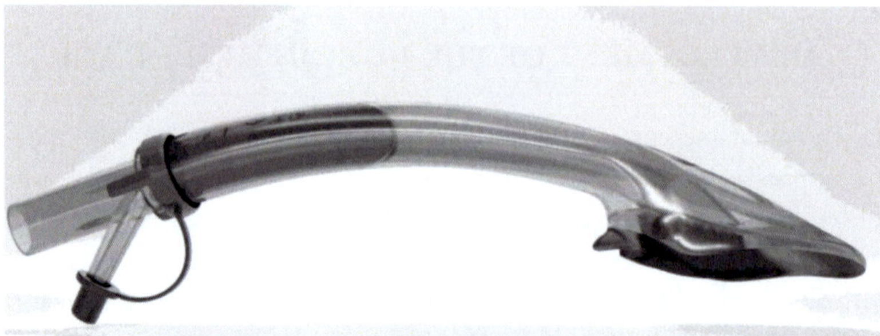

Figure 2. i-gel O_2 – side view of the device (courtesy of Intersurgical® Ltd., UK).

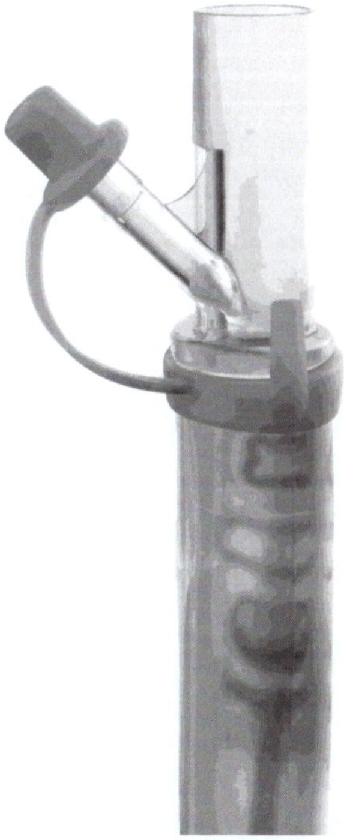

Figure 3. i-gel O_2 – additional channel for passive O_2 insufflation (courtesy of Intersurgical® Ltd., UK).

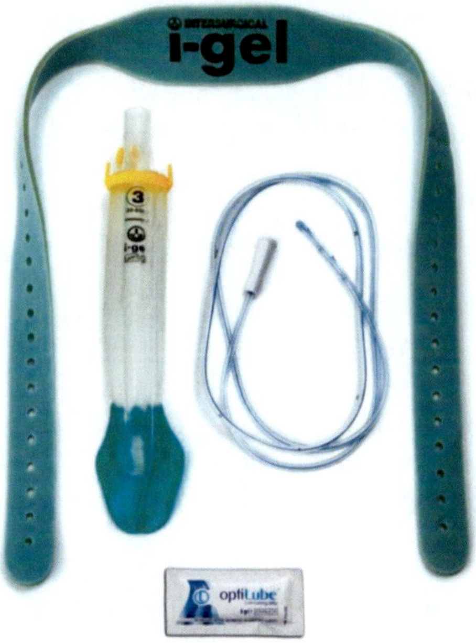

Figure 4. i-gel O_2 Resus Pack contains the i-gel device, sachet of lubricant, suction tube and airway support strap (courtesy of Intersurgical® Ltd., UK).

REFERENCES

[1] J. P. Nolan and D. Lockey, Airway management for out-of-hospital cardiac arrest – More data required, *Resuscitation* 80: 1333-4 (2009).

[2] Resuscitation Council UK, Adult Advanced Life Support. Chapter 7 [online] Available from: http://www.resus.org.uk/pages/als.pdf (2010).

[3] M. C. White, T. M. Cook and P. A. Stoddart PA, A critique of elective pediatric supraglottic airway devices, *Paediatr. Anaesth.* 19, 55-65 (2009).

[4] H. Idris and A. Gabrielli, Advances in airway management, *Emerg. Med. Clin. N. Am.* 20, 843-57 (2002).

[5] UK Resuscitation Council, Advanced Life Support Guide. 5th Ed., *London: UK Resuscitation Council* (2010).

[6] P. A. Baker and J. B. Webber, Failure to ventilate with supraglottic airways after drowning, *Anaesth. Intensive Care* 39, 675-7 (2011).

[7] O. A. Bamgbade, W. R. Macnab and W. M. Khalaf, Evaluation of the i-gel® airway in 300 patients, *Eur. J. Anaesthesiol.* 25, 865-6 (2008).

[8] B. Richez, L. Saltel, F. Banchereau, R. Torrielli and A. M. Cros, (2008) A new single use supraglottic airway with a noninflatable cuff and an esophageal vent: An observational study of the i-gel®, *Anaesthesia* 106, 1137-9 (2008).

[9] N. M. Wharton, B. Gibbison, D. A. Gabbott, G. M. Haslam, N. Muchatuta and T. M. Cook, i-gel® insertion by novices in manikins and patients. *Anaesthesia* 63, 991-5 (2008).

[10] J. J. Gatward, M. J. Thomas, J. P. Nolan and T. M. Cook TM, Effect of chest compressions on the time taken to insert airway devices in a manikin, *Br. J. Anaesth.* 100, 351-6 (2008).

[11] J. J. Gatward, T. M. Cook, C. Seller, J. Handel, T. Simpson, V. Vanek and F. Kelly, Evaluation of the size 4 i-gel® airway in one hundred non-paralysed patients, *Anaesthesia* 63, 1124-30 (2008).

[12] B. Sharma, R. Sehgal, C. Sahai and J. Sood, PLMA vs i-gel®: a comparitive evaluation of respiratory mechanics in laparoscopic cholecystectomy, *J. Anaesth. Clin. Pharmacol.* 26, 451-7 (2010).

[13] D. A. Gabbott and R. Beringer R., The i-gel® supraglottic airway: A potential role for resusctiation? *Resuscitation* 73, 161-2 (2007).

[14] C. D. Deakin, J. P. Nolan, J. Soar, K. Sunde, R. W. Koster, G. B. Smith and G. D. Perkins, European Resuscitation Council Guidelines for Resuscitation 2010 Section 4. Adult advanced life support, *Resuscitation* 81, 1305-52 (2010).

[15] J. Soar, The i-gel® supraglottic airway and resuscitation – some initial thoughts, *Resuscitation* 74, 197 (2007).

[16] K. M. Jackson and T. M. Cook, Evaluation of four airway training manikins as patient simulatros for the insertion of eight types of supraglottic airway devices, *Anaesthesia* 62, 388-93 (2007).

[17] W. Schmidbauer, S. Bercker, T. Volk, G. Bogusch, G. Mager and T. Kerner, Oesophageal seal of the novel supralaryngeal airway device i-gel® in comparison with the laryngeal mask airways Classic and ProSeal using a cadaver model, *Br. J. Anaesth.* 102, 135-9 (2009).

[18] C. J. Acott, Extraglottic airway devices for use in diving medicine – part 3: the i-gel®, *Diving Hyperbar. Med.* 38, 124-7 (2008).

[19] Fourth National Audit Project of the Royal College of Anaesthetists and the Difficult Airway Society, Major complications of airway management in the UK. Report and Findings (2011).

[20] J. P. Nolan, J. Soar, D. A. Zideman, D. Biarent, L. L. Bossaert, C. Deakin, R. W. Koster, J. Wyllie and B. Bottiger B, European Resuscitation Council Guidelines for Resuscitation 2010 Section 1. Executive summary. *Resuscitation* 81:1219-76 (2010).

[21] E. Piraccini, R. M. Corso, V. Agnoletti, S. Maitan and G. Gambale, Use of the i-gel for tracheal intubation without the interruption of chest compressions, *J. Emerg. Med.* 43, e67-8 (2012).

[22] J. Tiesmeier and M. Emmerich, Successful use of the i-gel supraglottic airway as a conduit for blind pre-hospital intubation during resuscitation, *Resuscitation* (2011).

[23] C. Larkin, B. King, A. D´Agapeyeff and D. Gabbott, iGel supraglottic airway use during hospital cardiopulmonary resuscitation, *Resuscitation* 83, e141 (2012).

[24] M. Thomas and J. Benger, Pre-hospital resuscitation using the iGEL, *Resuscitation* 80, 1437 (2009).

[25] K. Ruetzler, C. Gruber, S. Nabecker, P. Wohlfarth, A. Priemayr, M. Frass, O. Kimberger, D. I. Sessler and B. Roessler, Hands-off time during insertion of six airway devices during cardiopulmonary resuscitation: a randomized manikin trial, *Resuscitation* 82, 1060-3 (2011).

[26] C. H. Wiese, J. Bahr, A. F. Popov, J. M. Hinz and B. M. Graf BM, Influence of airway management strategy on 'no-flow'time' in a standardized single rescuer manikin scenario – a comparison between LTS-D and i-gel®, *Resuscitation* 80, 100-3 (2009).

[27] C. L. Yang, J. Wen, Y. P. Li and Y. K. Shi, Cardiocerebral resuscitation vs cardio-pulmonary resuscitation for cardiac arrest: a systematic review, *Am. J. Emerg. Med.* 30, 784-93 (2012).

[28] American Heart Association in collaboration with International Liaison Committee on Resuscitation, Guidelines 2000 for cardiopulmonary resuscitation and emergency cardiovascular care: international consensus on science, *Circulation* 102, 1-348 (2000).

[29] J. P. Nolan, Prehospital and resuscitative airway care: should the gold standard be reassessed? *Curr. Opin. Crit. Care* 7, 413-21 (2001).

[30] J. P. Nolan and J. Soar J, Airway techniques and ventilation strategies, *Curr. Opin. Crit. Care* 14, 279-86 (2008).

[31] T. Kitamura, T. Iwami, T. Kawamura, K. Nagao, H. Tanaka and A. Hiraide, Bystander-initiated rescue breathing for out-of-hospital cardiac arrests of noncardiac origin, *Circulation* 122, 293-9 (2010).

[32] M. M. Hayes, G. A. Ewy, N. D. Anavy, R. W. Hilwig, A. B. Sanders, R. A. Berg, C. W. Otto and K. B. Kern, Continuous passive oxygen insufflation results in a similar outcome to positive pressure ventilation in a swine model of out-of-hospital ventricular fibrillation, *Resuscitation* 74, 357-65 (2007).

[33] S. Steen, Q. Liao, L. Pierre, A. Paskevicius and T. Sjoberg, Continuous intratracheal insufflation of oxygen improves the efficacy of mechanical chest compressions - active decompression CPR, *Resuscitation* 62, 219-27 (2004).

[34] B. J. Bobrow, G. A. Ewy, L. Clark, V. Chikani, R. A. Berg, A. B. Sanders, T. F. Vadeboncoeur, R. W. Hilwig and K. B. Kern, Passive oxygen insufflation is superior to bag-valve-mask ventilation for witnessed ventricular fibrillation out-of-hospital cardiac arrest, *Ann. Emerg. Med.* 54, 656-62 (2009).

Conflict of interest: Amy L. Williams and Rebecca M. Anderson are employees of Intersurgical Ltd. Dr Muhammed A. Nasir is the inventor of the i-gel supraglottic airway.

In: The i-gel Supraglottic Airway
Editors: Pavel Michalek and William Donaldson
ISBN: 978-1-62417-897-9

Chapter 13

Complications Related to the i-gel Airway

***William Donaldson*[1,*] *and Pavel Michalek*[1,2]**
[1]Department of Anaesthesia, Antrim Area Hospital, UK
[2]Department of Anesthesia and Intensive Medicine,
First Medical Faculty of the Charles University and
General University Hospital, Prague, Czech Republic

Abstract

The incidence of complications associated with the i-gel and other supraglottic airway devices (SADs) is low when used in accordance with manufacturers' guidelines, and generally lower for SADs than for the endotracheal tube. Some complications can carry with them a significant degree of morbidity such as (regurgitation leading to) aspiration of gastric contents, laryngospasm and trauma associated with insertion of the device, or its position. 'Minor' complications include sore throat, dysphonia, and dysphagia, are more common and, although they carry less morbidity with them, impact on the patient experience and should not be discounted as trivial.

This chapter reviews complications associated with SADs in general and specifically those reported with the i-gel airway.

Introduction

The classic Laryngeal Mask Airway (LMA Classic®, cLMA, LMA company, Mahe, Seychelles) is the prototypical supraglottic airway device (SAD). It was invented by Dr Brain, and was conceived as an alternative to either the facemask or the tracheal tube for both spontaneous and controlled ventilation [1]. It was introduced into the clinical arena in 1988. Its use has been extensively studied: it is the most studied SAD with over 2500 publications [2]. To date, over 300 million insertions of the device have been carried out [3].

* Corresponding author: William Donaldson. E-mail address: willdonaldson@mac.com.

The i-gel is a second-generation device, introduced into clinical practice in 2007. It differs from most other SADs in that it lacks an inflatable cuff – a feature that has led some authors to suggest that it may cause less complications related to compression of the larynx and pharynx [4]. In common with other 2nd generation SADs, the i-gel possesses a gastric channel. This feature allows the device to separate the respiratory and gastrointestinal tracts and may confer an advantage when dealing with regurgitated fluid.

Complications

National Audit Project 4 (NAP4)

The fourth National Audit Project (NAP4), a joint prospective study into major complications of airway management between the Royal College of Anaesthetists and the Difficult Airway Society in the United Kingdom, was published in March 2011 [5].

The report estimated that 2.9 million general anesthetics are carried out each year in the UK. There were 133 complications reported that related to anesthesia (the Intensive Care and the Emergency Departments were considered separately), giving an incidence of complications related to general anesthesia of 1:22000. The authors note that a wide degree of under-reporting most likely occurred and that the true incidence is probably much higher.

NAP4 found that in 56% of general anesthetics, the airway was managed with a SAD. Complications relating to the use of SADs were examined in detail in Section 2: chapter 11 of the report [6]. The types of complications associated with these devices are shown in table 1:

There were three common themes that the report's authors found in complications relating to SAD use: poor patient selection, poor operation selection and inexpert use.

Regurgitation and Aspiration

Regurgitation of gastric contents is a distinct entity from, and may not necessarily lead to, aspiration of gastric contents. It is a phenomenon that is multifactorial [7] (see Table 2). Whether regurgitation leads to aspiration depends on the amount of gastric content regurgitated and the degree of protection of the respiratory tract, either by the presence of active laryngeal reflexes in an awake patient or with a device such as a SAD or a cuffed endotracheal tube in a patient undergoing general anesthesia.

Table 1. Airway complications associated with SADs reported to NAP4

• Aspiration
• Airway trauma
• Loss of airway on insertion
• Failed insertion
• Displacement after insertion
• Loss of airway during maintenance
• Extubation-related problems

Table 2. factors predisposing to regurgitation (after Asai [7])

Patient factors	Full stomach Diabetes Mellitus Increased intracranial pressure Gastrointestinal obstruction Recurrent regurgitation Raised intra-abdominal pressure
Operation factors	Upper abdominal surgery Lithotomy/ head-down positions Laparoscopic surgery
Anesthesia factors	Insufficient depth of anesthesia Gastric insufflation Early removal of airway device
Device factors	SADs decrease lower esophageal sphincter tone SADs may increase gastric insufflation

NAP4 found that primary aspiration of gastric contents led to eight deaths and two cases of brain damage. In the cases reviewed by the project, primary aspiration of gastric contents was the leading cause of these outcomes - accounting for 50% of anesthesia-related deaths and 53% of outcomes of death and brain damage. The primary method of airway management in these patients was recorded as: laryngeal mask airway 13, i-gel 1, tracheal tube 8 and none 1.

The NAP4 report looked in detail at complications associated with the use of supraglottic airways [6]. Two of the key findings regarding aspiration were that:

1 Patients were poorly assessed for their risk of regurgitation: patients invariably had risks factors for regurgitation that were overlooked.
2 The choice of airway management in some patients was poor: many had SADs inserted where there were clear indications for endotracheal intubation.

1st Generation Supraglottic Airways

The prototypical SAD is the cLMA. It is an example of a first-generation SAD and, as such, consists of a stem and an inflatable cuff with no separate gastric channel. Its use is indicated for airway maintenance during routine and emergency anesthetic procedures in fasted patients using either spontaneous or controlled ventilation [3].

The incidence of regurgitation with the classic LMA in early studies was found to be as high as 25% [8]. A large meta-analysis by Brimacombe and Berry in 1995 showed this to be a gross overestimate. In this analysis (involving 12901 patients) the incidence of aspiration was found to be 0.02% [9]. The incidence of aspiration with laryngeal masks has been found to be comparable to that with endotracheal tubes, when precautions regarding patient selection with these devices are followed [10]. However, SADs that are incorrectly positioned, particularly those through which positive-pressure ventilation is undertaken may lead to gastric insufflation and an increased risk of regurgitation of gastric contents [11].

The idea of providing-positive pressure through a SAD has polarized opinion leading to an editorial in the British Journal of Anaesthesia [12], although this editorial predated the emergence of many of the 2nd generation SADs that have been specifically designed to overcome some of the problems that beset the previous generation.

2nd Generation Supraglottic Airways

Second-generation devices were developed with features designed to decrease the risk of aspiration: in general, these devices have a separate gastric channel or have a compartment designed to contain any regurgitated material.

Devices with a dedicated second gastric channel include:

- Proseal-laryngeal mask airway® (PLMA, Intavent Direct, Maidenhead, UK)
- LMA-Supreme® (Intavent Direct, Maidenhead, UK)
- Laryngeal tube suction II (LTS-II) which has a disposable version (LTS-D, VBM Mediztechnik GmBH, Sulz, Germany)
- i-gel® (Intersurgical Ltd., Wokingham, UK)

Devices designed to trap and store regurgitated material:

- The Streamlined Liner of the Pharynx Airway (SLIPA, SLIPA medical, Douglas, Isle of Man, UK) is a cuffless airway device, with a large compartment intended to trap and store regurgitated fluid.

The net result of either design feature is the intended protection of the respiratory tract from regurgitated gastric content. As an additional benefit to their design features many 2nd generation devices generate a better airway sealing pressure, rendering them more suitable as devices through which controlled ventilation may be undertaken.

Do second generation devices offer greater protection against regurgitation and aspiration of gastric contents?

The answer is unclear, in part, due to the low incidence of regurgitation. For example, if a clinical trial that was adequately powered was set up to detect a 50% reduction in aspiration between the PLMA and cLMA, 1.3 million patients would be required in each arm [2].

It is well recognized that gastric insufflation increases the risk of regurgitation. Schmidbauer et al. recently published the results of a cadaveric study which examined the performance of several devices, all of which were 2nd generation SADs, in a simulated airway obstruction model. The authors studied the degree of gastric insufflation when each of the devices was exposed to airway pressures of 20, 40 and 60mbar.

The authors found that all devices withstood gastric insufflation at 20mbar, but that each of the devices tested was associated with gastric insufflation at pressures of 40 and 60mbar [13]. They concluded that airway pressures of greater than 20mbar should be avoided when using SADs. The findings cannot, however, be related directly to clinical practice and this is commented upon by the authors.

Regurgitation and Aspiration: The i-gel

As a second-generation device, the i-gel possesses a separate gastric channel, which is designed to separate the respiratory and gastrointestinal tracts. Despite, and in some cases because of, these features there have been cases described in the literature of both regurgitation and aspiration of gastric contents:

Gibbison et al described a case series of three patients who regurgitated under anesthesia [14]. In two of these cases, the authors stated that the i-gel protected the patients from aspiration. The third case did aspirate, but with no complications and was discharged the same day. The authors state that the drain tube allowed recognition of regurgitation, which they suggest may have gone undiscovered with the use of a first generation device. They conclude that the incidence of regurgitation and aspiration for the device is low, and noted that – at the time – no patients appeared to have come to harm from such episodes.

This phenomenon of 'recognition of regurgitation' is also described in a case by Liew et al [15]. The authors present the case of a young fit male who was adequately fasted. Halfway through the patient's operation they noted that yellow gastric contents were dripping from the gastric channel of the i-gel on to the floor. Despite efforts to pass a suction catheter, the regurgitation continued and a rapid sequence induction and intubation was performed, as per the manufacturer's recommendations [16]. The patient later confessed to the consumption of a can of a carbonated drink a few hours before induction, which he did not volunteer at the preoperative visit. The patient recovered with no adverse sequelae.

The i-gel has been found to have a lower esophageal seal than the cLMA and PLMA, but together with the PLMA was found to drain away regurgitated fluid effectively [17]. The lower esophageal seal is likely due to the fact that the tip of the i-gel is narrower – which was a deliberate design intended to decrease dysphagia associated with the SADs [2].

There is still a paucity of high-quality evidence associated with the i-gel and other 2nd generation SADs with regard to their ability to deal with the risk of regurgitation and aspiration and large, well-conducted trials are needed in this area. Despite this, the authors of NAP4 made recommendations regarding the use of a 2nd generation SAD, including: "If tracheal intubation is not considered to be indicated but there is some (small) increased concern about regurgitation risk a second generation supraglottic airway is a more logical choice than a first generation one." [6].

TRAUMA

Microscopic trauma associated with SAD insertion is thought to be relatively common but of little consequence and, in any case, difficult to detect. Macroscopic trauma, however, may lead to significant morbidity. It may occur at a number of sites and be caused by a number of mechanisms (Table 3).

The main areas are the pharyngeal mucosa, laryngeal apparatus, epiglottis, uvula, tongue, teeth and lips. Trauma may result in laceration and bleeding, ischemic injuries, or neurological injuries as a result of compression of nerves and may be caused directly through forceful placement, or indirectly by compression.

Minor trauma associated with device insertion is often evidenced by the presence of blood on the device upon its removal. The reported incidence of this for the cLMA is between 12-15% [18] and 10% in association with the PLMA [19]. Studies have reported an incidence of this phenomenon with the i-gel as low as 0% [20,21] and as high as 20% [22].

Despite the high incidence of blood in their study, Ragazzi et al. found that more patients complained of pharyngolaryngeal pain in the comparator group (LMA-Supreme). The typical incidence of blood on the i-gel at removal is between 4% and 13% in most published studies [23-27].

Lacerations to the pharynx associated with the cLMA have been reported; In one case this led to the pulmonary aspiration of blood [28]. Arytenoid dislocation has been reported after airway maintenance with a cLMA [29].

A response to the report highlighted methods that may lead to arytenoid trauma (direct contact with arytenoids, insertion with cuff inflated, insertion with rotation) but emphasized that when LMA was inserted using standard techniques, and when malpositioning was recognized and dealt with, the risk to the arytenoids was minimal [30]. This advice had already been dispensed by the device's inventor [31]. Despite Brain's advice – which reaffirmed the importance of adhering to the standard method of insertion - both uvular [32, 33] and epiglottic injuries [34] have been associated with LMA use. Injury to the lingual frenulum during insertion has been reported with use of the PLMA [35, 36], and the i-gel (discussed below). The mechanism of injury is usually backward folding of the tongue on insertion, stretching the frenulum.

Ischemia of the tongue has been described in association with the intubating laryngeal mask airway (ILMA) after prolonged insertion [37].

Table 3. sites, types and mechanisms of traumatic injuries associated with SADs

Site of injury	Type(s) of injury	Mechanism(s) of injury
Pharyngeal mucosa	Laceration Bruising	Forceful insertion, inadequate lubrication Prolonged insertion, too high cuff pressures
Laryngeal apparatus	Arytenoid dislocation Recurrent laryngeal nerve injury	Direct trauma Compression of the nerve in pirifom fossa
Uvula	Trauma leading to ischemia and necrosis	Direct trauma Prolonged compression
Epiglottis	Bruising Laceration	Incorrect or forceful insertion, anatomical abnormalities
Tongue	Frenular injury Lingual nerve injury	Incorrect or forceful insertion Compression of inferior or lateral surface of the tongue by cuff or tube of SAD
Teeth	Displacement Fracture of roots	Direct trauma Biting on SAD/ bite block
Lips	Laceration Nerve injury	Direct trauma Compression by device, taping to device

Dental injuries occur in about 1% of anesthetics, and are responsible for a significant proportion of legal claims against practitioners [38,39]. Dental injuries occur less frequently with SAD insertion than they do with direct laryngoscopy [40], and are also associated with removal of these devices. Few studies have looked for or mentioned dental damage in association with the i-gel, but where they have the incidence is very low [41-43]. Interestingly, Theiler's recently published cohort study cites poor dentition as an identifier for i-gel failure [44].

Dental damage is not all one way traffic: a letter to Anaesthesia described how a sharp crown exposed by decay tore the cuff of two cLMAs during insertion [45]. Particular care should be taken to assess the patient's dentition at the preoperative visit [40].

Trauma Associated with the i-gel

The technique of insertion of the i-gel differs to that of other SADs. Though insertion is usually straightforward, in cases of difficulty a few maneuvers are recommended by the manufacturer to aid insertion: deep rotation, jaw thrust and the triple maneuver. Inserting the device with an off-midline approach has been suggested [46]. Taxak and Gopinath noted in a letter to Anesthesiology that insertion of the i-gel may be hindered by obstruction caused by pushing the tongue back into the pharynx, stopping further advancement of the device [47]. The authors stated that they had followed the manufacturer's guidelines but that they had to reinsert the device having pulled out and stabilized the patient's tongue. In a reply to this letter, Theiler agrees that this may offer a solution and also points out that the base of the tongue may be displaced by the i-gel – advising that the position of the tongue should be checked after device insertion.

Michalek et al. described a series of two cases where there was trauma to the lingual frenulum following insertion of an i-gel, one of which required the use of electrical diathermy to stop the bleeding [48]. The authors noted that the deep bowl of the i-gel was likely to trap the tongue on insertion if due care was not taken to prevent this, and suggested the thumb technique: the gloved thumb of the non-dominant hand is inserted into the mouth. It is used to depress the tongue and can be used to provide traction for jaw thrust. The i-gel can then be passed over the operator's thumb.

A case where a size five i-gel was associated with massive laryngeal hemorrhage has been described by Dangelser and colleagues [49]. In this case, traumatic injury to an aryepiglottic fold was thought to be the source of the bleeding. The patient in whom the device was inserted was on steroid therapy for interstitial pneumonitis and the authors question whether the i-gel should be inserted in patients with mucosal fragility.

Nerve Injury

Nerve injuries associated with supraglottic airway devices have been well described in the literature. Injuries to the lingual nerve, hypoglossal nerve, inferior alveolar nerve and recurrent laryngeal nerves have been described in association with several different SADs [50-55]. Whilst the etiology of neurological injury by SADs is multifactorial, in many of these cases the inflatable cuff of the devices were implicated – either by rendering the device as being too rigid on insertion or by direct compression whilst the device was in situ.

Despite its lack of a cuff, nerve injury in association with the i-gel has been described; Theron described a case where a patient complained of a numb lower lip postoperatively. The cause was attributed to pressure on the mental nerve, either by taping the lower lip so that it came to lie against the bite block of the i-gel or by folding of the lower lip against the device and not noticing this [56]. The patient's symptoms subsided over a few days. In a reply to this letter, Chapman stresses the importance of taping the device correctly, size selection, lubrication and insertion technique [57].

Renes presented a case in which a patient complained of tongue numbness and loss of taste, following anesthesia where an i-gel was used to maintain the airway. After review by a neurologist, a diagnosis of bilateral lingual nerve injury was made. The authors postulated that the nerves could have been subjected to pressure by the buccal stabilizer of the device or by the proximal ridge in the bowl against the inferior surface of the tongue or at the lateral edge of the tongue (the most common site of injury to the lingual nerve) [58].

In their case series where they describe cases of i-gel associated trauma to the tongue, Michalek et al. also refer to symptoms in one of the cases consistent with an injury to the lingual nerve [48].

A recently published article describes cases of tongue numbness in association with both the i-gel and the LMA-Supreme, assumed to be secondary to lingual nerve injuries [59]. Symptoms resolved completely in both patients within two weeks. In their cohort study, Theiler et al. reported two instances of neurological damage [44]. In one case a patient described numbness of the tongue that resulted from it having been trapped between the device and the patient's lower teeth, with full resolution of symptoms within two months. A second case, this time of glossopharyngeal nerve injury, was attributed to having selected too large a size of i-gel (size 5) – basing this on the actual weight of the patient. The authors state that they should perhaps have taken into consideration the patient's height, sex and age. They go on to emphasize that device selection should involve choosing the smallest device that provides an adequate airway seal – particularly where patients are overweight or scheduled for longer procedures.

'Routine Complications' (Minor Adverse Events)

Less severe complications such as sore throat, dysphonia, dysphagia and pharyngeal dryness are well described and occur with greater frequency with SAD use than the complications already discussed in this chapter. Though they may not be associated with the same degree of morbidity, these 'routine complications' impact on patients' satisfaction [60].

Sore Throat

The term postoperative sore throat (POST) in the context of anesthesia is a blanket term [61]. On further questioning, patients often complain of one or more of the following symptoms: pharyngeal dryness, continuous throat pain (mild, moderate or severe), dysphagia, dysphonia, or odynophagia – pain on swallowing or eating.

The etiology of sore throat is unclear. Factors associated with increased incidences include female sex, use of succinylcholine, younger patients and gynecological surgery [61]. Trauma to different areas by different devices (SADs and endotracheal tubes) cause a similar incidence of POST[62].

The incidence of POST associated with use of the LMA ranges from 5.8% - 34% compared with 14.4% to 53% in association with endotracheal intubation [61]. Use of a facemask alone is associated with an incidence of sore throat of 3-8% [63]. There are differences in the sites of forces applied by a supraglottic airway (posterior pharynx) and endotracheal tubes (glottic entrance) which explain the different nature of complaints associated with them; dysphonia is more common with an endotracheal tube, and dysphagia more common with SADs [64].

There are several factors that may lead to the development of a sore throat with SAD use (Table 4):

Sore Throat and the i-gel Airway

Eschertzhuber and colleagues conducted a study where the mucosal pressures exerted by the LMA-Supreme and the i-gel over four anatomical locations were measured. The authors found that the mucosal pressures exerted by both devices were low, but that pressures exerted by the LMA-Supreme were highest in the hypopharynx [25]. They found that the i-gel exerted pressure evenly across all locations studied.

The soft nature of the cuff of the i-gel might lead one to expect a lower incidence of sore throat than with other SADs [4] – and in some comparative studies this is the case [21, 43, 65, 66]. Other studies have demonstrated a higher incidence of sore throat with the i-gel [23, 26, 27]. In the of the studies by Kleine-Bruegenney and Theiler which looked at blind intubation, the authors stated that passage of the harder (Rüsch and Magill) PVC tubes through the i-gel may have contributed to the higher incidence of sore throat seen with the i-gel [26, 27].

Table 4. Factors implicated in the development of POST with SADs

Factor	Mechanism
Insertion technique	Leading edge of deflated cuff may cause trauma Inflated cuff causes more epiglottic downfolding, which increases POST Repeated attempts are associated with increased POST
Size of device	Smaller sizes of SAD are associated with less POST
Use of lubricants	Adequate lubrication is essential Lidocaine gel is associated with an increase in POST
Over inflation of the cuff	Some studies have shown decreased POST with intracuff pressure monitoring
Duration of surgery	Increased POST in operations of over 60min duration
Airway gases	Lack of humidification can dry mucosal surfaces and increase POST

The comparator in each of these studies was the single-use intubating LMA, which has a softer tracheal tube. Theiler's large prospective cohort study, that involved 2049 i-gel insertions, reported an incidence of sore throat of 2.3%, although the authors acknowledge that this is likely to be an underestimate [44]. The size of the i-gel used has been implicated in the etiology of sore throat, with one study finding a 50% incidence of sore throat where a size 5 i-gel was used and an incidence of only 7% where a size 4 was used [67]. Similar results have been found for the cLMA, where selection of a smaller sized device led to a decrease in the incidence of sore throat [68].

Management of POST

The majority of cases of sore throat associated with SADs are self-limiting. Patients should be reassured and asked to rest their voices. Pain may be treated with gargles containing anti-inflammatory and analgesic agents, or with systemic agents. Where sore throat persists, particularly if it associated with hoarseness – referral to an otolaryngologist for further investigation may be warranted [63].

AVOIDING COMPLICATIONS WITH THE I-GEL

Given the complications described above, there are a number of areas that the anesthesiologist can focus on in order to decrease the chances of adverse events when using the i-gel airway. These are summarized below (Table 5):

Table 5. Areas of focus to prevent complications with use of the i-gel airway

Area of focus	Key points
Airway assessment	Check mouth opening and dentition Mallampatti III patients contraindicated Watch for neck shape and thyroid/cricoid cartilage dimensions
Assessment of risk of regurgitation	Check for risk factors (see Table 1)
Patient selection	Care with patients with central obesity, may require device selection based on ideal weight
Device selection	Use smaller device if seal acceptable and for prolonged surgery
Head positioning	Neck flexion, head extension: "sniffing the morning air" for insertion Maintain head and neck neutral or in flexion, avoid neck extension
Device insertion	Lubricate all aspects of device as per manufacturer's guidance Ensure adequate depth of anesthesia Insert until definitive resistance (with the incisor marking approximate to the incisors) Avoid forceful insertion May consider paramidline approach or using a thumb to depress the tongue
Post insertion checks	Check tongue after insertion Ensure that lips/tongue are not taped to teeth or bite block Ensure that air leaks are not apparent, either gastric or through the gastric channel of the i-gel
Review of gastric channel	Regularly check the gastric channel intraoperatively

Conclusion

The i-gel airway is associated with a low incidence of complications, which is similar to other second-generation SADS. Careful adherence to the manufacturer's guidelines with regard to device selection, lubrication, insertion and fixation will limit the occurrence of some of the issues that have been described in this chapter.

Of particular importance with the use of any SAD is appropriate patient assessment. Scrupulous attention should be made to airway (including dental) assessment and the assessment of the risk of regurgitation.

References

[1] A. I. Brain, The laryngeal mask—a new concept in airway management, *Br. J. Anaesth.* 55, 801–6 (1983).

[2] T. M. Cook and B. Howes, Supraglottic airway devices: recent advances, *Cont. Educ. Anaesth. Crit. Care Pain* 11, 56-61 (2011).

[3] Instructions for use - LMA Classic, LMA Flexible single use and LMA Unique. The LMA Company pp. 1–2. 2011

[4] R. M. Levitan and W. C. Kinkle, Initial anatomic investigations of the i-gel airway: a novel supraglottic airway without inflatable cuff, *Anaesthesia* 60, 1022–6 (2005).

[5] T. M. Cook, N. Woodall and C. Frerk, on behalf of the Fourth National Audit Project, Major complications of airway management in the UK: results of the Fourth National Audit Project of the Royal College of Anaesthetists and the Difficult Airway Society. Part 1: Anaesthesia, *Br. J. Anaesth.* 106, 617–631 (2011).

[6] Section 2 of the NAP 4 report. 4th National Audit Project (NAP4): Major complications of airway management in the United Kingdom - Report and Findings – March 2011. http://www.rcoa.ac.uk/node/1413

[7] T. Asai, Editorial II: Who is at increased risk of pulmonary aspiration? *Br. J. Anaesth.* 93, 497–500 (2004).

[8] P. Barker, J. A. Langton, P. J. Murphy and D. J. Rowbotham, Regurgitation of gastric contents during general anaesthesia using the laryngeal mask airway, *Br. J. Anaesth.* 69, 314–315 (1992).

[9] J. R. Brimacombe and A. Berry, The incidence of aspiration associated with the laryngeal mask airway: a meta-analysis of published literature, *J. Clin. Anesth.* 7, 297–305 (1995).

[10] A. Bernardini and G. Natalini G, Risk of pulmonary aspiration with laryngeal mask airway and tracheal tube: analysis on 65712 procedures with positive pressure ventilation, *Anaesthesia* 64, 1289–1294 (2009).

[11] J. H. Devitt, R. Wenstone, A. G. Noel and M. P. O'Donnell, The laryngeal mask airway and positive-pressure ventilation, *Anesthesiology* 80, 550–5 (1994).

[12] G. Sidaras and J. M. Hunter, Is it safe to artificially ventilate a paralysed patient through the laryngeal mask? The jury is still out, *Br. J. Anaesth.* 86, 749–753 (2001).

[13] W. Schmidbauer, H. Genzwürker, O. Ahlers, H. Proquitte and T. Kerner, Cadaver study of oesophageal insufflation with supraglottic airway devices during positive pressure ventilation in an obstructed airway, *Br. J. Anaesth.* 109, 454–8 (2012).

[14] B. Gibbison, T. M. Cook and C. Seller, Case series: protection from aspiration and failure of protection from aspiration with the i-gel airway, *Br. J. Anaesth.* 100, 415–417 (2008).

[15] G. Liew, B. John and S. Ahmed, Aspiration recognition with an i-gel airway, *Anaesthesia* 63, 786 (2008).

[16] i-gel user guide 2012. Intersurgical Ltd., Wokingham, UK.

[17] W. Schmidbauer, S. Bercker, T. Volk, G. Bogusch, G. Mager and T. Kerner, Oesophageal seal of the novel supralaryngeal airway device i-gel™ in comparison with the laryngeal mask airways Classic™ and ProSeal™ using a cadaver model, *Br. J. Anaesth.* 102, 135–9 (2009).

[18] M. R. Parker and C. J. Day, Visible and occult blood contamination of laryngeal mask airways and tracheal tubes used in adult anaesthesia, *Anaesthesia* 55, 388–390 (2000).

[19] T. M. Cook, G. Lee and J. P. Nolan, The proseal™ laryngeal mask airway: a review of the literature, *Can. J. Anesth.* 52, 739–60 (2005).

[20] M. Ibrahim, A. Ragab and H. El Shamaa, i-gel vs cuffed tracheal tube during volume controlled ventilation in elective laparoscopic cholecystectomy, *Egypt. J. Anaesth.* 27, 7–11 (2011).

[21] B. Sharma, R. Sehgal, C. Sahai and J. Sood, PLMA vs. i-gel: a comparative evaluation of respiratory mechanics in laparoscopic cholecystectomy, *J. Anaesthesiol. Clin. Pharmacol.* 26, 451–7 (2010).

[22] R. Ragazzi, L. Finessi, I. Farinelli, R. Alvisi and C. A. Volta, LMA Supreme™ vs i-gel™: a comparison of insertion success in novices, *Anaesthesia* 67, 384–8 (2012).

[23] T. C. Van Zundert and J. R. Brimacombe, Similar oropharyngeal leak pressures during anaesthesia with i-gel, LMA-ProSeal and LMA-Supreme laryngeal masks, *Acta Anaesthesiol. Belg.* 63, 35–41 (2012).

[24] J. R. Lee, M. S. Kim, J. T. Kim, H. J. Byon, Y. H. Park, H. S. Kim and C. S. Kim, A randomised trial comparing the i-gel™ with the LMA Classic™ in children, *Anaesthesia* 67(6), 606–611 (2012).

[25] S. Eschertzhuber, J. Brimacombe, M. Kaufmann, C. Keller and W. Tiefenthaler, Directly measured mucosal pressures produced by the i-gel™ and laryngeal mask airway Supreme™ in paralysed anaesthetised patients, *Anaesthesia* 67(4), 407–410 (2012).

[26] M. Kleine-Brueggeney, L. Theiler, N. Urwyler, A. Vogt A and R. Greif, Randomized trial comparing the i-gel™ and Magill tracheal tube with the single-use ILMA™ and ILMA™ tracheal tube for fibreoptic-guided intubation in anaesthetized patients with a predicted difficult airway, *Br. J. Anaesth.* 107, 251–7 (2011).

[27] L. Theiler, M. Kleine-Brueggeney, N. Urwyler, T. Graf, C. Luyet and R. Greif, Randomized clinical trial of the i-gel™ and Magill tracheal tube or single-use ILMA™ and ILMA™ tracheal tube for blind intubation in anaesthetized patients with a predicted difficult airway, *Br. J. Anaesth.* 107, 243–50 (2011).

[28] A. Norton, J. Germonpré and T. Semple, Pulmonary aspiration of blood following traumatic laryngeal mask airway insertion, *Anaesth. Intensive Care* 26(2), 213–215 (1998).

[29] M. K. Rosenberg, E. Rontal, M. Rontal and M. Lebenbom-Mansour, Arytenoid cartilage dislocation caused by a laryngeal mask airway treated with chemical splinting, *Anesth. Analg.* 83, 1335-6 (1996).

[30] J. R. Brimacombe, Arytenoid dislocation and the laryngeal mask airway, *Anesth. Analg.* 85, 463 (1997).

[31] A. Brain, Laryngeal mask misplacement—causes, consequences and solutions, *Anaesthesia* 47, 531–532 (1992).

[32] J. J. Lee, Laryngeal mask and trauma to uvula, *Anaesthesia* 44, 1014–1015 (1989).

[33] S. R. Emmett, S. D. Lloyd and M. N. Johnston, Uvular trauma from a laryngeal mask, *Br. J. Anaesth.* 109, 468-9 (2012).

[34] B. McKinney and R. Grigg, Epiglottitis after anaesthesia with a laryngeal mask, *Anaesth. Intensive Care* 23, 618–619 (1995).

[35] Z. M. Haris, W. T. Loo and J. Brimacombe, Frenular injury during insertion of the ProSeal laryngeal mask airway using the introducer tool technique, *Anesth. Analg.* 102, 1906–1907 (2006).

[36] M.-J. Park, H.-S. Kim, J.-T. Kim, C.-S. Kim, and S.-D. Kim, Tearing of the lingual frenulum caused by insertion of the ProSeal LMA in a child - a case report. *Korean J. Anesthesiol.* 57, 644 (2009).

[37] N. S. Gerstein, D. Braude, J. S. Harding, and A. Douglas, Lingual ischemia from prolonged insertion of a fastrach laryngeal mask airway, *West J. Emerg. Med.* 12, 124–127 (2011).

[38] T. M. Cook, S. Scott, and R. Mihai, Litigation related to airway and respiratory complications of anaesthesia: an analysis of claims against the NHS in England 1995-2007, *Anaesthesia* 65, 556–563 (2010).

[39] N. M. Cass, Medicolegal claims against anaesthetists: a 20 year study, *Anaesth. Intensive Care* 32, 47-58 (2004).

[40] J. S. Yasny, Perioperative dental considerations for the anesthesiologist, *Anesth. Analg.* 108, 1564–1573 (2009).

[41] P. Jindal, A. A. Rizvi, G. Khurana and J. P.Sharma, Safety and efficacy of insertion of supraglottic device in anaesthetised patients by first-time users, *S. Afr. J. Anaesthesiol. Analg.* 16, 23-6 (2010).

[42] I. Singh, M. Gupta and M. Tandon, Comparison of clinical performance of i-gel with LMA-Proseal in elective surgeries. *Indian J. Anaesth.* 53, 302–5 (2009).

[43] W. H. Teoh, K. M. Lee, T. Suhitharan, Z. Yahaya, M. M. Teo and A. T. Sia, Comparison of the LMA Supreme vs the i-gel™ in paralysed patients undergoing gynaecological laparoscopic surgery with controlled ventilation, *Anaesthesia* 65, 1173–9 (2010).

[44] L. Theiler, M. Gutzmann, M. Kleine-Brueggeney, N. Urwyler, B. Kaempfen and R. Greif, i-gel™ supraglottic airway in clinical practice: a prospective observational multicentre study, *Br. J. Anaesth.* (2012). [Epub. ahead of print]

[45] H. A. McLure, Dental damage to the laryngeal mask, *Anaesthesia* 51, 1078–1079 (1996).
[46] L. G. Theiler, M. Kleine-Brueggeney, D. Kaiser, N. Urwyler, C. Luyet, A. Vogt and R. Greif, Crossover comparison of the laryngeal mask supreme and the i-gel in simulated difficult airway scenario in anesthetized patients, *Anesthesiology* 111, 55–62 (2009).
[47] S. Taxak and A. Gopinath, Insertion of the i-gel™ airway obstructed by the tongue, *Anesthesiology* 112, 500-1 (2010).
[48] P. Michalek, W. J. Donaldson and J. D. Hinds, Tongue trauma associated with the i-gel supraglottic airway, *Anaesthesia* 64, 692-3 (2009).
[49] G. Dangelser, A. S. Dincq, G. Lawson and E. Collard, Case report: severe laryngeal hemorrhage after withdrawal of a size 5 i-gel in elective surgery, *Acta Anaesthesiol. Belg.* 60, 255–257 (2009).
[50] A. Stewart and W. A. Lindsay, Bilateral hypoglossal nerve injury following the use of the laryngeal mask airway, *Anaesthesia* 57, 264–265 (2002).
[51] D. Hanumanthaiah, S. Masud and A. Ranganath, Inferior alveolar nerve injury with laryngeal mask airway: a case report, *J. Med. Case Rep.* 5, 122 (2011).
[52] J. Brimacombe, G. Clarke and C. Keller, Lingual nerve injury associated with the ProSeal laryngeal mask airway: a case report and review of the literature, *Br. J. Anaesth.* 95, 420–423 (2005).
[53] P. Trümpelmann and T. Cook, Unilateral hypoglossal nerve injury following the use of a ProSeal™ laryngeal mask, *Anaesthesia* 60, 101–102 (2005).
[54] K. Endo, Y. Okabe, Y.Maruyama, T, Tsukatani and M. Furukawa, Bilateral vocal cord paralysis caused by laryngeal mask airway, *Am. J. Otolaryn.* 28, 126–129 (2007).
[55] K. Nagai, C. Sakuramoto and F. Goto, Unilateral hypoglossal nerve paralysis following the use of the laryngeal mask airway, *Anaesthesia* 49, 603–604 (1994).
[56] S. Baxter, Phenomenon with i-gel airway? *Anaesthesia* 63, 1265 (2008).
[57] D. Chapman, Nerve damage following the use of an i-gel supraglottic airway device. A reply, *Anaesthesia* 63(4), 441–2 (2008).
[58] S. H. Renes, R. Zwart, G. J. Scheffer, and S. Renes, Lingual nerve injury following the use of an i-gel laryngeal mask, *Anaesthesia* 66, 226–227 (2011).
[59] P. Rujirojindakul, C. Prechawai and E. Watanayomnaporn, Tongue numbness following laryngeal mask airway Supreme™ and i-gel™ insertion: two case reports, *Acta Anaesthesiol. Scand.* (2012). [Epub ahead of print]
[60] A. Macario, M. Weinger, S. Carney and A. Kim, Which clinical anesthesia outcomes are important to avoid? The perspective of patients, *Anesth. Analg.* 89, 652–652 (1999).
[61] F. E. McHardy and F. Chung, Postoperative sore throat: cause, prevention and treatment, *Anaesthesia* 54, 444–453 (1999).
[62] P. E. Scuderi, Postoperative sore throat: more answers than questions, *Anesth. Analg.* 111, 831–832 (2010).
[63] L. Zuccherelli, Postoperative upper airway problems, *S. Afr. J. Anaesthesiol. Analg.* 9, 1–5 (2007).
[64] M. Chandler, Tracheal intubation and sore throat: a mechanical explanation, *Anaesthesia* 57, 155–161 (2002).

[65] J. F. Heuer, M. Stiller, J. Rathgeber, C. Eich, K. Züchner, M. Bauer and A. Timmermann, Evaluation der neuen Kehlkopfmasken Ambu AuraOnce™ und Intersurgical i-gel™, *Anaesthesist* 58, 813–20 (2009). [Article in German, abstract in English.]

[66] C. Keijzer, D. R. Buitelaar, K. M. Efthymiou, M. Šrámek, J. ten Cate, M. Ronday, T. Stoppa, J. M. Huitink and P. F. Schutte, A comparison of postoperative throat and neck complaints after the use of the i-gel® and the La Premiere® disposable laryngeal mask: a double-blinded, randomized, controlled trial, *Anesth. Analg.* 109, 1092–5 (2009).

[67] D. Cattano, L. Ferrario, V. Maddukuri, S. Sridhar, Y. Khalil and C. A. Hagberg, A randomized clinical comparison of the Intersurgical i-gel and LMA Unique in non-obese adults during general surgery, *Minerva Anestesiol.* 77, 292–7 (2011).

[68] D. M. Grady, F. McHardy, J. Wong, F. Jin, D. Tong, and F. Chung, Pharyngolaryngeal morbidity with the laryngeal mask airway in spontaneously breathing patients: does size matter? *Anesthesiology* 94, 760 (2001).

Conflict of interest: Dr Donaldson has delivered lectures on the i-gel for Intersurgical.

In: The i-gel Supraglottic Airway
Editors: Pavel Michalek and William Donaldson
ISBN: 978-1-62417-897-9

Chapter 14

COMPARISON OF THE I-GEL WITH OTHER SUPRAGLOTTIC AIRWAY DEVICES

***Francis P. McAleavey*[1,*] *and Pavel Michalek*[1,2]**
[1]Department of Anaesthesia, Antrim Area Hospital, UK
[2]Department of Anaesthesia and Intensive Care,
First Medical Faculty of the Charles University and
General University Hospital, Prague, Czech Republic

ABSTRACT

Supraglottic airway devices are routinely used to maintain airway patency in a variety of in and out-of-hospital scenarios. There is a wide range of supraglottic airway devices available to the clinician, each with unique design features which set it apart from its competitors.

The i-gel is a supraglottic airway device, which differs from familiar laryngeal mask airways in that it lacks an inflatable cuff - the oropharyngeal seal instead being maintained by the presence of a cuff formed from a thermoplastic elastomer. Among the reported advantages which the i-gel enjoys over its competitors are: greater ease of use, higher oropharyngeal seal pressures, reduced leak and a reduced incidence of post-operative throat pain. The wider profile of its integrated airway lumen and bite block should also render it less likely to malrotate while in situ.

INTRODUCTION

Supraglottic airway devices are routinely used to maintain airway patency in anesthetized patients where there is no clear indication for endotracheal intubation [1, 2]. Their rise in popularity has led to the production of several different devices which may be used to fulfil this role.

* Corresponding author: Francis P. McAleavey. E-mail address: fpmcaleavey@gmail.com.

Recently, pediatric sizes of the i-gel airway have become available. The manufacturers feel that design features specific to the i-gel as compared to more conventional supraglottic airways (i.e. more closely related to the original model as conceived by Brain) may confer some benefit in the management of pediatric airways. Children are known to be more susceptible to complications arising from the use of supraglottic airway devices. The supraglottic airway device has a role in the management of the difficult airway, whether anticipated or unforeseen; as a rescue airway in a Plan B scenario or as a dedicated airway in cases where, for example, a patient's neck movement is restricted. In this situation the supraglottic airway device can act as a conduit for an endotracheal tube railroaded over an intubating catheter or a fiberoptic laryngoscope [3]. It is in the clinician's interest to know which of the pieces of equipment available is most suited to a given situation from an ease of use, patient safety and cost effectiveness standpoint.

Randomized Controlled Trials

The randomized controlled trial (RCT) is a clearly defined type of scientific experiment. The RCT is, in the medical sciences, a cornerstone of evidence-based medicine [4]. In relation to SADs, RCTs provide useful information about efficacy of the device, insertion parameters, selected adverse effects and complications.

The main feature of the RCT is that the subjects of the trial (patients) are randomly allocated into two or more groups of treatment. This allocation is called randomization and it is performed after the evaluation of patient eligibility, his/her recruitment but before starting the treatment or intervention [5]. Unlike audits, all RCTs are classified as research projects and must receive an appropriate ethical approval by a responsible body (Regional Ethical Committee – REC or Institutional Review Board – IRB) [6]. This approval must be in written form. All participants should receive a detailed written information leaflet in advance of recruitment and must sign to indicate that they have given informed consent.

Participants have the right to withdraw their consent during any stage of the study (Table 1). All RCTs must be performed in accordance with the Helsinki declaration.

Two types of RCTs are usually employed in testing SADs:

a Parallel groups – participants are randomly allocated to the different groups (usually by using sealed envelopes or a computerized database). Each patient in the group receives an intervention.

b Cross-over design – each participant receives two (or more) consecutive interventions in a randomly assigned order.

Study Power

The power of any statistical method is the probability of rejecting the null hypothesis (no statistical difference between the groups) when this hypothesis is incorrect. The power is the probability of not revealing a false negative result (type II error). The chance of making this type II error is called false negative rate (β).

Table 1. The phases of a randomized controlled trial [4]

Trial phase	Process
1. Enrollment	Assessment for eligibility Randomization
2. Allocation	Allocated to intervention Received intervention
3. Follow up	Followed up
4. Analysis	Analyzed

Power may be calculated as:

$1 - \beta$ (power = sensitivity)

Power analysis should be performed prior to study in order to calculate the study sample size (number of participants required to exclude type II error at some reasonable level). Power of 80% (0.8) at a significance level of 5% is usually calculated to detect a difference in the primary outcome (5-20%).

Blinding the Study

Blinding means that operators and/or participants or even study results assessors do not know which intervention was used in which patient. RCTs exploring SADs may be blinded for participants and assessors but blinding is almost impossible for the operators performing the interventions.

Primary Outcomes

In studies concerning SADs, the following primary outcomes are usually evaluated: total insertion success rate/failure rate, 1st attempt insertion success rate, insertion times, oropharyngeal seal (leak) pressures and leak fractions (Table 2). A few studies have assessed changes in hemodynamic parameters after the insertion of SAD as their primary outcome.

Secondary Outcomes

The most commonly assessed secondary outcomes with studies into SADs include the incidence of postoperative complications – sore throat, difficulty swallowing, cough, hoarseness, neck pain or temporary tongue numbness following the procedures. Other secondary outcomes may be the quality of fibreoptic views through the devices, incidence of gastric insufflation, ease of gastric tube insertion or blood staining of the devices on removal.

Table 2. Parameters evaluated with the SADs

Parameter (units)	Explanation
Oropharyngeal seal/leak pressure (cmH_20) (OSP/OLP)	Maximal airway pressure which can withstand an SAD without an audible leak
Leak volume (mL)	Volume leaking at given inspiratory pressure or volume
Leak fraction (%)	Leak volume divided by inspired volume
Esophageal seal pressure (cmH_20)	Maximal pressure measured in esophagus which can withstand an SAD without contamination of the airway

SUPRAGLOTTIC DEVICES DESCRIBED IN THIS CHAPTER

A range of supraglottic airway devices are available. These may be broadly classified into 1st generation and 2nd generation devices (absence or presence of an additional channel for drainage of gastric contents) or those with an inflatable cuff for an oropharyngeal seal, and those without.

SADs which have been trialled against the i-gel and i-gel itself are described briefly in the following paragraphs.

1st Generation SADs

LMA Classic®/LMA Unique® (Orthofix Ltd., Maidenhead, UK)

The LMA Classic (classic LMA - cLMA) was introduced in 1988 as an alternative to facemask anesthesia and intubation for airway maintenance. The LMA Unique (LMA-U) is the single-use version, introduced in 1997 (Figure 1). The cLMA is manufactured from silicone rubber and is latex-free. It may be autoclaved. The LMA-U is manufactured from clear medical grade PVC.

The LMA has an inflatable cuff, the tip of which sits in the hypopharynx, between the respiratory and gastrointestinal tract. Bars at the terminus of the device prevent obstruction of the aperture by the epiglottis.

Unlike some of its second-generation counterparts it does not allow access to the gastrointestinal tract.

Laryngeal Mask Auraonce™ (Ambu A/S, Ballerup, Denmark)

The AuraOnce is a disposable 1st generation SAD introduced into clinical practice in the United Kingdom in February 2004 (Figure 2). Its design is based on the cLMA.

Differences between these two SADs include an angulated breathing tube (similar to the ILMA) and softer, thinner cuff with the AuraOnce mask.

Laryngeal Mask (LM) Solus™ (Intersurgical Ltd., Wokingham, UK)

The LMA solus is produced by Intersurgical. It is a single-use 1st generation supraglottic airway device. The device is based on the LMA-Unique.

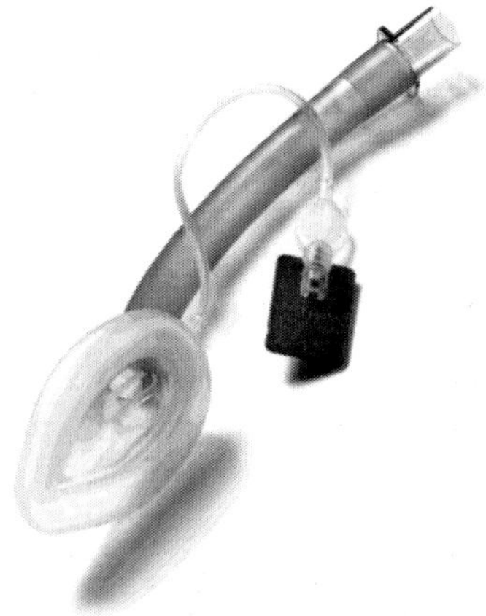

Figure 1. The LMA-Unique.

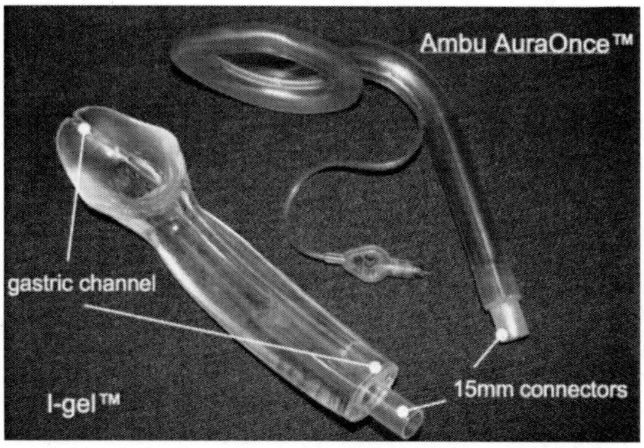

Figure 2. Ambu AuraOnce and i-gel.

La Premiere® Laryngeal Mask (Armstrong Medical Ltd., Coleraine, Northern Ireland)

The La Premiere is a standard disposable laryngeal mask based on the LMA-Classic. The mask employs the "inflate to fit" insertion technique. The pilot balloon has an over-pressure indicator – if the cuff pressure/volume is too high the pilot balloon overinflates and vice versa.

Intubating LMA™ (ILMA), LMA Fastrach™ (Orthofix Ltd., Maidenhead, UK)

The ILMA is a laryngeal mask airway designed to facilitate the placement of a tracheal tube via its lumen. It has a unique modification at the terminus of its airway lumen designed to direct a tube anteriorly towards the glottis. It is available in single-use and reusable versions.

2nd Generation SADs

i-gel® (Intersurgical Ltd., Wokingham, UK)

The i-gel is a second-generation supraglottic airway device introduced by Intersurgical in 2007. It has several features that distinguish it from the laryngeal mask airway. The device is manufactured from a thermoplastic elastomer (styrene ethylene butadiene styrene), which is soft and has a gel-like consistency to the touch. It does not rely on the inflation of a cuff to provide a perilaryngeal seal.

Schmidbauer et al. found in a cadaveric study that the "cuff" of the device conformed well to laryngopharyngeal anatomy.

The device incorporates a bite block, which should prevent occlusion of the i-gel's lumen in the event of a patient biting down at emergence. The extra width that this feature provides may also reduce the incidence of rotation of the device while in situ. At the distal end of the device, there is an epiglottis blocker, the purpose of which is to prevent downfolding of the epiglottis over the glottic opening.

A gastric channel allows the placement of a nasogastic tube with the device in situ.

Proseal™ LMA (PLMA) (Intavent Orthofix Ltd., Maidenhead, UK)

The PLMA has a double tube arrangement with an inflatable cuff (Figure 3). The airway lumen is wire reinforced and flexible. The second lumen permits access to the alimentary tract. The device may be positioned with the aid of a removable metal introducer. The device also possesses a bite block.

The PLMA's manufacturers claim that the design of the device permits the attainment of seal pressures of up to 30cmH_2O for positive pressure ventilation.

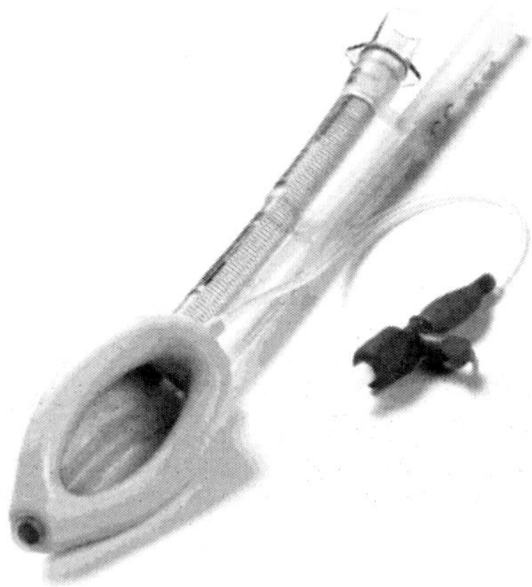

Figure 3. ProSeal Laryngeal Mask Airway (courtesy of Chemelek Ltd., Czech Republic).

LMA Supreme™ (LMA-S) (Laryngeal Mask Company, Mahé, Seychelles)

The LMA Supreme is similar in some respects to the i-gel. It is single-use, permits access to the gastrointestinal tract via a drain tube and incorporates a bite block.

However it is constructed from medical grade silicone, possesses an inflatable cuff with a reinforced tip and its airway tube is both anatomically shaped and semi-rigid (Figure 4).

Streamlined Liner of the Pharynx Airway – SLIPA™ (Curveair Ltd., London, UK)

This device represents a new concept in the 2nd generation SADs. It is a cuffless disposable pre-shaped pharyngeal sealing device (Figure 5). Design of SLIPA allows storage of regurgitated gastric fluid thus limiting the potential for aspiration.

COMPARISON OF CLINICAL PERFORMANCE DURING ELECTIVE PROCEDURES

Supraglottic airways have a range of applications in the elective clinical setting. They are used as a convenient alternative to facemask anesthesia, and as an alternative to endotracheal intubation. All high-quality RCTs, comparing the i-gel with other SADs are analyzed in this chapter (you may see the complete list of published studies in Table 3 - Appendix).

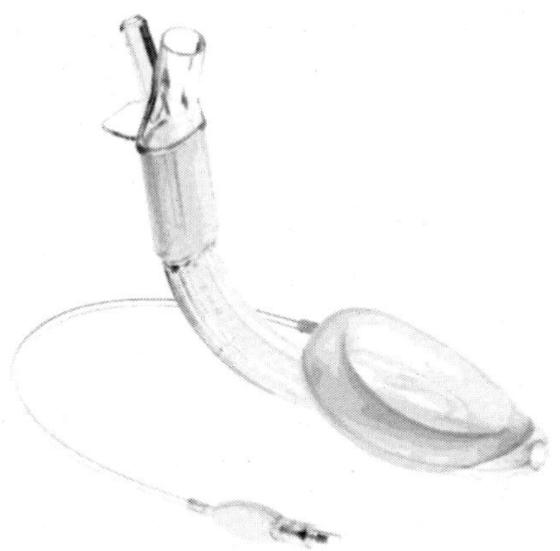

Figure 4. Supreme Laryngeal Mask (courtesy of Chemelek Ltd., Czech Republic).

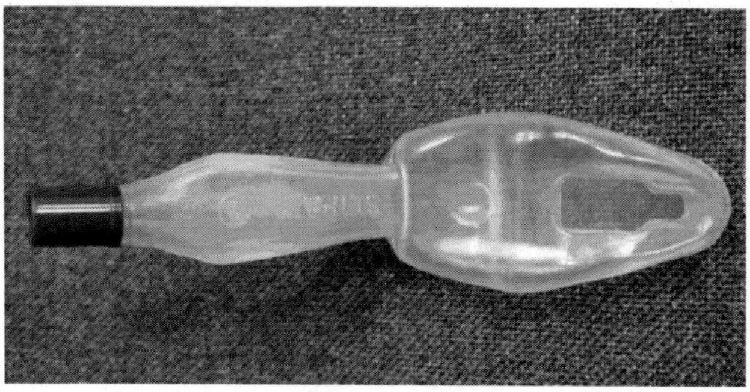

Figure 5. SLIPA (Streamlined Liner of the Pharynx Airway).

Comparison of i-gel with 1st Generation SADs

The i-gel airway has been compared with various 1st generation SADs – LMA-Classic, LMA-Unique, Aura Once LM, La Premiere LM and the Solus LM.

The performance of the i-gel against the LMA classic has been assessed by more researchers. Janakiraman et al. [7] set up a randomized crossover trial, involving 50 healthy, spontaneously breathing anesthetized patients. Their primary outcome measure was successful insertion in one attempt. The i-gel did not fare well when used in accordance with the manufacturer's guidelines (54% success vs 86%; p=0.01). However, overall success with the i-gel improved to 84% vs 92% on the second attempt, when an alternative, larger, size of i-gel was used. The authors also noted a significantly better fiberoptic view of the glottis from the terminus of the i-gel. The authors felt at the time that they could not recommend the i-gel as an alternative to the cLMA without revision of the sizing guidelines.

Shin et al. compared the i-gel with the ProSeal LMA and cLMA in 167 patients scheduled for orthopedic surgery [8]. The airway leak pressures were significantly higher with both of the 2nd generation SADs than with the cLMA. Postoperative complaints were similar in all three groups apart from sore throat, which was highest in the cLMA group.

Another study was carried out by Helmy and colleagues [9] in 2010, which compared the performance of the i-gel and cLMA in 80 spontaneously ventilated patients. They found significantly higher seal pressures with the i-gel in situ. However, in contrast to the earlier study, they found the i-gel significantly faster and easier to insert than the cLMA. They also found that there was a low incidence of gastric insufflation associated with the use of the i-gel in comparison with its competitor. The authors estimated that there was probably no statistically significant difference in the occurrence of postoperative complications associated with the use of either device, except perhaps in the incidence of PONV, being lower with the i-gel.

Danha and colleagues [10] compared the i-gel with the LMA-U in healthy patients undergoing elective orthopedic, general or middle ear surgery requiring positive pressure ventilation. Their findings demonstrated little difference between the two devices with respect to effectiveness in the delivery of positive pressure ventilation. Mean leak volumes for the two devices were 30 and 23 ml respectively. They found no significant difference between peak airway pressures or expired tidal volumes. Interestingly, there was a significant difference in the number of manipulations required for device insertion, favouring the i-gel. The authors also noted that there was a significant difference in the mean time to successful insertion of the devices, 13 seconds for the i-gel and 19 for the LMA-U. This study was powered but sample size of 15 patients in each group appears to be very low.

The performance of the LMA-U compared to that of the i-gel in mild to moderately obese patients undergoing CMV in elective surgery was studied by Weber et al. [11]. They found that, while there was no difference in the ease of insertion of the two devices, the use of the i-gel was associated with significantly higher leak pressures in both mild and moderately obese patients undergoing short elective surgery in the supine position.

The study conducted by Francksen and colleagues assessed the performance of the i-gel and LMA-Unique in 80 females scheduled for minor gynecological procedures under conditions of controlled ventilation [12]. The authors found significantly higher airway leak pressures in the i-gel group (29 cmH_2O vs. 18 cmH_2O, $p < 0.0001$). Views of the vocal cords through the devices using a fiberscope were better in the i-gel group, while the incidence of postoperative sore throat and dysphagia was similar in both groups.

A similar study with a cross-over design studied the i-gel and LMA-U in 39 patients receiving muscle relaxation [13]. The authors did not note any statistical difference between airway leak pressures, leak volumes or leak fractions during controlled ventilation. Insertion times were shorter for the i-gel.

The reverse was found in the study by Amini and Khoshfetrat, who compared i-gel with the Solus™ laryngeal mask [14].

The authors reported higher seal pressures and fiberoptic scores with the Solus™ LM. Insertion times were similar for those devices. The authors admit that their experience with the i-gel was limited prior to commencing the study. Regarding airway assessment parameters, patients in the i-gel group were assessed as having higher Mallampati classes than LM group patients.

Donaldson and colleagues [15] compared the i-gel to the Ambu AuraOnce LM in 204 healthy patients undergoing elective surgery while anesthetized and using a standardized protocol. Muscle relaxants were given to all patients. Their primary outcome measure was the difference in airway seal pressures between the two devices. They showed that seal pressure with the i-gel was significantly higher (30.4 cmH_2O vs 27.8 cmH_2O; $p=0.007$). They showed no difference, however, in the overall ease of insertion or ventilatory pressures for a given tidal volume. The incidence of complications arising from the use of either device was low, however the patients who had received the i-gel demonstrated a lower incidence of sore throat and difficulty swallowing at 24h, despite a higher (albeit still low) incidence of bloodstaining on the i-gel at removal.

Keijzer and colleagues compared the incidence of postoperative sore throat and neck pain in 218 patients allocated to the i-gel or La Premiere LM groups [16]. Airway management using i-gel was associated with a significantly lower frequency of both adverse effects at 1, 24 and 48 hours. Regarding secondary outcomes leak pressures were higher with the i-gel as well as fiberoptic views through the device.

Three studies evaluated hemodynamic responses after insertion of the i-gel in comparison with other airway devices. Ismail et al. studied hemodynamic parameters following insertion of three airway devices [17]. The i-gel caused lower increase in blood pressure and heart rate than the endotracheal tube or cLMA. Placement of the i-gel also did not influence perfusion index on the periphery (Table 2).

There was no increase in the intraocular pressure (IOP) as a response to the i-gel insertion while IOP elevated with remaining devices. Jindal and colleagues found the i-gel to be quicker to insert than the cLMA by novice users and that it did not cause any significant hemodynamic response [18]. Another study by the same authors showed that insertion and removal of the i-gel was associated with significantly lower hemodynamic response than the same maneuvers with the cLMA and SLIPA [19].

Conclusions Arising from the Studies i-gel Vs. 1st Generation SADs

Comparison of the i-gel with 1st generation SADs does not compare similar devices. 1st generation SADs place an emphasis on high esophageal seal pressures achieved by cuff inflation and placement of the cuff tip into the esophageal inlet. The i-gel has a different sealing mechanism and, as a 2nd generation device with a gastric channel, allows separation of the respiratory and gastrointestinal tracts. This drainage channel allows easy recognition and drainage of gastric contents. In comparison with the 1st generation SADs the i-gel has demonstrated significanly higher pharyngeal seal pressures with a reported range between 19.3 – 30.4 cmH_2O [14, 15] (1st generation SADs seal pressures varied between 17 – 27.8 cmH_2O).

Insertion times were similar or shorter in i-gel patients, whilst the incidence of postoperative complaints was fairly similar apart from for sore throat and neck pain. Hemodynamic parameters and intraocular pressures were not changed in association with i-gel insertion or removal.

Comparison of the i-gel with Other 2nd Generation SADs

The design features of the 2nd generation SADs are more or less similar. Several studies have compared i-gel either with ProSeal LMA or with the LMA Supreme (LMA-S).

The mechanics of ventilation during laparoscopic cholecystectomy in which a supraglottic airway was used was studied by Sharma et al. [20] in 2010. They compared the performance of the i-gel with that of the Proseal LMA in a randomised comparative study involving sixty patients. The authors concluded that the PLMA had a slight edge over the i-gel in a laparoscopic setting. The PLMA was found to have a greater seal pressure than the i-gel, and it was felt that the larger drainage channel present on the PLMA was advantageous. On fiberoptic examination, the incidence of malrotation was lower with the PLMA. However, while ventilatory mechanics were adequate with both devices, dynamic compliance was less impaired in the patients who were ventilated through the i-gel.

Singh et al. evaluated oropharyngeal seal pressures and other parameters in sixty patients who were randomized to receive either an i-gel or a PLMA in elective surgical procedures [21]. Seal pressures were higher in the PLMA group while the first attempt insertion rate, ease of gastric tube insertion and postoperative complication profiles were better with the i-gel.

Placement of ProSeal LMA may be guided by using a bougie or duodenal tube inserted into the gastric channel. A study by Gasteiger and colleagues compared guided insertion using the i-gel and PLMA [22]. They found guided insertion easy and quick for both SADs, however the PLMA provided a better oropharyngeal seal (30 cmH_2O vs. 23 cmH_2O, $p < 0.0001$).

Van Zundert and Brimacombe evaluated oropharyngeal leak pressures, ease and time of insertion, fiberoptic scores and postoperative complaints in 150 patients randomly allocated to receive an i-gel, PLMA or LMA Supreme [23]. There was no significant difference reported in the oropharyngeal leak pressures with all three devices withstanding pressures over 30 cmH_2O. The LMA Supreme was quicker and easier to insert than the PLMA. The study did not show any differences in postoperative complications.

The use of supraglottic airway devices may have several benefits in the ambulatory surgery setting. Teoh et al. [24] studied the use of the i-gel and LMA-S in 100 paralysed patients undergoing gynecological laparoscopic surgery. In accordance with other studies comparing a supraglottic airway device with an inflatable cuff to the i-gel, they found a lower incidence of postoperative sore throat in the i-gel group. Interestingly, they found the two devices to be roughly equivalent in terms of ventilatory parameters and no difference in the mean time to insertion or first successful ventilation.

Chew et al. evaluated the performance of the i-gel and LMA Supreme in 90 spontaneously breathing adult patients under general anesthesia [25]. The oropharyngeal leak pressures were higher and insertion was easier in the LMA Supreme group but fiberoptic views were better in the patients anesthetized with the i-gel.

Lorenz Theiler's group from Switzerland compared the i-gel and LMA Supreme in a simulated difficult laryngoscopy scenario (application of a neck collar reducing neck extension and mouth opening) in sixty anesthetized patients [26]. There was no difference in the primary outcome – overall success rate. Tidal volumes and oropharyngeal leak pressures were similar between the groups wheras the i-gel demonstrated better fiberoptic scores and less epiglottic downfolding.

On the other hand, the LMA Supreme required shorter insertion times.

Controlled ventilation with the i-gel vs. LMA Supreme without the use of muscle relaxants was assessed in 85 patients scheduled for day surgery procedures. There was no difference between the devices in terms of insertion success rate, oropharyngeal seal pressures, insertion times, placement of a gastric tube through the drainage channel and incidence of postoperative complaints [27].

An Egyptian study [28] investigated the performance of the i-gel vs. the LMA Supreme in elective surgery. Sixty healthy patients were randomly assigned to either device, and were mechanically ventilated post-induction.

The authors found no significant difference in ease of insertion of the devices. However, in contrast to the work of Danha with the broadly similar LMA-U, they found that leak pressures were significantly higher with the i-gel (25.5 cmH_2O vs. 21.1 cmH_2O) and for the same tidal volumes, peak and plateau airway pressures were significantly lower with the i-gel. Hemodynamic stability in both groups was commented upon as excellent.

Ragazzi et al. evaluated insertion success rates of the i-gel and LMA Supreme by novice operators [29]. The authors found better first time insertion success rate, higher oropharyngeal seal pressures and fewer failures in the LMA Supreme group but a lower incidence of the postoperative sore throat associated with the i-gel. They suggest that LMA Supreme might be a preferable SAD in airway emergencies managed by novice anesthesiologists.

Eschertzhuber et al. evaluated directly measured oropharyngeal and hypopharyngeal mucosal pressures following the i-gel or LMA Supreme insertions [30]. They found that pressures exerted on the mucosa were low in both devices (0-10.7 cmH_2O) and did not compromise oropharyngeal mucosal perfusion. Distribution of the pressures was more symmetrical with the i-gel, suggesting sealing mechanism of the device based on matching the perilaryngeal anatomy.

Conclusions Arising from the Studies i-gel Vs. 2nd Generation SADs

Published evidence shows that the i-gel is a reliable 2nd generation SAD. Documented oropharyngeal leak pressures are 20.7-35.6 cmH_2O [25, 20], which is lower than those for the PLMA (29.6-38.9 cmH_2O) but comparable with the LMA Supreme (21.1-32 cmH_2O). Insertion time, success rate and the incidence of postoperative complications is comparable with other 2nd generation SADs.

Comparison of the i-gel with Tracheal Intubation

Two studies evaluated the differences between airway management in elective procedures under general anesthesia using i-gel or tracheal intubation.

Uppal, Fletcher and Kinsella investigated the potential of the i-gel as an alternative to tracheal intubation during PCV in 2009 [31]. In their study of 25 ASA I-II patients, they found that there was no statistically significant difference in leak volumes or tidal volumes at pressures of up to 25 cmH_2O.

They also found no evidence of gastric insufflation at these pressures. Their findings supported the use of the i-gel as an alternative method of maintaining airway patency during PCV at reasonable inspired pressures.

Ibrahim et al. compared the i-gel with the tracheal tube in sixty elective patients scheduled for laparoscopic cholecystectomy [32]. Muscle relaxation and volume-controlled ventilation (VCV) were employed for the procedures. No differences in leak fractions were found before pneumoperitoneum. Significant differences were recorded after the initiation of pneumoperitoneum and with the use of higher inspiratory volumes (8 and 10 $ml.kg^{-1}$).

Use of the i-gel in Children

The use of supraglottic airways in pediatric anesthesia is increasing [33]. Relatively few studies of the use of the i-gel in pediatric populations have been published at the time of writing. In total, 10 studies involving 5 RCTs [34-38] and five descriptive studies can be found in the databases (as of September 2012). These studies are analyzed in detail in Chapters 7 and 8.

USE IN PREDICTED DIFFICULT AIRWAYS AND AS A DEDICATED AIRWAY

The use of the laryngeal mask airway in cases where management is difficult is well established, and has been incorporated into the emergency algorithms of the Difficult Airway Society [39]. Use of the reusable intubating LMA has been shown to be highly successful and safe [40] but the attendant costs are also high, limiting its use for training purposes.

The supraglottic airway has also been used where difficulty in airway management has been predicted.

There are several studies comparing the performance of the i-gel as a dedicated airway with more conventional laryngeal mask airways, both in mannequins and in humans.

Again, because of the high cost of the reusable ILMA, clinicians may be more inclined to use an alternative such as the i-gel in their everyday practice, and in the event of an emergency may require converting to a tracheal tube.

The studies of Theiler [41], Kleine-Brueggeney [42], Halwagi [43] and Wadhwa [44] are presented in Chapters 9 and 10. These studies show that i-gel may be used as a conduit for endotracheal tube insertion. However, fiberscope-guided techniques have a significantly higher success rate than do blind insertions.

EMERGENCY USE

Theiler et al. [26] simulated a difficult airway scenario in 60 anesthetised patients in a randomised crossover comparison of the LMA-S with the i-gel. The patients were anesthetised while wearing an extrication collar, which limited neck movement and mouth opening. Although the study could not prove equivalence of the performance of the two devices, there was no statistically significant difference between the devices in terms of ease of insertion, ventilatory success leak pressures or tidal volumes. It is worth noting that the i-gel failed on two occasions because of insertion difficulty, and twice because of inadequate ventilation, whereas the LMA-S' three failures in this study were due to ventilatory difficulties. The only statistically significant differences between the devices demonstrated was in the fiberoptic view of the glottis, which was significantly better with the i-gel, and in the reduced rate of epiglottic downfolding, where again the i-gel performed better.

Outside of the hospital setting, there have been several studies comparing the performance of the i-gel with other supraglottic airway devices. Supraglottic airway devices may be advantageous in an out-of-hospital setting, as bag mask ventilation and tracheal intubation are difficult skills which require training to acquire and must be practised regularly to maintain proficiency. Indeed, at least one in-hospital study on anesthetized patients [15] suggested that there was no learning curve in the insertion of supraglottic airway devices.

Studies exploring the role of i-gel in pre-hospital airway management and as an airway device in cardiac arrest and cardiopulmonary resuscitation (CPR) are mostly experimental, using mannequins as study subjects. These studies are analyzed in Chapter 16.

Conclusion

The i-gel performs well as a supraglottic airway. Its ease of use and reliable placement together with acceptably high seal pressures make it ideally suited to a range of applications in elective anesthetic scenarios. It has been shown to be comparable to other available supraglottic airway devices in terms of ventilatory mechanics. The device is probably outperformed by the PLMA in laparoscopic cases, however, as this device achieves significantly higher seal pressures.

Postoperative safety profile of the i-gel is very good, showing a low incidence of postoperative sore throat, swallowing difficulties and neck pain.

The pediatric version of the i-gel performs well in a clinical setting. It has been shown to perform as well as the classic LMA in children, but was significantly more quickly inserted and gave a better fiberoptic view of the glottis when a scope was employed.

The i-gel has a role in the management of the predicted and unanticipated difficult airway. It is a useful conduit for a tracheal tube when a fiberoptic-guided technique is employed. In mannequin studies, it was as reliable in this application as the ILMA. These findings have been corroborated in live patients in further studies. However, blind intubation through the i-gel airway is not likely to be successful and is not recommended apart from in emergency, life-saving situations where the fiberscope is not immediately available.

In an out-of-hospital setting, the i-gel performs well in the hands of practitioners with low amounts of exposure to airway management. It has been shown that it is easy to use, and the level of skill retention of non-practising volunteers appears to be higher than those for its competitors. Again, however, the PLMA appears to be more a reliable conduit for ventilation.

Table 3. Published RCTs comparing the i-gel airway with other SADs or with an endotracheal tube

Study (adult patients)	Design	No. of participants (receiving i-gel)	Other device	Primary outcome	Power analysis	Success rate(%)	1st time success	OSP (cmH_20)	Insertion (sec)
Shin[8]	Comp.	167 (64)	cLMA,PLMA	OSP	Yes	100	78	27.1	-
Helmy[9]	Comp.	80 (40)	cLMA	Success	Yes*	100	90	25.6	15.6
Uppal[13]	Comp.	39 (39)	uLMA	OSP	Yes	100	97.4	25	12.2
Siddiqui[45]	Comp.	100 (50)	cLMA	Success	No	100	90	-	-
Cattano[46]	Comp.	50 (25)	uLMA	Ins.time	No	100	68	23.1	21
Francksen[12]	Comp.	80 (40)	uLMA	Success	Yes	100	90	29	15
Danha[10]	Comp.	30 (15)	uLMA	LeakVol.	Yes	100	100	20.0	13
Donaldson[15]	Comp.	204 (103)	AuraO	OSP	Yes	96.3	86.4	30.4	11.0
Janakiraman[7]	Crossover	50 (50)	cLMA	1st time s.	Yes	84	54	20	-
Amini[14]	Comp.	120 (60)	Solus	OSP	Yes	93.3	77	19.3	20
Weber[11]	Crossover	50 (50)	LMA-S	OSP	Yes	100	92	23.7	18.3
Keijzer[16]	Comp.	218 (109)	LaPrem	Postop.	Yes	100	-	26.8	8.5
Singh[21]	Comp.	60 (30)	PLMA	OSP	Yes	100	100	25.3	-
Sharma[20]	Comp.	60 (30)	PLMA	Dyn.C	Yes	100	93.3	35.6	13.7
Gasteiger[22]	Comp.	152 (75)	PLMA	OSP	Yes	100	97.3	23.0	-
Van Zundert[23]	Comp.	150 (50)	PLMA,LMA-S	OSP	Yes	94	80	30.0	44*
Teoh[24]	Comp.	100 (50)	LMA-S	OSP	Yes	100	96	25.0	15.4
Chew[25]	Comp.	90 (45)	LMA-S	OSP	Yes	100	93.3	20.7	20
Ragazzi[29]†	Comp.	80 (40)	LMA-S	1st time s.	Yes	85	54	24.0	28
Fernandez[27]	Comp.	85 (43)	LMA-S	Success	Yes	100	86	25.2	32.5*
Theiler[26]	Crossover	60 (60)	LMA-S	Success	Yes	93	85	27.0	42*
Erchertzhuber[30]	Comp.	30 (15)	LMA-S	MP	Yes	100	100	27.3	-
Ali[28]	Comp.	60 (30)	LMA-S	Success	No	100	73	25.5	-
Ibrahim[32]	Comp.	60 (30)	ET	Leak fraction	Yes	100	86.7	25.8	-
Jindal[19]	Comp.	75 (25)	cLMA,SLIPA	Success	No	100	96	-	3.5
Uppal,b) [31]	Crossover	25 (25)	ET	Leak fraction	Yes	100	100	28	-

Study (intubation)	Design	No. of participants (receiving i-gel)	Other device	Primary outcome	Power analysis	Success rate	1st time success	OSP (cmH_20)	Insertion (sec)
Theiler[41]	Comp.	80 (40)	sILMA	TIsuccess	Yes	98	90	26	33
Halwagi[43]	Comp.	160 (80)	ILMA	1st TIsuc.	Yes	96	84	-	26
Wadhwa[44]	Comp.	60 (30)	ILMA	TISuccess	No	100	-	-	10.5
Kleine-Brueg.[42]	Comp.	160 (80)	sILMA	TISuccess	Yes	98.8	94	24	23
Lee[36]	Comp.	99 (50)	cLMA	OSP	Yes	100	96	22	17
Goyal[37]	Comp.	120 (40)	PLMA,cLMA	Success	No	100	95	26	-
Theiler[38]	Comp.	208 (106)	AuraO	OSP	Yes	93	91	22	27
Fukuhara[34]	Comp.	134 (67)	PLMA	OSP	Yes	100	94	24	13
Gasteiger[35]	Crossover	51 (51)	PLMA	OSP	Yes	100	92	21	28

Legends: Comp. = comparative (two or more groups), cLMA = Laryngeal Mask Airway Classic®, uLMA = Laryngeal Mask Airway Unique®, PLMA = Pro Seal® Laryngeal Mask Airway, AuraO = AuraOnce® Laryngeal Mask, Solus = Solus® Laryngeal Mask, LMA-S = Laryngeal Mask Airway Supreme®, ET = endotracheal tube, ILMA = Intubating Laryngeal Mask Airway®, sILMA = single-use Intubating Laeyngeal Mask Airway, OSP = oropharyngeal seal pressure, Leak Vol. = leak volume, 1st time s. = success rate at the 1st insertion, Postop. = postoperative complications, Dyn. C. = dynamic compliance, MP = mucosal pressure, TIsuccess = success rate of tracheal intubation.

* = power analysis not performed for a primary outcome, † = only novice operators involved.

REFERENCES

[1] T. Cook and B. Howes, Supraglottic airway devices: recent advances, *Cont. Ed. Anaesth. Crit. Care Pain 2*, 56-61 (2011).

[2] M. R. Hernandez, P. A. Clock jr. and A. Ovassapian, Evolution of the extraglottic airway: a review of its history, applications, and practical tips for success, *Anesth. Analg*. 114, 349-68 (2012).

[3] Timmermann, Supraglottic airways in difficult airway management: successes, failures, use and misuse, *Anaesthesia* 66, S45-56 (2011).

[4] S. E. Strauss, W. S. Richardson, P. Glasziou and R. B. Haynes, *Evidence-based medicine: how to practice and teach EBM*, 3rd ed. Elsevier, New York (2005).

[5] K. F. Schulz, D. G. Altman, D. Moher; for the CONSORT Group, Consort 2010 statement : updated guidelines for reporting parallel group randomised trials, *Br. Med. J*. 340, c332 (2010).

[6] S. J. Edwards, R. J. Lilford and J. Hewison, The ethics of randomised controlled trials from the perspectives of patients, the public and healthcare professionals, *Br. Med. J*. 317, 1209-12 (1998).

[7] C. Janakiraman, D. B. Chethan, A. R. Wilkes, M. R. Stacey and N. Goodwin, A randomised crossover trial comparing the i-gel supraglottic airway and classic laryngeal mask airway, *Anaesthesia* 64, 674-8 (2009).

[8] W. J. Shin, Y. S. Cheong, H. S. Yang and T. Nishiyama, The supraglottic airway i-gel in comparison with ProSeal laryngeal mask airway and classic laryngeal mask airway in anaesthetized patients, *Eur. J. Anaesthesiol*. 27, 598-601 (2010).

[9] M. Helmy, H. M. Atef, E. M. El-Taher and A.M. Henidak, Comparitive study between i-gel, a new supraglottic airway device, and classical laryngeal mask airway in anesthetised spontaneously ventilated patients, *Saudi J. Anaesth*., 4,131-6 (2010).

[10] R. F. Danha, S. Sreevathsa, N. Crombie, C. Hillermann and C. Mendonca, Positive pressure ventilation with i-gel versus LMA-Unique: a randomised comparative study, *J. Anesth. Clinic. Res*, 2, 11 (2011).

[11] U. Weber, R. Oguz, L. A. Potura, O. Kimberger, A. Kober and E. Tschernko, Comparison of the i-gel and LMA-Unique laryngeal mask airway in patients with mild to moderate obesity during elective short-term surgery, *Anaesthesia* 66, 481-7 (2011).

[12] H. Francksen, J. Renner, R. Hanss, J. Scholz, V. Doerges and B. Bein, A comparison of the i-gelTM with the LMA-UniqueTM in non-paralysed anaesthetised adult patients, *Anaesthesia* 64, 1118-24 (2009).

[13] V. Uppal, S. Gangaiah, G. Fletcher and J. Kinsella, Randomised crossover comparison between the i-gel and the LMA-Unique in anaesthetised, paralysed adults, *Br. J. Anaesth*. 103, 882-5 (2009).

[14] S. Amini and M. Khosfetrat, Comparison of the Intersurgical Solus™ laryngeal mask airway and the i-gel supralaryngeal device, *Anaesthesia* 65, 805-9 (2010).

[15] W. Donaldson, A. Abraham, M. Deighan and P. Michalek, i-gel™ vs. AuraOnce™ laryngeal mask for general anaesthesia with controlled ventilation in paralysed patients. *Biomed. Pap*. 155, 155-64 (2011).

[16] C. Keijzer, D. R. Buitelaar, K. M. Efthymiou, M. Šrámek, J. ten Cate, M. Ronday, T. Stoppa, J. M. Huitink and P. F. Schutte, A comparison of postoperative throat and neck

complaints after the use of the i-gel® and the La Premiere® disposable laryngeal mask: a double-blinded, randomized, controlled trial, *Anesth. Analg.* 109, 1092-4 (2010).

[17] S. A. Ismail, N. A. Bisher, H. W. Kandil, H. A. Mowafi and H. A. Atawia, Intraocular pressure and haemodynamic responses to insertion of the i-gel, laryngeal mask airway or endotracheal tube, *Eur. J. Anaesthesiol.* 28, 443-8 (2011).

[18] P. Jindal, A. A. Rizvi, G. Khurana and J. P. Sharma, Safety and efficacy of insertion of supraglottic devices in anaesthetised patients by first time users, *S. Afr. J. Anaesthesiol. Analg.* 16, 23-6 (2010).

[19] P. Jindal, A. Rizvi and J. P. Sharma, Is i-gel a new revolution among supraglottic airway devices? *Middle East J. Anesth.* 20, 53-8 (2009).

[20] B. Sharma, R. Sehgal, C. Sahai and J. Sood, PLMA vs. i-gel: a comparative evaluation of respiratory mechanics in laparoscopic cholecystectomy. *J. Anaesth. Clin. Pharmacol.* 26, 451-7 (2010).

[21] Singh, M. Gupta and M. Tandon, Comparison of clinical performance of i-gel™ with LMA-ProSeal™ in elective surgeries, *Indian J. Anaesth.* 53, 302-5 (2009).

[22] L. Gasteiger, J. Brimacombe, D. Perkhofer, M. Kaufmann and C. Keller, Comparison of guided insertion of the LMA ProSeal™ vs. the i-gel™, *Anaesthesia* 65, 913-6 (2010).

[23] T. C. van Zundert and J. R. Brimacombe, Similar oropharyngeal leak pressures during anaesthesia with i-gelTM, LMA-ProSeal™ and LMA-Supreme™ laryngeal masks, *Acta Anaesth. Belg.* 63, 35-41 (2012).

[24] W. H. Teoh, K. M. Lee, T. Suhitharan, Z. Yayha, M. M. Teo and A. T. Sia, Comparison of the LMA Supreme vs the i-gel in paralysed patients undergoing gynaecological laparoscopic surgery with controlled ventilation, *Anaesthesia* 65, 1173-9 (2010).

[25] E. F. Chew, N. H. Hashim and C. Y. Wang, Randomised comparison of the LMA Supreme™ with the i-gel™ in spontaneously breathing anaesthetised adult patients, *Anaesth. Intensive Care* 38, 1018-22 (2010).

[26] L. G. Theiler, M. Kleine-Brueggeney, D. Kaiser, N. Urwyler, C. Luyet, A. Vogt, R. Greif and M. M. Unibe, Crossover comparison of the Laryngeal Mask Supreme and the i-gel in simulated difficult airway scenario in anesthetized patients, *Anesthesiology* 111, 55-62 (2009).

[27] Fernandez Diez, A. Perez Villafane, J. C. Bermejo Gonzalez and J. M. Marcos Vidal, Supreme larnygeal mask airway vs the i-gel supraglottic airway in patients under general anesthesia and mechanical ventilation with no neuromuscular block: a randomized clinical trial, *Rev. Esp. Anestesiol. Reanim.* 56, 474-8 (2009). [Article in Spanish, English abstract]

[28] M. Z. Ali, R. S. Ebied, A. F. El-Tawdy, A. I. Refaat and N. M. Kamal, Controlled mechanical ventilation with LMA Supreme versus i-gel in anesthetized adult patients, *J. Egypt. Soc. Parasitol.* 41, 365-78 (2011).

[29] R. Ragazzi, L. Finessi, I. Farinelli, R. Alvisi and C. A. Volta, LMA Supreme™ vs i-gel™ – a comparison of insertion success in novices, *Anaesthesia* 67, 384-8 (2012).

[30] S. Eschertzhuber, J. Brimacombe, M. Kaufmann, C. Keller and W. Tiefenthaler, Directly measured mucosal pressures produced by the i-gel™ and laryngeal mask airway Supreme™ in paralysed anaesthetised patients, *Anaesthesia* 67, 407-10 (2012).

[31] V. Uppal, G. Fletcher and J. Kinsella, Comparison of the i-gel with the cuffed tracheal tube during pressure controlled ventilation, *Br. J. Anaesth.* 102, 264-8 (2009).

[32] M. Ibrahim, A. Ragab and H. ElShamaa, i-gel vs cuffed tracheal tube during volume controlled ventilation in elective laparoscopic cholecystectomy, *Egypt. J. Anaesth.* 27, 7-11 (2011).

[33] M. C. White, T. M. Cook and P. A. Stoddart, A critique of elective paediatric supraglottic airway devices, *Paediatr. Anaesth.* 19, S55-65 (2009).

[34] Fukuhara, R. Okutani and Y. Oda, A randomized comparison of the i-gel and the ProSeal laryngeal mask airway in pediatric patients: performance and fibreoptic findings, *J. Anesth.* (2012), [Epub. ahead of print].

[35] L. Gasteiger, J. Brimacombe, E. Oswald, D. Perkhofer, A. Tonin, C. Keller and W. Tiefenthaler, LMA ProSeal™ vs i-gel™ in ventilated children: a randomised crossover study using the size 2 mask, *Acta Anaesthesiol. Scand.* (2012), [Epub. ahead of print].

[36] J. R. Lee, M. S. Kim, J. T. Kim, H. J. Byon, Y. H. Park, H. S. Kim and C. S. Kim, A randomised controlled trial comparing the i-gel with the LMA classic in children, *Anaesthesia* 67, 606-611 (2012).

[37] R. Goyal, R. N. Shukla and G. Kumar, Comparison of size 2 i-gel™ supraglottic airway with LMA-ProSeal™ and LMA-Classic™ in spontaneously breathing children undergoing elective surgery, *Paediatr. Anaesth.* 22, 355-9 (2012).

[38] L. G. Theiler, M. Kleine-Brueggeney, B. Luepold, F. Stucki, S. Seiler, N. Urwyler and R. Greif, Performance of the pediatric-sized i-gel compared with the Ambu AuraOnce laryngeal mask in anesthetized and ventilated children, *Anesthesiology* 115, 102-10 (2011).

[39] J. J Henderson , M. T. Popat, I. P. Latto and A. C. Pearce. Difficult Airway Society guidelines for the management of unanticipated difficult intubation, *Anaesthesia* 59, 675-94 (2004).

[40] N. S. Gerstein, D. A. Braude, O. Hung, J. C. Sanders, M. F. Murphy, The Fastrach intubating laryngeal mask airway: an overview and update, *Can. J. Anaesth,* 57, 588-601 (2010).

[41] L. Theiler, M. Kleine-Brueggeney, N. Urwyler, T. Graf, C. Luyet and R. Greif, Randomized clinical trial of the i-gel™ and Magill tracheal tube or single-use ILMA™ and ILMA™ tracheal tube for blind intubation in anaesthetized patients with a predicted difficult airway, *Br. J. Anaesth.* 107, 243-50 (2011).

[42] M. Kleine-Brueggeney, L. Theiler, N. Urwyler, A.Vogt and R.Greif, Randomised controlled trial comparing the i-gel and Magill tracheal tube with the single-use ILMA and ILMA tracheal tube for fibreoptic guided intubation in anaesthetized patients with a predicted difficult airway. *Br. J. Anaesth.* 107, 251-7 (2011).

[43] L. Halwagi, N. Massicotte, A. Lallo, A. Gauthier, D. Boudreault, M. Ruel and F. Girard, Tracheal intubation through the i-gel™ supraglotttic airway versus the LMA Fastrach™: a randomised controlled trial. *Anesth. Analg.* 114, 152-6 (2012).

[44] R. Wadhwa and S. Kalra, Comparison of hemodynamic changes and ease of endotracheal intubation through i-gel vs ILMA. *J. Anaesthesiol. Clin. Pharmacol.* 26, 379-82 (2010).

[45] S. Siddiqui, U. S. Raees, S. Z. Siddiqui, S. Haider and S. A. Raza, Comparison of performance and safety of i-gel with laryngeal mask airway (classic) for general anaesthesia with controlled ventilation, *Anaesth. Pain and Intensive Care* 14, 17-20 (2010).

[46] D. Cattano, L. Ferrario, V. Maddukuri, S. Sridhar, Y. Khalil and C. A. Hagberg, A randomized clinical comparison of the Intersurgical i-gel and LMA Unique in non-obese adults during general surgery, *Minerva Anestesiol.* 77, 292-7 (2011).

Conflict of interest: Dr Francis McAleavey declares no conflict of interest; Prof. Pavel Michalek has lectured for several companies manufacturing supraglottic airway devices inluding Intersurgical Ltd., AMBU Ltd. and Intavent Orthofix Ltd.

In: The i-gel Supraglottic Airway
Editors: Pavel Michalek and William Donaldson

ISBN: 978-1-62417-897-9

Chapter 15

TEACHING AIRWAY SKILLS AND THE ROLE OF THE AIRWAY SKILLS LABORATORY

Pavel Michalek[1,2,*] and Pavel Herda[1]

[1]Department of Anesthesia and Intensive Medicine,
First Medical Faculty of the Charles University and
General University Hospital, Prague, Czech Republic
[2]Department of Anaesthesia, Antrim Area
Hospital, Antrim, UK

ABSTRACT

Education plays a very important role in the acquisition of airway management skills. These skills can be learned using various methods. Basic and routine airway management skills such as: bag-mask ventilation, insertion of supraglottic airway devices and direct laryngoscopy are key parts of ordinary anesthetic procedures. They are usually taught by an experienced supervisor on patients directly in the operating room. Some less frequently used and special airway skills, such as fiberoptic intubation or surgical access to the trachea are best learned using airway simulators, mannequins, animals or cadavers. Because access to laboratory animals and fresh cadavers is difficult in many departments, airway mannequins play a key role in learning these specialized skills. Airway mannequins may also be used for practising insertion of various supraglottic airway devices, including the i-gel, and for direct laryngoscopy or videolaryngoscopy.

A well-structured airway management curriculum should be a part of anesthetic training worldwide. This training, led by a designated specialist, should include regular practice in an airway skills laboratory, management of cases with difficult airways under direct supervision in the operating room, theoretical teaching sessions, assessment and audit of performance. Airway management programs should be coordinated at national and international level with regular airway courses and conferences.

* Corresponding author: Pavel Michalek. E-mail address: pafkamich@yahoo.co.uk.

INTRODUCTION

Education in airway management is an integral part of the curricula in anesthesia and critical care medicine. Inability to maintain the patent airway and adequate oxygenation can lead to brain damage or the death of a patient within minutes [1, 2].

The 4th National Audit, a joint project of the Royal College of Anaesthetists (RCoA) and the Difficult Airway Society (DAS) in the United Kingdom, looked at complications during airway management over a one year period [3].

In total, 184 major airway complications were reported in this audit. Patient abnormalities such as disturbed craniofacial anatomy or trauma were the most common causative and contributory factors, found in 77% of complications.

Unfortunately, operator factors such as incorrect judgement and insufficient education/training contributed in approximately half of the cases of life-threatening airway complications [3].

The closed claims analysis system in the United States (American Society of Anesthesiologists) showed that 6% of all claims were related to airway injuries. Patient care in these cases was judged to be below an acceptable standard in 21% of claims [4].

The situation is worse in pre-hospital emergency care and regarding intubations performed by non-anesthetic medical professionals. Wang et al. looked at the success rates and complications of out of hospital airway management in the United States. They reported that tracheal intubation was attempted in 82% of all airway cases but with only a 77% success rate. The authors found a 0.1% incidence of esophageal intubation [5].

All these reports have raised concerns about the quality of education and airway management training amongst medical professionals. The first formal airway training curriculum in the United Kingdom was published by Stringer et al. in 2002 [2]. Previously, the Royal College of Anaesthetists had published obligatory skills in airway management for anesthesia trainees in its official documents (Table 1). At the moment, three different bodies in the UK have airway management training modules published on their websites and offer airway courses and workshops.

In conclusion, all professional bodies agree that airway management training is a vitally important part of basic anesthetic training and that it should be delivered regularly, professionaly and using multiple learning tools.

Table 1. Skills included in the RCoA competency-based training documents in 2000 and 2002 [2]

Skills to be learned in a clinical environment	Skills to be learned in a non-clinical environment with some clinical experience
Basic airway skills with airway and facemask Use of the laryngeal mask airway Direct laryngoscopy and tracheal intubation Rapid sequence induction (RSI) Use of alternative blades and bougies Failed intubation drill Placement of double lumen tubes (DLT)	Intubation through a LMA (blind and fiberoptic) Fiberoptic intubation via the nose and mouth Awake intubation Use of other airway devices, e.g. Combitube Elective transtracheal ventilation Retrograde intubation Emergency cricothyrotomy

THE AIRWAY SKILLS LABORATORY

Some anesthetic departments have their own airway skills laboratory for practising routine and difficult airway skills [6]. Such a laboratory should have different adult and pediatric mannequins (Figure 1) and simulators for teaching and practising the following tasks – bag-mask ventilation [7], insertion of supraglottic airway devices [8, 9], tracheal intubation through SADs, training of fiberoptic intubation through the nose and mouth, insertion of optical stylets, videolaryngoscopy and managing the difficult pediatric airway (Figure 2). Basic phantoms for practising infraglottic surgical approaches to the airway such as cricothyrotomy, mini-tracheotomy and tracheostomy should be also available.

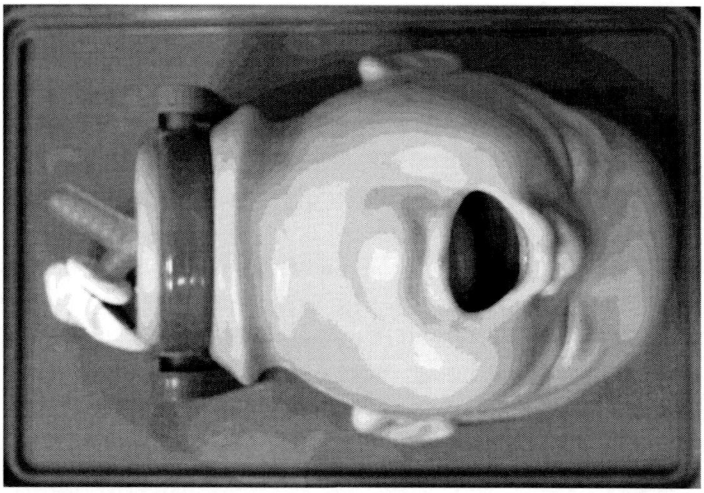

Figure 1. Pediatric airway trainer.

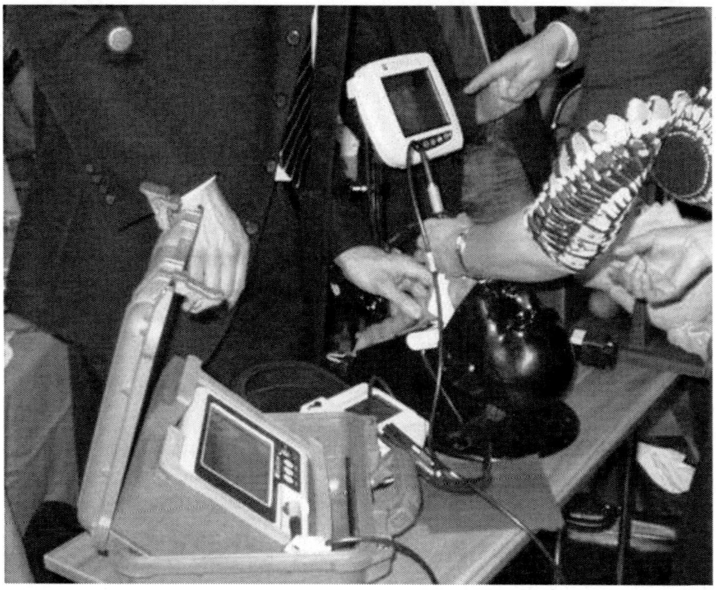

Figure 2. Airway skills laboratory.

Regular sessions in this laboratory should be formally led by a designated person with a board certification in anesthesia and intensive care and, ideally, with an airway management fellowship. These sessions in the laboratory should be run for paramedics and nursing staff, teaching them how to perform bag-mask ventilation or the insertion of SADs. Anesthesia and Emergency Medicine trainees should be taught the tasks discussed above and also how to intubate the trachea using various devices.

The airway skills laboratory should also be used by consultants and other airway specialists for the simulation of difficult cases and for trialling novel equipment and methods.

All of the airway equipment available in the operating rooms as well as devices or aids available on Difficult Airway Trolleys in the theatres and ICU should also be included in the airway skills laboratory inventory.

Teaching Insertion of Supraglottic Airways

The insertion techniques of various SADs [8] are taught on airway mannequins usually only for non-medical staff. Paramedics, operating department practitioners, nursing staff and medical or nursing students are initially instructed how to insert the device (videotape, DVD) and then practise the technique of insertion on an appropriate training mannequin [9]. Insertion of the classic LMA, intubating LMA, i-gel and AuraOnce (Aura-i) laryngeal mask is practised in this way in our department. Junior trainees usually practice the insertion of SADs into mannequins only in special conditions. Such conditions might include: simulation of the difficult airway (cervical spine immobilization, inflation of the tongue, fixation of the neck in flexion), unusual positions (lateral, prone) or on pediatric airway mannequins.

Mannequin studies relevant to the i-gel airway are described in Chapter 16 of this monograph.

Teaching Video-Laryngoscopy and Insertion of Optical Stylets

Direct laryngoscopy has been the method of choice for locating the vocal cords for more than seven decades. Some patients, however, cannot be intubated using a classical laryngoscope because establishing a direct line of sight between the operator´s eye and the patient's vocal cords is impossible. New optical and video technologies have been developed within recent years to help overcome this problem [10].

Videolaryngoscopes have a similar design to the classical Macintosh blade and a special micro-video camera incorporated close to the tip of the blade. Various reusable (Glidescope, Pentax AWS, McGrath laryngoscope) and fully disposable (Airtraq) devices are available on the market [10].

Videolaryngoscopes contain an attached or wireless monitor for direct viewing of the process of intubation. These devices are a very useful tool in cases where the larynx lies anteriorly. They are also a very good instructive tool for understanding the processes of direct laryngoscopy and tracheal intubation [11]. Training sessions with videolaryngoscopes use different airway models including a newly developed pediatric head simulating a child with Pierre-Robin syndrome [12].

Rigid optical stylets are another tool that can be used in the management of the difficult airway [13]. More than ten optical stylets are commercially available at the moment. In experienced hands, rigid stylets can be more successful and less traumatic than direct laryngoscopy [14]. The Bonfils optical stylet was developed for a retromolar approach to tracheal intubation in patients with limited mouth opening, cervical spine immobility or neck trauma. The Shikani stylet combines the features of a fiberoptic bronchoscope and a rigid lightwand and it has been used for both anticipated and unpredicted difficult intubations. Both stylets may even be inserted in awake patients. Their use is not easy for beginners and must be practised on mannequins prior to using them in real patients.

Teaching How to Use the Bougie, Aintree and Frova Airway Catheters

The bougie, Aintree intubating catheter (AIC) and Frova catheter are elastic or semi-rigid introducers which are inserted into the trachea through the vocal cords in cases where direct insertion of a tracheal tube is not possible – anterior larynx position, narrowing or edema of vocal cords, large epiglottis. These introducers serve as a guide for the endotracheal tube, which is then railroaded over it to enter the trachea. Both the Aintree and Frova catheters are hollow and allow the anesthesiologist to oxygenate through them using a standard circuit and a neonatal tracheal tube connector [6].

The gum-elastic bougie was introduced into clinical anesthetic practice shortly after the Second World War [15, 16]. It was first used by Robert Macintosh in 1949. Several types of bougies are commercially available. Tracheal intubation over the bougie should be more successful than with an intubating stylet. Success rate after two attempts was 96% for the bougie yet only 66% with a stylet in a simulated difficult airway scenario [17]. Use of a combination of the gum elastic bougie with the application of BURP (backward upwards and right external pressure on the larynx) showed a 94.3% success rate of tracheal intubation when the cords could not be seen (larynx grade 3 according to Cormack and Lehane) [18]. Tracheal intubation using the McCoy laryngoscopic blade and a gum elastic bougie can be a very useful technique in prehospital medicine in patients with suspected cervical spine trauma who are immobilized in a neck collar [15]. Gum elastic bougies and other introducers may be also inserted blindly through supraglottic airway devices including the i-gel (Figure 3) if a fiberscope is not readily available [19]. The Aintree intubating catheter is the most commonly used introducer for insertion through SADs [19]. Both the standard (Eschmann, reusable Portex) bougie and the Aintree catheter have been very effective as aids to tracheal intubation. The disposable Portex bougie has a lower success rate and sufficient data is not available to support the routine use of the Frova catheter.

Insertion of a gum elastic bougie and other introducers into the trachea is a key part of any difficult airway management syllabus. Anesthetic trainees and paramedics are taught how to use these tools using mannequins, initially under normal circumstances and then in simulated difficult airway scenarios [20]. To simulate difficulty, the mannequins have their necks immobilized either by using a cervical spine collar, fixing the mannequin's neck in flexion or by introducing air to inflate the mannequin's tongue (AirSim mannequin) (Figure 4). These maneuvers serve to recreate a situation where the larynx lies anteriorly.

Learning how to use the bougie can be combined with use of the McCoy laryngoscopic blade, videolaryngoscopy or by blind insertion of the bougie through SADs (cLMA, ILMA or i-gel airway).

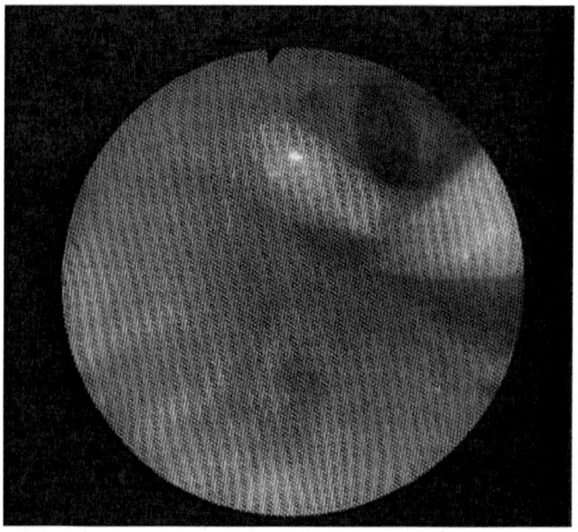

Figure 3. Insertion of gum elastic bougie through the i-gel supraglottic airway.

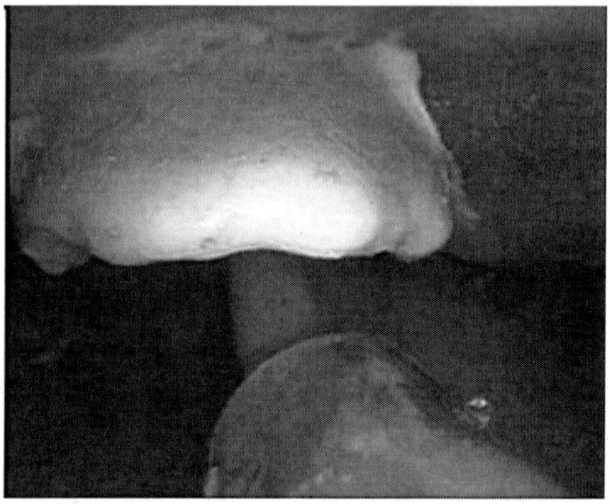

Figure 4. Simulated grade 3 laryngeal view and insertion of bougie.

Teaching Fiberoptic Intubation

Awake fiberoptic intubation is still considered as the gold standard technique for expected or predicted difficult laryngoscopy scenarios [6]. As part of the learning process, several tasks have to be completed. Firstly, trainees should learn how to safely manipulate and control an intubating bronchoscope. This equipment is very expensive and damage to the fibers or other parts of the scope can cost a significant amount of money to repair. The Oxford fiberoptic teaching box (Figure 5) was developed by Popat, Kapila and Gale in 1995 and allows first time and inexperienced users to learn how to manipulate the fiberscope.

The second task for the beginner consists of the identification of key human anatomical structures important for fiberoptic intubation. This task is best achieved by using intubating airway mannequins. Several such mannequins are commercially available, with the AirSim (TruCorp, Belfast, Northern Ireland) and the Airway Trainer (Laerdal, Stavanger, Norway) being most realistic [21].

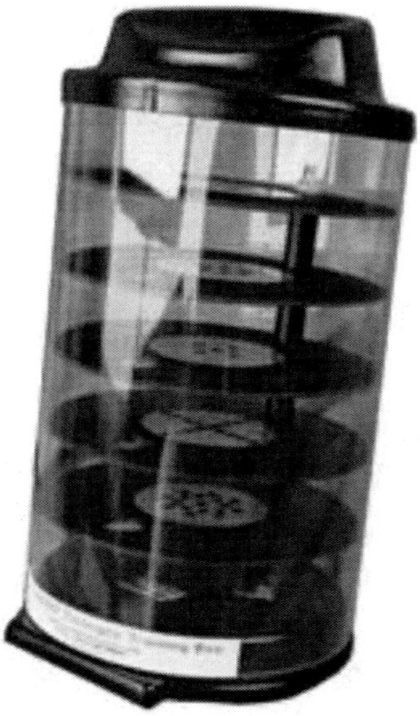

Reprinted with permission of John Wiley and sons from Stringer et al., Anaesthesia 2005;60:1022-6.

Figure 5. Oxford fiberoptic teaching box.

Trainees must learn how to identify the epiglottis and vocal cords during nasal fiberoptic intubation and how to locate the uvula, epiglottis and laryngeal inlet during the intraoral approach [22, 23]. The next step should be fiberoptic intubation through SADs – intubating laryngeal mask airway, i-gel or Aura-i laryngeal mask in patients scheduled for elective procedures and without predicted difficult laryngoscopy.

Fiberoptic intubation through SADs is technically easier than the classical approaches - the cords are a short distance from the bowl of the device and are usually easily located. There is little pressure on the trainee: patients are asleep and can be oxygenated and have volatile agent administered via the SAD between intubation attempts. Patients should be consented for fiberoptic technique prior to anesthesia. The final step is training in awake or asleep oral or nasal fiberoptic intubation in patients with predicted or known difficult laryngoscopy. Trainees should always perform this task under the direct supervision of an experienced teacher. One course in the United Kingdom even teaches participants to intubate each other with a fiberscope [24].

Simulation of the Surgical Airway

While difficult or failed laryngoscopies are relatively common scenarios in routine anesthetic practice, indications for emergency surgical airways are extremely rare. The main circumstance is the "cannot intubate, cannot ventilate" (CICV) situation which has an estimated incidence of less than 1: 5.000 cases [6].

This circumstance may, however, be quite frequent in combat medicine and guidelines for advanced life support in military trauma patients (BATLS) recommend cricothyrotomy as the method of choice in maxillofacial and neck traumas [25].

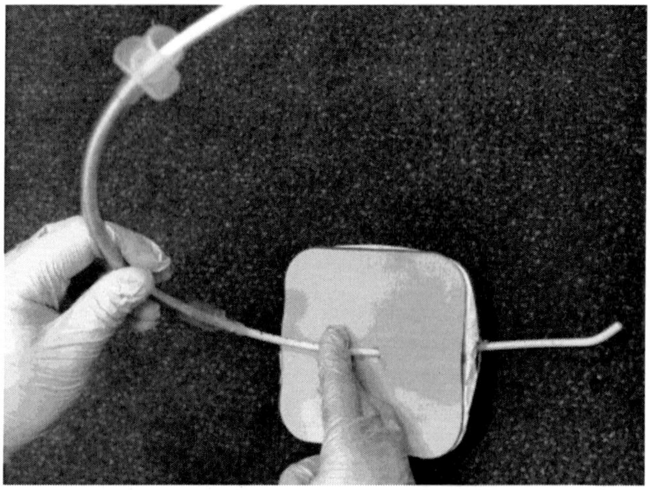

Figure 6. Bougie-assisted cricothyrothomy (BACT) on a tracheal model.

In normal anesthetic practice, this method should always be performed if the oxygenation fails after attempting conventional methods (bag-mask ventilation, tracheal intubation, insertion of SADs). However, many trainees and even consultants are not comfortable using emergency surgical access to the airways [26]. The techniques include transtracheal jet ventilation, puncture minicricothyrotomy sets (Quick Trach, Mini Trach, etc.) and bougie-assisted cricothyrotomy (BACT). In our institution, we prefer to teach trainees BACT due to its relative ease, the short time to perform the procedure and because a cuffed 6.0 mm tracheal tube is inserted into the trachea providing secure airway.

There are two options available for teaching trainees to perform surgical airways. Commercial or home-made models of the larynx and trachea may be used (Figure 6) [2].

Another possibility is using fresh, non-embalmed cadavers for practising puncture cricothyrotomy and BACT, but this option is becoming more and more difficult due to legal regulations. Trainees in our institution have to complete practical surgical airways training at least twice a year and all specialists must complete the training once a year.

ALTERNATIVE METHODS OF TEACHING

Practising on mannequins and simulators are the most common and most simple methods of how to acquire and practice airway skills. Other simulation methods are rarely used in clinical settings. Animal models may be used for airway management simulations. Pigs have a similar airway anatomy to humans for direct laryngoscopy and their tracheas may be used for practising surgical cricothyrotomies and tracheostomies. However, performing surgery on animals is strictly regulated and this method is also quite expensive. Isolated pig tracheas are sometimes used during airway workshops for surgical airway simulation.

An important and useful aspect of airway training is the use of audiovisual material – videotapes, DVDs, interactive CD-ROMs, etc. [1, 2, 6]. They should be provided to trainees as a first learning tool before commencing practical sessions on airway mannequins.

Postgraduate lectures, case presentations, case-based discussions, workshops, assessments of performance, audit and research projects relating to airway management are also an integral part of any airway management program run by a department or trust [6].

CONCLUSION

Complex education in airway management involves multiple tasks performed in differing situations. Whilst most of routine skills, such as bag-mask ventilation, placement of oral and nasal airways, insertion of supraglottic airway devices and tracheal intubation using direct laryngoscopy are effectively taught and learned in the operating rooms, less frequent procedures have to be practised using experimental methods [27, 28].

Airway simulators and mannequins play an extremely important role in practising fiberoptic intubation, intubation through supraglottic airways and in learning surgical infraglottic airway techniques. Although some authors argue that there is a difference between man and mannequin [29, 30], they provide airway anatomy that is somewhat similar to human anatomy and they help trainees to gain familiarity and experience with airway equipment and its use.

Most anesthetic departments should have a designated anesthesiologist who is responsible for running airway management education and who is accountable for the quality and safety of airway procedures within the department. Regular practice on real patients and airway mannequins is necessary in order to gain and maintain the airway skills of any professional involved in airway management.

Future directions in airway management should include development of the Master of Science (MSc) program and regular airway fellowships recognizing airway skills as a separate anesthetic sub-specialty.

REFERENCES

[1] K. R. Stringer, S. Bajenov and S. M. Yentis, Training in airway management, *Anaesthesia* 57, 967-983 (2002).

[2] P. A. Baker, J. M. Weller, K. B. Greenland, R. H. Riley and A. F. Merry, Education in airway management, *Anaesthesia* 66, S101-S111 (2011).

[3] T. M. Cook, N. Woodall and C. Frerk, Major complications of airway management in the UK: results of the Fourth National Audit Project of the Royal College of Anaesthetists and the Difficult Airway Society, Part 1: anaesthesia, *Br. J. Anaesth.* 106, 617-31 (2011).

[4] C. Hagberg, R. Georgi and C. Krier, Complications of managing the airway, *Best Pract. Res. Clin. Anaesthesiol.* 19, 641-59 (2005).

[5] H. E. Wang, N. C. Mann, G. Mears, K. Jacobson and D. M. Yealy, Out-of-hospital airway management in the United States, *Resuscitation* 82, 378-85 (2011).

[6] T. Strang and P. Michalek, Difficult airways – prediction and management. *Anest. Intenziv. Med.* 17, 195-202 (2006).

[7] H. Soleimanpour, C. Gholipouri, J. R. Panahi, M. R. Afhami, R. R. Ghafouri, S. E. Golzari, M. Soleimanpour and R. M. Esfanjani, Role of anesthesiology curriculum in improving bag-mask ventilation and intubation success rates of emergency medicine residents: a prospective descriptive study, *BMC Emerg. Med.* 11, 8 (2011).

[8] D. M. Miller, A proposed classification and scoring system for supraglottic sealing airways: a brief review, *Anesth. Analg.* 99, 1553-9 (2004).

[9] E. Laiou, T. H. Clutton-Brock, R. J. Lilford and C. A. Taylor, The effects of laryngeal mask airway passage stimulation training on the acquisition of undergraduate clinical skills: a randomised controlled trial, *BMC Med. Educ.* 11, 57 (2011).

[10] J. C. Sakles, R. Rodgers and S. M. Keim, Optical and videolaryngoscopes for emergency airway management, *Intern. Emerg. Med.* 3, 139-43 (2008).

[11] B. H. Boedeker, K. A. Boedeker, M. A. Bernhagen, D. J. Miller and T. Lacy, Battlefield tracheal intubation training using virtual simulation: a multi center operational assessment of video laryngoscope technology, *Stud. Health. Technol. Inform.* 163, 74-76 (2011).

[12] D. White, A new tool for pediatric intubation training, *EMS Pediatric Equipment*, Dec. 19 (2001). [available on: www.ems1.com]

[13] E. B. Liem, D. G. Bjoraker and D. Gravenstein, New options for airway management: intubating fibreoptic stylets, *Br. J. Anaesth.* 91, 408-18 (2003).

[14] B. E. McGuire and R. A. Younger, Rigid indirect laryngoscopy and optical stylets, *Cont. Educ. Anaesth. Crit. Care Pain* 10, 148-51 (2010).

[15] J. D. Hinds and P. Michalek, The gum elastic bougie: one of anaesthesia´s best-kept secrets, *J. Paramed. Practice* 1, 21-25 (2008).

[16] Hodzovic, A. R. Wilkes and I. P. Latto, Bougie assisted difficult airway management in a manikin – the effect on position held on placement and force exerted by the tip, *Anaesthesia* 59, 38-43 (2003).

[17] P. S. Gataure, R. S. Vaughan and I. P. Latto, Simulated difficult intubation. Comparison of the gum elastic bougie and the stylet, *Anaesthesia* 51, 935-8 (1996).

[18] J. P. Nolan and M. E. Wilson, An evaluation of the gum elastic bougie. Intubation times and incidence of sore throat, *Anaesthesia* 47, 878-81 (1992).

[19] D. T. Wong, J. J. Yang, H. Y. Mak and N. Jagannathan, Use of intubation introducers through a supraglottic airway to facilitate tracheal intubation: a brief review, *Can. J. Anaesth.* 59, 704-15 (2012).

[20] Hodzovic, A. R. Wilkes and I. P. Latto, To shape or not to shape… simulated bougie-assisted difficult intubation in a manikin, *Anaesthesia* 58, 792-797 (2003).

[21] J. H. Yang, Y. M. Kim, H. S. Chung, J. Cho, H. M. Lee, G. H. Kang, E. C. Kim, T. Lim and Y. S. Cho, Comparison of four manikins and fresh frozen cadaver models for direct laryngoscopic orotracheal intubation training, *Emerg. Med. J.* 27, 13-6 (2010).

[22] P. G. Dalal, G. B. Dalal, L. Pott, D. Bezinover, J. Prozesky and W. Bosseau Murray, Learning curve of novice anesthesiology residents performing simulated fibreoptic upper airway endoscopy, *Can. J. Anaesth.* 58, 802-809 (2011).

[23] U. Raveendra, Teaching and training in fibreoptic bronchoscope-guided endotracheal intubation, *Indian J. Anaesth.* 55, 451-455 (2011).

[24] V. Patil, G. L. Barker, R. J. Harwood and N. M. Woodhall, Training course in local anaesthesia of the airway and fibreoptic intubation using course delegates as subjects, *Br. J. Anaesth.* 89, 586-593 (2002).

[25] N. H. Fraser and W. F. De Mello, Oxygenate rather than intubate, *Anesth. Analg.* 105, 1167-8 (2007).

[26] K. B. Greenland, C. Acott, R. Segal, G. Goulding, R. H. Riley and A. F. Merry, Emergency surgical airway in life-threatening acute airway emergencies – why are we so reluctant to do it? *Anaesth. Intensive Care* 39, 578-584 (2011).

[27] K. E. Lucisano and L. A. Talbot, Simulation training for advanced airway management for anesthesia and other healthcare providers: a systematic review, *AANA J.* 80, 25-31 (2012).

[28] G. B. Drummond, Controlling the airway: skill and science, *Anesthesiology* 97, 771-773 (2002).

[29] M. R. Rai, M. T. Popat, Evaluation of airway equipment: man or manikin? *Anaesthesia* 66, 1-3 (2011).

[30] K. Schebesta, M. Hüpfl, B. Rössler, H. Ringl, M. P. Müller and O. Kimberger, Degrees of reality: airway anatomy of high-fidelity human patient simulators and airway trainers, *Anesthesiology* 116, 1204-9 (2012).

Conflict of interest: Prof. Pavel Michalek has lectured for several companies manufacturing supraglottic airway devices inluding Intersurgical Ltd., AMBU Ltd. and Intavent Orthofix Ltd. Dr Pavel Herda declares no conflict of interest.

In: The i-gel Supraglottic Airway
Editors: Pavel Michalek and William Donaldson
ISBN: 978-1-62417-897-9

Chapter 16

EXPERIMENTAL STUDIES RELATED TO THE I-GEL

Pavel Michalek[1,2,*]
[1]Department of Anesthesia and Intensive Medicine,
First Medical Faculty of the Charles University and
General University Hospital, Prague, Czech Republic
[2]Department of Anaesthesia, Antrim Area
Hospital, Antrim, UK

ABSTRACT

Mannequin studies are an important part of the evaluation of any supraglottic airway device. Airway simulators are used as a teaching tool for paramedics, medical students, nursing staff and also for anesthetic trainees. Mannequin studies related to the i-gel are focused on three different areas – insertion of the device by novices, paramedics and nurses, insertion of the i-gel in simulated difficult airway scenarios and tracheal intubation through the device.

The i-gel airway has demonstrated a shallow insertion learning curve when inserted by inexperienced users. It is also one of quickiest devices to insert in mannequins. Most novices prefer i-gel over other SADs in mannequin studies. The i-gel has also showed high success rates in mannequin studies as a conduit for fiberoptic tracheal intubation.

The i-gel has been also investigated in some cadaver studies exploring the position of the device in relationship to the vocal cords. Other studies have explored esophageal seal pressures on the cadaver model.

INTRODUCTION

Airway mannequins and simulators are a very important component of education schemes in airway management [1]. Sophisticated airway models possess anatomical

* Corresponding author: Pavel Michalek. E-mail address: pafkamich@yahoo.co.uk.

structures that are very similar to human tissues. These mannequins usually consist of a head with a complete oral cavity, nostrils allowing the passage of an intubating fiberscope, an epiglottis, laryngeal structures, trachea and main bronchi. They are frequently used for practising tracheal intubation including fiberoptic techniques and for the insertion of various supraglottic airway devices (SADs). Modern airway mannequins, such as the Airsim (Trucorp Ltd., Belfast, UK) (Figure 1), allow simulation of difficult airway scenarios – by inflation of the tongue and the ability to fix the neck in the neutral position or in flexion [2, 3].

Airway trainers are widely used and accepted for training and teaching purposes, however some recent articles have questioned their similarity with the real patients [4, 5]. When compared with computed tomography (CT) scans, the pharyngeal airspace was found to be quite different between airway mannequins and adult patients [5].

Novices in anesthesia, paramedics, policemen, firemen and other people involved in out-of-hospital emergency situations are often taught basic airway skills on mannequins [6-8]. The main reason for this is to gain familiarity with the airway equipment used and with basic and advanced techniques of airway management. They are taught how to perform bag-mask ventilation, how to insert oral and nasal airways, various supraglottic airway devices, Combitube. Trainee anesthesiologists and paramedics also learn how to intubate the trachea using mannequin-based teaching.

Genuine difficult airway situations are quite rare, occurring with incidences of 1:260 for failed intubation with Macintosh blades and 1:5000 for "cannot intubate, cannot ventilate" situations [9, 10]. Simulation of difficult laryngoscopy scenarios in mannequins help to practise strategies in how to deal with these situations. Airway trainers can be used for practising oral and nasal fiberoptic intubation as well as for blind or fiberscope-guided intubation through various SADs [1, 2].

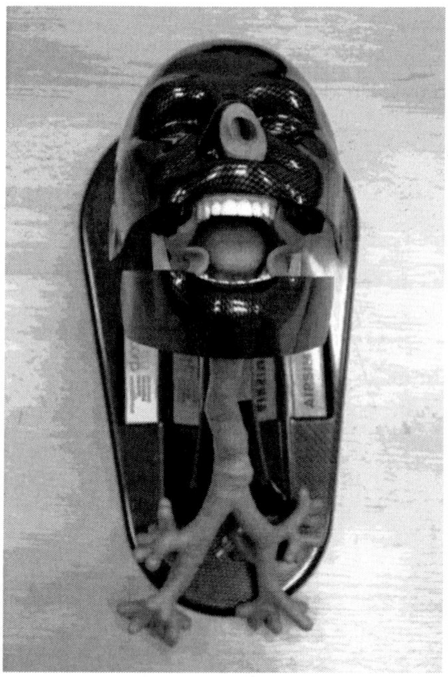

Figure 1. "Airsim" airway management trainer.

MANNEQUIN STUDIES EXPLORING INSERTION PARAMETERS OF THE I-GEL

The first mannequin study of the i-gel was published by Jackson and Cook in 2007. They evaluated the insertion of eight different SADs (Airway Management Device™ – AMD, Cobra Perilaryngeal Airway, Combitube™, i-gel™, Laryngeal Tube®, Laryngeal Tube Disposable – LTD, Laryngeal Tube Suction II – LTS II and Streamlined Liner of the Pharynx Airway – SLIPA) into four different airway mannequins. Insertion of the i-gel supraglottic airway was found to be the easiest when compared with other SADs [11].

Wharton et al. evaluated i-gel insertion by inexperienced users in both mannequins and human subjects. Fifty novices in airway management (physicians of different specialties than anesthesia, medical students and operating department practitioners) inserted a size 4 i-gel into the Airsim airway trainer. Insertion was attempted following a demonstration by an experienced operator. All fifty devices were successfully inserted (100% success rate) with an 88% success rate on the first attempt with a median insertion time of 14 seconds. Some additional airway maneuvers were required in more than 50% of attempts – most commonly neck extension and chin lift [12].

Another study with a crossover design evaluated differences between the i-gel and LMA Unique insertion parameters in a mannequin. Fifty-nine medical students placed both devices into a mannequin (SimMan, Laerdal Medical, UK). The i-gel required a significantly shorter insertion time and demonstrated more effective ventilation than the LMA Unique [13, 14].

Six different SADs were evaluated in a simulated chemical, biological, nuclear, radiation (CBNR) scenario using the Advanced Airway Trainer (Laerdal Medical, UK). The Combitube, classic laryngeal mask airway, intubating laryngeal mask airway, i-gel, Laryngeal Tube and ProSeal LMA were inserted by fifty-eight paramedics wearing either CBNR personal protective equipment (CBNR-PPE) or their standard uniform. The i-gel had the shortest insertion time under all circumstances. Wearing CBNR-PPE significantly increased the insertion times for all SADs [15].

The i-gel and classic LMA (cLMA) were compared using a mannequin for success rate and speed of insertion when placed by experienced anesthesiologists or novice physicians. The i-gel showed a significantly higher overall first insertion attempt success rate (90.5% vs. 63.8% for the cLMA), faster insertion times and better first attempt insertion rates by the novice physicians [16].

SIMULATED CARDIOPULMONARY RESUSCITATION SCENARIOS AND I-GEL INSERTION

The i-gel has also been trialled using airway mannequins in several studies related to cardiopulmonary resuscitation (CPR). The device was usually easy to insert, demonstrated short insertion times and high first attempt success rates.

The effect of insertion of two SADs – i-gel and Laryngeal Suction Tube (LTS-D) – on "no-flow-time" during single-rescuer CPR in mannequins was evaluated with paramedics as operators. Insertion time for each SAD was around 10 seconds and time to the first effective breath was 40 seconds. The authors concluded that each SAD might be a good tool for airway management in a cardiac arrest scenario [17].

Ruetzler and colleagues compared the insertion of six different airway devices in a mannequin during CPR [18]. They studied the effect of airway device insertion on the interruption of chest compression. All SADs scored better than tracheal intubation. However, the insertion time for i-gels in this study was longer than for other SADs.

Tracheal intubation and the insertion of six other different airway devices by paramedics was evaluated using a mannequin in another study [19]. Paramedics and novices in airway management were educated using an audio-visual lecture and practical demonstration with a mannequin and subsequently performed airway interventions.

Their performance was re-assessed after 3 months having not performed any other training or practise in airway management skills. Success rates of SADs insertion were significantly higher than success rates of tracheal intubation.

Fischer et al. assessed the insertion of four SADs and bag-mask ventilation (BMV) using the airway trainer. The operators in this study were third-year medical students.

Time to achieve effective ventilation was shortest with BMV and the i-gel. At twelve months the study was repeated and the same methods also performed best. BMV was associated with significantly higher level of gastric insufflation than i-gel [20].

Use of the i-gel as an alternative to tracheal tube in pre-hospital care has been trialled in a mannequin also by Tiesmeier and Emmerich [21].

INTUBATION THROUGH THE I-GEL IN MANNEQUINS

Three studies have evaluated use of the i-gel as a conduit for tracheal intubation in mannequin settings. They were set up following the first successful case reports from the describing the use of the device as a conduit for insertion of tracheal tubes in difficult laryngoscopy situations. Two SADs – the i-gel and intubating laryngeal mask airway (ILMA) were inserted in three different airway trainers by 25 anesthesiologists of different grades (Figure 2). The efficacy of ventilation and fiberoptic views through the devices were assessed by an independent person (Figure 3).

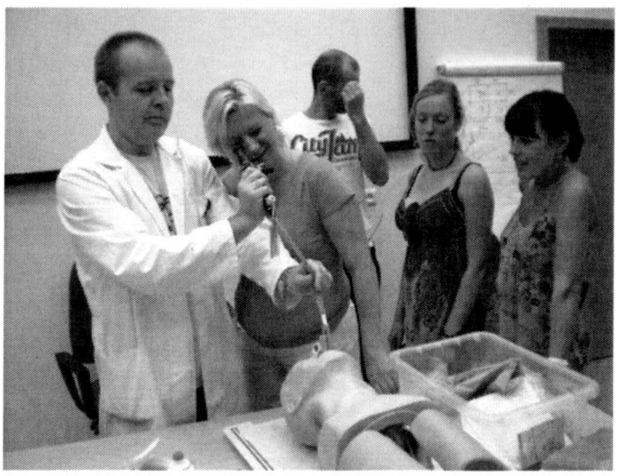

Figure 2. Fiberoptic intubation through the i-gel in a mannequin.

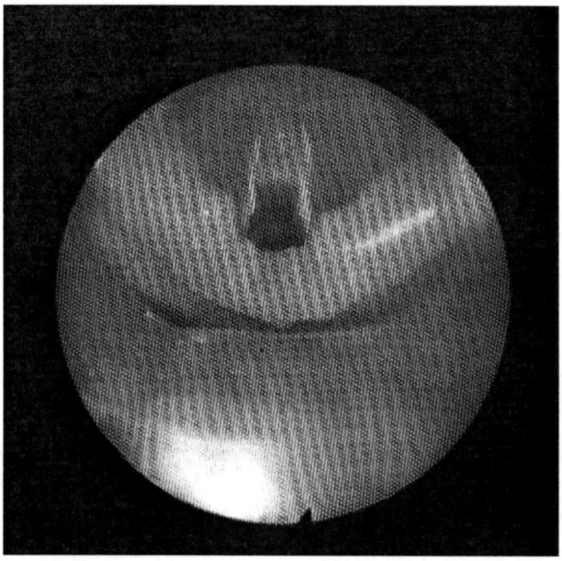

Figure 3. View through the i-gel of the vocal cords of a mannequin.

All participants then attempted to insert a gum-elastic bougie, an Aintree intubating catheter (AIC) and a soft tracheal tube blindly into a mannequin´s trachea through the SADs, as well as passing an intubating fiberscope through the devices into the trachea. Fiberoptic intubation was highly successful through both the ILMA and i-gel, whilst blind intubation through the i-gel showed a significantly lower success rate than through the ILMA [22].

De Lloyd et al. compared the cLMA and i-gel as conduits for fiberoptic tracheal intubation in mannequin settings. The participants railroaded an Aintree catheter or tracheal tube over the fiberscope into the manequin´s trachea. Total success rate, time taken for tracheal intubation, ease of insertion and operator preference were recorded. Tracheal intubation through the i-gel was faster and participants preferred it to the cLMA [23].

A single-use intubating bronchoscope (Ambu aScope^{TM}, Ambu A/S, Ballerup, Denmark) has been evaluated for tracheal intubation through three different SADs – i-gel, cLMA and ILMA. The i-gel was the fastest intubation conduit followed by the ILMA and cLMA [24].

Evaluation of the i-gel on Cadavers

Dr Muhamed Nasir and his team carried out the first cadaver studies evaluating the i-gel at the Cambridge University, Department of Anatomy in 2002. Following this, a study was performed using fresh cadavers at the University of Maryland (US). This study evaluated the placement, definitive position and seal mechanisms of the i-gel supraglottic airway in 65 non-embalmed cadavers. Fiberoptic views through the device were performed, as well as neck dissections and neck and head radiographs. A full view of the glottic opening through the i-gel was achieved in more than 60% of cadavers, with a Percentage of Glottis Opening (POGO) score of greater than 50% in all cadavers. All radiographs and neck dissections revealed correct positioning of the device, covering the vocal cords and the perilaryngeal area (Figure 4) (Figure 5) [25].

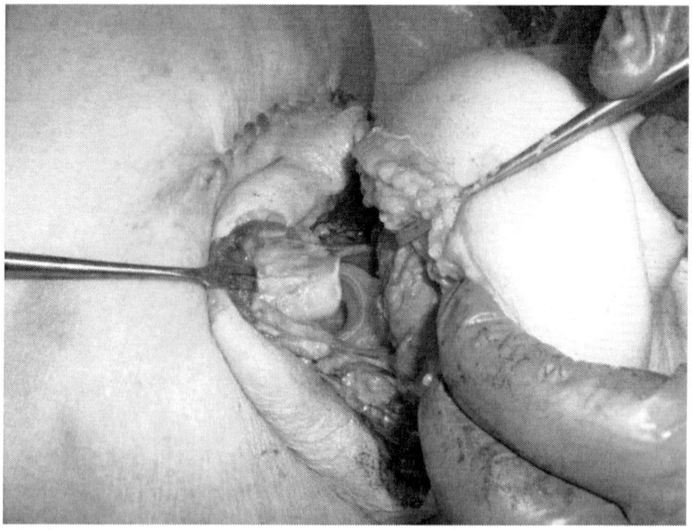

Figure 4. Neck dissection with the i-gel inserted in situ (courtesy of Intersurgical® Ltd., UK).

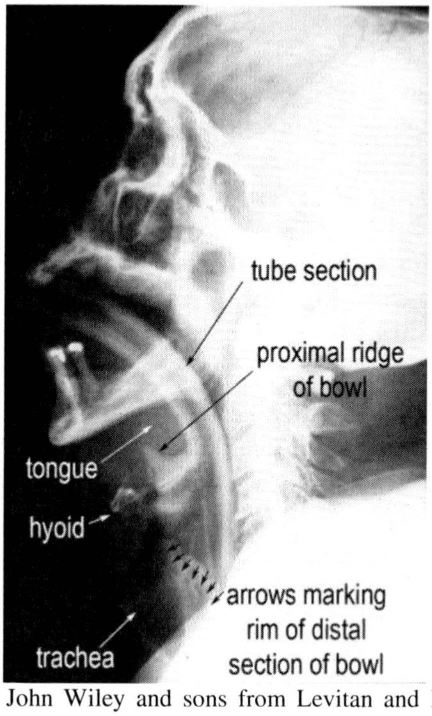

Reprinted with permission of John Wiley and sons from Levitan and Kinkle, Anaesthesia 2005;60: 1022-6.

Figure 5. Lateral head and neck radiograph with the i-gel inserted.

Two cadaver studies have evaluated esophageal seal pressures and mechanisms of gastric insufflation:

Schmidbauer et al. studied the esophageal seal of the i-gel, cLMA and LMA ProSeal on non-embalmed cadavers. They simulated slowly and quickly increasing pressures through distal esophagus upwards, simulating regurgitation and vomiting scenarios. Both of the laryngeal mask airways withstood higher esophageal pressures than i-gel. However, the drainage channels of i-gel and LMA ProSeal were able to drain away the esophageal fluid effectively. This study suggested that the drainage channel of the i-gel is able to drain away fluid effectively and that this may compensate for the lower esophageal pressure tolerance of the device [26].

The effect of inspiratory pressure on esophageal insufflation was studied in fresh cadavers during simulated complete airway obstruction.

All six airway devices (LMA ProSeal, LMA Supreme, LTS-D, LTS II, Combitube and i-gel) withheld peak inspiratory pressures of 20 mbar while at higher pressures (of 40 and 60 mbars) esophageal insufflation occurred in all of the airway devices [27].

Other Experimental Studies Related to i-gel

The i-gel airway has also been tested in vitro for its physical properties, changes of consistency during pressure and temperature changes and creation of artefacts during magnetic resonance imaging (MRI).

In one study, the i-gel was exposed to hyperbaric pressures (203, 284 and 608 kPa) and fast decompression. There were no changes recorded in either its structure or consistency following these pressure changes [28]. In another study, the cuff volume of the i-gel remained stable after exposure to simulated high altitude (4572 m above the sea level) using an altitude chamber [29].

Zaballos et al. studied artefacts associated with different SADs during MRI examination. Neither the i-gel airway nor the Ambu Aura laryngeal mask were responsible for any artefacts during MRI imaging whereas the cLMA, LMA Unique and LMA ProSeal produced artefacts related to the ferromagnetic material contained in the pilot balloon valve [30].

Conclusion

Most published mannequins studies have showed that the i-gel is an ideal tool for learning airway skills by inexperienced users. Its insertion is highly successful, rapid and the skills to insert it are well retained over time. In addition, novices have been shown to prefer the i-gel to other supraglottic airway devices.

Fiberoptic intubation through the i-gel is quite straightforward using mannequins and airway trainers and should be a part of advanced airway skill training in every department. Blind intubation through the i-gel is difficult in mannequins and has showed relatively low success rates. However, the situation in real human patients may be different and blind intubation through the device might succeed in the absence of fiberoptic equipment.

Cadaver studies show that the i-gel covers the perilaryngeal area well and that the opening of the bowl corresponds to the glottic opening in the majority of cases. i-gels also might be used in the future under non-standard conditions, such as high altitude, diving and air transfers due to the stability of its cuff.

The device is also not responsible for artifact formation during MRI imaging and could theoretically replace the LMA for this indication.

REFERENCES

[1] K. R. Stringer, S. Bajenov and S. M. Yentis, Training in airway management, *Anaesthesia* 57, 967-83 (2002).

[2] G. M. Jordan, J. Silsby, G. Bayley and T. M. Cook, Evaluation of four manikins as simulators for teaching airway management procedures specified in the Difficult Airway Society guidelines and other advanced airway skills, *Anaesthesia* 62, 708-12 (2007).

[3] J. H. Yang, Y. M. Kim, H. S. Chung, J. Cho, H. M. Lee, G. H. Kang, E. C. Kim, T. Lim and Y. S. Cho, Comparison of four manikins and fresh frozen cadaver models for direct laryngoscopic orotracheal intubation training, *Emerg. Med. J.* 27, 13-6 (2010).

[4] P. A. Klock jr, Airway simulators and mannequins: a case of high infidelity? *Anesthesiology* 116, 1179-80 (2012).

[5] K. Schebesta, M. Hüpfl, B. Rössler, H. Ringl, M. P. Müller and O. Kimberger, Degrees of reality: airway anatomy of high-fidelity human patient simulators and airway trainers, *Anesthesiology* 116, 1204-9 (2012).

[6] F. Thomas, J. Carpenter, C. Rhoades, R. Holleran and G. Snow, The usefulness of design of experimentation in defining the effect difficult airway factors and training have on simulator oral-tracheal intubation success rates in novice intubators, *Acad. Emerg. Med.* 17, 460-3 (2010).

[7] R. Nakstad and M. Sandberg, Airway management in simulated restricted access to a patient – can manikin-based studies provide relevant data? *Scand. J. Trauma Resusc. Emerg. Med.* 19, 36 (2011).

[8] M. J. Larsen, F. X. Guyette and J. Suyama, Comparison of three airway management techniques in a simulated tactical setting, *Prehosp. Emerg. Care* 14, 510-4 (2010).

[9] C. M. Burkle, M. T. Walsh, B. A. Harrison, T. B. Curry and S. H. Rose, Airway management after failure to intubate by direct laryngoscopy: outcomes in a large teaching hospital, *Can. J. Anaesth.* 52, 634-40 (2005).

[10] T. Strang and P. Michalek, Difficult airways – prediction and management, *Anest. Intenziv. Med.* 17, 195-202 (2006).

[11] K. M. Jackson and T. M. Cook, Evaluation of four airway training manikins as patient simulators for the insertion of eight types of supraglottic airway devices, *Anaesthesia* 62, 388-93 (2007).

[12] N. M. Wharton, B. Gibbison, D. A. Gabbott, G. M. Haslam, N. Muchatuta and T. M. Cook, i-gel insertion by novices in manikins and patients, *Anaesthesia* 63, 991-5 (2008).

[13] S. Sreevathsa, C. Hillermann. C. Mendonca, A. Ruhnke and P. Kothare, A randomised crossover comparison between the i-gel supraglottic airway and the LMA-unique: a manikin study. *Eur. J. Anaesthesiol.* 25, S238-9 (2008) [abstract].

[14] R. Sachdeva, S. Sreevathsa, C. Hillermann and C. Mendonca, A randomised crossover comparison of two supraglottic airway devices in novices: a manikin study, *Anaesthesia Product News* 18-19 (2010).

[15] N. Castle, Y. Pillay and N. Spencer, Insertion of six different supraglottic airway devices whilst wearing chemical, biological, radiation, nuclear-personal protective equipment: a manikin study, *Anaesthesia* 66, 983-8 (2011).

[16] K. Stroumpoulis, C. Isaia, E. Bassiakou, I. Pantazopoulos, G. Troupis, A. Mazarakis, T. Demestiha and T. Xanthos, A comparison of the i-gel and classic LMA insertion in manikins by experienced and novice physicians, *Eur. J. Emerg. Med.* 19, 24-7 (2012).

[17] C. H. Wiese, J. Bahr, A. F. Popov, J. M. Hinz and B. M. Graf, Influence of airway management strategy on "no flow time" in a standardized single rescuer manikin scenario (a comparison between LTS-D and i-gel), *Resuscitation* 80, 100-3 (2009).

[18] K. Ruetzler, C. Gruber, S. Nabecker, P. Wohlfarth, A. Priemayr, M. Frass, O. Kimberger, D.I. Sessler, B. Roessler, Hands-off time during insertion of six airway devices during cardiopulmonary resuscitation: a randomised manikin trial, *Resuscitation* 82, 1060-3 (2011).

[19] K. Ruetzler, B. Roessler, L. Potura, A. Priemayr, O. Robak, E. Schuster and M. Frass, Performance and skill retention of intubation by paramedics using seven different airway devices – a manikin study, *Resuscitation* 82, 593-7 (2011).

[20] H. Fischer, E. Hochbrugger, A. Fast, H. Hager, B. Steinlechner, H. Konig, P. Eisenburger, S. Frantal and R. Greif, Performance of supraglottic airway devices and 12 month skill retention: a randomized controlled study with manikins, *Resuscitation* 82, 326-31 (2011).

[21] J. Tiesmeier and M. Emmerich, The i-gel supraglottic airway as an alternative in the preclinical medical aid? A comparative study on a manikin, *Crit. Care* 14, Suppl. 1, P311 (2010) [abstract].

[22] P. Michalek, W. Donaldson, C. Graham and J.D. Hinds, A comparison of the i-gel supraglottic airway as a conduit for tracheal intubation with the intubating laryngeal mask airway: a manikin study, *Resuscitation* 81, 74-7 (2010).

[23] L. de Lloyd, I. Hodzovic, S. Voisey, A. R. Wilkes and I. P. Latto, Comparison of fibrescope guided intubation via the classic laryngeal mask airway and i-gel in a manikin, *Anaesthesia* 65, 36-43 (2010).

[24] S. Scutt, N. Clark, T. M. Cook, C. Smith, T. Christmas, L. Coppel and K. Crewdson, Evaluation of a single-use intubating videoscope (Ambu aScope^{TM}) in three airway training manikins for oral intubation, nasal intubation and intubation via three supraglottic airway devices, *Anaesthesia* 66, 293-9 (2011).

[25] R. M. Levitan and W. C. Kinkle, Initial anatomic investigation of the i-gel airway: a novel supraglottic airway without inflatable cuff, *Anaesthesia* 60, 1022-6 (2005).

[26] W. Schmidbauer, S. Bercker, T. Volk, G. Bogusch, G. Maher and T. Kerner, Oesophageal seal of the novel supralaryngeal airway device i-gel^{TM} in comparison with the laryngeal mask airways Classic^{TM} and ProSeal^{TM} using a cadaver model, *Br. J. Anaesth.* 102, 135-9 (2009).

[27] W. Schmidbauer, H. Genzwürker, O. Ahlers, H. Proquitte and T. Kerner, Cadaver study of oesophageal insufflation with supraglottic airway devices during positive pressure ventilation in an obstructed airway, *Br. J. Anaesth.* 109, 454-8 (2012).

[28] J. Law, A. Bair, J. Capra, A. Holder and R. Allen, Characterization of airway device cuff volumes at simulated altitude, *Aviat. Space Environment. Med.* 82, 555-8 (2012).
[29] C. J. Acott, Extraglottic airway devices for use in diving medicine – part 3: the i-gel™, *Diving and Hyperbaric Medicine* 38, 124-7 (2008).
[30] M. Zaballos, E. Bastida, T. del Castillo, J. G. de Villoria and C. Jimenez, In vitro study of magnetic resonance imaging artefacts of six supraglottic airway devices, *Anaesthesia* 65, 569-72 (2010).

Conflict of interest: Prof. Pavel Michalek has lectured for several companies manufacturing supraglottic airway devices inluding Intersurgical Ltd., AMBU Ltd. and Intavent Orthofix Ltd.

List of Authors

Yukako Abukawa, MD

Assistant Professor
Department of Anesthesiology and Intensive Care Medicine
Tokyo Women's Medical University
Tokyo, Japan

William Donaldson, MB FRCA

Consultant Anaesthetist
Department of Anesthesia, Antrim Area Hospital
Antrim, United Kingdom/Northern Ireland

Robert Greif, MD MME FERC

Professor of Anesthesiology and Pain Medicine
Director Peripheral Anaesthesia Division
Director Medical Education Program
Department of Anaesthesiology and Pain Therapy
Bern University Hospital, Inselspital and University of Bern
Bern, Switzerland

Mjr. Tomas Henlin, MD

Staff Consultant Anesthesiologist
Department of Anesthesia and Intensive Medicine,
1st Medical Faculty of Charles University and
Central Military Hospital, Prague, Czech Republic

Pavel Herda, MD

Staff Consultant Anesthesiologist, Lead of Dental and Maxillofacial Perioperative Care
Department of Anesthesia and Intensive Medicine,
1st Medical Faculty of Charles University and General University Hospital,
Prague, Czech Republic

Kohichi Hiroki, MD

Associate Professor,
Department of Anesthesiology and Intensive Care Medicine
Tokyo Women's Medical University
Tokyo, Japan

Jiri Malek, MD PhD

Associate Professor and Senior Lecturer
Department of Anesthesia and Intensive Medicine, 3rd Medical Faculty of Charles University and University Hospital Kralovske Vinohrady, Prague, Czech Republic

Francis J. McAleavey, MBBCh BAO

Specialty Doctor in Anaesthesia,
Department of Anesthesia, Antrim Area Hospital
Antrim, United Kingdom/Northern Ireland

Pavel Michalek, MD PhD DESA

Associate Professor, Head of Pregraduate and Postgraduate Education
Department of Anesthesia and Intensive Medicine, 1st Medical Faculty of Charles University and General University Hospital, Prague, Czech Republic

Donald M. Miller, MB ChB FFA (SA) PhD

Consultant Anaesthetist and Senior Lecturer,
Department of Anaesthetics, Guy´s, King´s and St. Thomas´ School of Medicine, Kings College, London, United Kingdom

Makoto Ozaki, MD

Professor and Chair,
Department of Anesthesiology and Intensive Care Medicine
Tokyo Women's Medical University
Tokyo, Japan

Lorenz G. Theiler, MD

Staff Consultant Anaesthesiologist
Department of Anaesthesiology and Pain Therapy
Bern University Hospital, Inselspital and University of Bern,
Bern, Switzerland

INDEX

A

B

C

D

E

F

G

H

I

J

K

L

M

N

O

P

Q

R

S

T

U

V

W

X

Y